Handbook of Genetic Disorders

Handbook of Genetic Disorders

Edited by **Luke Stanton**

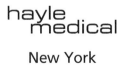

New York

Published by Hayle Medical,
30 West, 37th Street, Suite 612,
New York, NY 10018, USA
www.haylemedical.com

Handbook of Genetic Disorders
Edited by Luke Stanton

International Standard Book Number: 978-1-63241-237-9 (Hardback)

Printed in the United States of America.

Contents

Preface

In my initial years as a student, I used to run to the library at every possible instance to grab a book and learn something new. Books were my primary source of knowledge and I would not have come such a long way without all that I learnt from them. Thus, when I was approached to edit this book; I became understandably nostalgic. It was an absolute honor to be considered worthy of guiding the current generation as well as those to come. I put all my knowledge and hard work into making this book most beneficial for its readers.

As opposed to common belief, genetic disorders are not necessarily hereditary. The research on genetic diseases has been speedily advancing in recent years so as to be able to comprehend the causes behind genetic disorders. Diagnosis and management of the various unifactorial or unigenetic disorders are analyzed in this book. It is quite complicated to heal a genetic disorder in contemporary times. Fortunately, our information on genetic disorders is increasing rapidly, primarily due to the double stranded arrangement identified by Watson and Crick in the 1950s. Hence, it is possible nowadays to comprehend the reason behind the disorder. This book deals with the various aspects of complicated genetic disorders.

I wish to thank my publisher for supporting me at every step. I would also like to thank all the authors who have contributed their researches in this book. I hope this book will be a valuable contribution to the progress of the field.

Editor

Unifactorial or Unigenetic Disorder

Genomic Study in β-Thalassemia

Saovaros Svasti, Orapan Sripichai, Manit Nuinoon,
Pranee Winichagoon and Suthat Fucharoen
Thalassemia Research Center, Institute of Molecular Biosciences, Mahidol University,
Phutthamonthon, Nakhonpathom
Thailand

1. Introduction

β-Thalassemia is characterized by the reduced or absent production of β-globin chains in the hemoglobin molecule leading to an excess of α-globin chains. The clinical findings of thalassemia caused by the imbalanced α/non α-globin chains synthesis include many pathological changes of various organs and a lower-than-average life expectancy. Most β-thalassemia major patients who are homozygous or compound heterozygous for β^0-thalassemia mutations have a severe phenotype of β-thalassemia disease and suffer from chronic anemia and requiring regular blood transfusions. In contrast, β^0-thalassemia/HbE disease is a very heterogeneous disorder and patients who carry identical β-thalassemia genotypes may present with a remarkable variability in disease severity. Their hemoglobin levels range from 3 to 13 g/dL with an average level of 7.7 g/dL (Fucharoen et al., 1987). Patients with mild to moderate clinical symptoms usually have normal growth development and survive without regular blood transfusions. Whereas severely affected patients have marked anemia, growth retardation, severe bone changes, hepatosplenomegaly and heavy iron overload similar to that of β-thalassemia major patients.

However, the reasons for this extraordinary clinical heterogeneity are not fully understood. It has been proposed that there are three levels of genetic control of clinical phenotypes in β-thalassemia: 1) primary modifiers due to heterogeneity of the β-thalassemia alleles, 2) secondary modifiers related to the reduced free α-globin pool or increased γ-globin production in adulthood and 3) tertiary modifiers based on candidate genes that may be involved in several pathological alterations, for example, genes that are related to iron absorption, jaundice, cardiac failure and bone defects. However, the fact that many β-thalassemia/HbE patients who have the same β- and α-globin genotypes still have variable clinical symptoms, suggests that there are still some additional factors which influence the severity of the disease. Recently, genome-wide association studies (GWAS) were performed in order to search for other genetic modifying factors. In the first GWAS, approximately 110,000 gene-based single nucleotide polymorphism (SNPs) were initially screened in pooled DNA and then validated in individual samples (Sherva et al., 2010). The second GWAS was conducted using high density SNP arrays to evaluate approximately 600,000 SNPs in individual samples (Nuinoon et al., 2010). The two SNPs association analyses identified highly significant SNPs located in 3 genes/regions (*P-value* of 1.00×10^{-7} to $1.00 \times 10^{-}$

[13]): the β-globin gene cluster and olfactory receptor genes upstream of β-globin gene cluster on chromosome 11p15.5, the *HBS1L-MYB* intergenic region on chromosome 6q23 and *BCL11A* on chromosome 2p15 (Nuinoon et al., 2010; Sherva et al., 2010). The three regions have been shown to be associated with fetal hemoglobin (HbF) level by genetic linkage and association studies. Moreover, 101 SNPs on 69 genes also showed association with disease severity with *P-values* of 1.00×10^{-5} to 1.00×10^{-6}. These genes have been shown to have less effect on disease severity as compared to the three mentioned regions. However, their roles in modification of disease severity need further investigation.

2. Hemoglobinopathies

Hemoglobin (Hb) is the protein of the red blood cells that transports oxygen from the lungs to tissues, and carbon dioxide from the tissues back to the lungs. It is composed of four globin chains, two α-like and two β-like globin chains, and each globin contains iron-coordinated heme moieties. The hemoglobinopathies fall into two distinct groups, the structural hemoglobin variants and the thalassemias. Hemoglobin variants result from structural alterations in the globin chain, which are mostly due to single amino acid substitutions, thereby altering the function of the hemoglobin tetramer. The thalassemias are characterized by the absence or reduced synthesis of one of the globin chains. Some mutations also lead to both phenotypes. Hemoglobinopathies are the most common monogenic disorders and it has been estimated that approximately 5.2% of the world population are carriers. Around 1.1% of couples worldwide are at risk for having children with a hemoglobin disorder and 2.7 per 1000 conceptions are affected (Modell & Darlison, 2008).

Thalassemias can be divided according to the globin gene(s) defect into α-thalassemia, β-thalassemia, δβ-thalassemia, γ-thalassemia, δ-thalassemia and εγδβ-thalassemia. However, the major groups of this inherited disorder are α-thalassemia and β-thalassemia.

2.1 α-Thalassemia

The α-like globin locus is located on the short arm of chromosome 16 in band p13.3. It includes an embryonic gene (ζ2), two fetal/adult genes (α2 and α1), three pseudogenes (ψζ1, ψα2, ψα1) and a gene (θ) of unidentified function. α-Thalassemia is classified by a reduction or absence in synthesis of α-globin chains. Molecular defects of α-thalassemia are mainly associated with deletions or mutations of one or more of the α-globin genes, of which now more than 35 known deletional mutations have been discovered (Hardison et al., 1998). α-Thalassemia 1 (--/αα) occurs from a deletion of the duplicated α-globin genes, while deletion or mutation of one copy of the duplicated α-globin genes, which produces a reduced amount of α-globin leads to α-thalassemia 2 (-α/αα). The clinical pathology of the patients is heterogeneous depending mainly on the number of defective genes.

2.2 β-Thalassemia

The β-globin locus is located on the short arm of chromosome 11 in band p15.5. It includes an embryonic gene (ε), two fetal genes (Gγ and Aγ), two adult genes (δ and β) and a pseudogene (ψβ). β-Thalassemia occurs as a consequence of a quantitative reduction of β-globin chain production. More than 200 point mutations and, rarely deletions, have been reported (Hardison et al., 1998). These genetic defects lead to a variable reduction in β-globin output ranging from a minimal deficit, mild β^+-thalassemia alleles, to the complete absence, β^0-thalassemia.

2.3 Hemoglobin E

HbE, the most common Hb variant among Southeast Asian populations, results from a G to A substitution at codon 26 (GAG to AAG) in exon 1 of the β-globin gene, which substitutes an amino acid residue from Glu to Lys. This abnormal gene produces a structurally abnormal hemoglobin which consists of $\alpha_2\beta^E{}_2$-globin chains. Moreover, the abnormal gene also activates a cryptic 5' splice site that causes abnormal pre-mRNA splicing. The aberrant splicing leads to a 16 nucleotide deletion of the 3' end in exon 1 and creates a new inframe stop codon (Orkin et al., 1982). This new cryptic splice site competes with the normal doner splice site, consequently the level of correctly spliced β^E-globin mRNA is decreased. As a result, HbE is synthesized at a reduced rate and thus the β^E-globin gene behaves like a mild form of β^+-thalassemia.

3. β-Thalassemia/HbE disease

β-Thalassemia/HbE disease is the most common form of β-thalassemia in many Asian countries. In Thailand, approximately 3,000 children are born with this condition each year, and there are some 100,000 patients in the population (Fucharoen & Winichagoon, 2000). It accounts for over 50% of cases of severe β-thalassemia in Indonesia and Bangladesh and is also very common in Vietnam, Cambodia, Laos, and Malaysia. It also occurs frequently in the eastern side of Indian subcontinent, including Sri Lanka and Maldives (Fucharoen & Winichagoon, 1997).

The major mechanism underlying the pathophysiology of β-thalassemia/HbE is due to the absence or inadequate β-globin chain production, and can be related to the deleterious effects of imbalanced globin chain synthesis. The excess α-globin chains in β-thalassemia, which are highly unstable, precipitate and lead to oxidative damage in developing (causing dyserythropoiesis) and mature red cells (causing shortened red blood cell survival). Hemolysis and ineffective erythropoiesis cause anemia in β-thalassemia (Rund & Rachmilewitz, 2005). Ineffective erythropoiesis leads to the expansion of marrow cavities and the massive medullar cell proliferation, resulting in skeletal deformities. The erythroid hyperplasia and ineffective erythropoiesis are responsible for the increased iron absorption, which together with regular blood transfusions, results in chronic iron overload and death in these patients.

3.1 Clinical Heterogeneity of β-Thalassemia/HbE disease

β-Thalassemia/HbE is generally classified as thalassemia intermedia. The patients have inherited a β-thalassemia allele and hemoglobin E, which acts as a mild β^+-thalassemia. However, despite seemingly identical genotypes, β-thalassemia/HbE patients have a remarkably wide spectrum of clinical phenotypes. Notable are variations in anemia, growth development, hepatosplenomegaly, and transfusion requirements. The clinical features range from asymptomatic or mild clinical symptoms with normal growth development and survival without transfusions, to transfusion-dependent thalassemia major who have marked anemia, growth retardation, severe bone changes, hepatosplenomegaly and heavy iron overload. A study of 802 β-thalassemia/HbE patients showed that hemoglobin levels in the steady state range from 3 to 13 g/dL with an average level of 7.7 g/dL (Fucharoen et al., 1987). Interestingly, the discordant severity of anemia ranged from 0 to 8.6 g/dL, while the distribution of differences of hemoglobin levels in 216 sib pairs from 98 families showed a remarkable skewness toward the lower values with a mode at 0-0.5 g/dL. This suggests that multiple genetic factors must be involved in determining the clinical variability (Fucharoen et al., 1984). The reasons for this extraordinary clinical heterogeneity are not fully understood.

3.2 β-Thalassemia/HbE disease modifiers

The pathophysiologic change in homozygous β-thalassemia patients is predominantly determined by the amount of excess α-globin chains. *In vitro* globin chain synthesis techniques available in the 1960s revealed that the central mechanism underlying the pathophysiology of β-thalassemia was related to the excess α-globin chains and the degree of chain imbalance (Weatherall et al., 1965). Similar to homozygous β-thalassemia, the effect of imbalanced globin chain synthesis to disease severity of β-thalassemia/HbE patients has been demonstrated. The *in vitro* globin chain synthesis showed a significant difference between α/non α-globin chains ratio of 2.08±0.42 and 2.55±0.34 in mild and severe groups (*P-value*<0.005), respectively (Fucharoen et al., 1987). Interestingly, there were overlaps in the range of α/non α-globin chains ratio of 1.34-2.90 in the mild group and 2.23-3.30 in the severe group. This suggested that other factors also contributed to the clinical symptoms of these patients.

The well-characterized or possible genetic modifiers which influence the severity of β-thalassemia have been classified. As the amount of excess α-globin chains determined the pathophysiologic change in β-thalassaemia, the factors affecting the excess α-globin pools, which may lead to variable clinical phenotype of the patients are classified as primary and secondary modifying factors. While the tertiary modifying factors are genetic factors that do not affect globin imbalance directly but modify complications of the disease in several different ways (Thein, 2008).

Recently in order to explore disease modifying factors we recruited about 1,300 Thai β⁰-thalassemia/HbE patients and classified them into three groups, mild, moderate and severe using a scoring system based on criteria of 6 representative parameters; hemoglobin level, age onset, age at the first blood transfusion, requirement of blood transfusion, spleen size or splenectomy, and growth development (Sripichai et al., 2008a). The analysis of known genetic modifiers and genome-wide SNPs association studies (GWAS) were performed using MassARRAY platform (Sequenom, Inc., San Diego, CA, USA) and Illumina Human 610-Quad BeadChips array (Illumina, San Diego, CA, USA) (Nuinoon et al., 2010; Sherva et al., 2010).

3.2.1 Primary modifying factors

The primary modifying factor is described by expression of the β-globin alleles due to the nature of the underlying β-thalassemia mutation itself. β-Thalassemia mutations range from null mutations (β⁰-thalassaemia) that cause a complete absence of β-globin production, to those that cause a minimal deficit (β⁺-thalassemia). Generally, interaction of two β⁺-

thalassemia alleles, in which there is some β-globin production such as the mutations at -28 ATA box (A→G), codon 19 (A→G), results in a milder disease. A recent study in a Thai β-thalassemia/HbE cohort showed that all β+-thalassemia/HbE patients had mild clinical symptoms (Table 1). On the contrary, co-inheritance of a β0-thalassaemia mutation, which causes a complete absence of β-globin production from the allele, and HbE results in a wide spectrum of phenotypes.

Since mutation of the βE-globin gene leads to the alternative splicing of βE-globin pre-mRNA, the amount of alternative spliced βE-globin mRNA may play a role in the variability of disease severity. Analysis of *in vitro* globin chain synthesis showed α/βE-globin chains ratio of 2.69±0.58 and 3.18±0.36 in mild and severe groups respectively (Fucharoen et al., 1987). A study in the 1990s by the RT-PCR technique showed that aberrantly spliced βE-globin mRNA in patients with severe clinical phenotype was higher than those of mild cases and the level of aberrantly spliced βE-globin mRNA was correlated with the degree of anemia in the patients (Winichagoon et al., 1995). A recent study using allele specific RT-qPCR confirmed that there were differences in the alternative splicing of the βE-globin mRNA among the patients and the correctly/aberrantly spliced βE-globin mRNA ratio in the mild group was higher than that of the severe group (Tubsuwan et al., 2011). Excluding factors correlated to high HbF production, XmnI -158 Gγ-globin, HBS1L–MYB intergenic region and BCL11A, the alternative splicing of the βE-globin mRNA contributed to at least 7.8% of the mild group.

3.2.2 Secondary modifying factors

The severity of anemia in β-thalassemia reflects the degree of α- to non-α-globin chain imbalance and the excess of unmatched α-globin chains with all their deleterious effects on the erythroid precursor cells. Therefore secondary modifying factors are described as factors that affect the degree of globin chain imbalance and the size of the free α-globin chain pool, either via the co-inheritance of α-globin gene mutations or through genetic determinants which increase the level of HbF production.

β-Thalassemia patients who co-inherit α-thalassemia will have less excess α-globin chains and tend to have less severe symptoms (Sripichai et al., 2008b; Wainscoat et al., 1983). The different types of α-thalassemia mutations that predominate in different racial groups display a wide range of severity. The degree of amelioration depends on the number of functional α-globin genes. None of the patients carrying α-thalassemia were in the severe group. After exclusion of β+-thalassemia mutations, all patients who co-inherited with α-thalassemia 1 heterozygote or α-thalassemia 2 homozygote, who have only 2 functional α-globin genes had mild clinical symptoms. About 90% of the patients who have only one defecteive α-globin gene were in the mild group and 10% were in the moderate group (Table 2). Co-inheritance of α-thalassemia appears to be a major genetic factor underlying the mild clinical phenotype of β-thalassemia/HbE. Moreover, a considerable number of patients, especially those who have co-inheritance of α-thalassemia 1, may have not yet been diagnosed or not presented to hospitals. The prevalence of 0.5% α-thalassemia 1 and 6.9% α-thalassemia 2 in the patients was lower as compared to 4% α-thalassemia 1 and 16% α-thalassemia 2 in Thai population. We suggest that the presence of α-thalassemia genes should always be considered in apparently mild cases of β0-thalassemia/HbE in Southeast Asia and probably in other countries where α-thalassemia is also prevalent.

	Disease severity				
	Mild			Moderate	severe
β-globin genotype	β^+/β^E	β^0/β^E	β^0/β^E	β^0/β^E	β^0/β^E
α-globin genotype	αα/αα	α-thal	αα/αα	αα/αα	αα/αα
No. of patient[*]	36 (2.8)	104 (8.1)	278 (21.7)	373 (29.2)	489 (38.2)
Hemoglobin (g/dL)[**]	7.56±1.05	8.22±1.11	7.53±1.25	5.57±1.51	4.55±1.141
Hemoglobin F (g/dL)[**]	1.47±0.71	1.94±0.91	3.28±1.20	2.02±0.92	1.50±0.81
Age at first presentation[*]					
<3 yr	5 (13.9)	18 (17.3)	62 (22.3)	133 (35.7)	377 (77.1)
3-10 yr	10 (27.8)	52 (50.0)	175 (62.9)	220 (59.0)	112 (22.9)
>10 yr	21 (58.3)	34 (32.7)	41 (14.8)	20 (5.3)	0
Age at first transfusion[*]					
< 5 yr	0	2 (1.92)	11 (3.96)	121 (32.44)	403 (82.41)
5-10 yr	1 (2.78)	12 (11.54)	50 (17.99)	174 (46.65)	83 (16.97)
> 10 yr	35 (97.22)	90 (86.54)	217 (78.06)	78 (20.91)	3 (0.61)
Requirement for transfusions[*]					
regular	0	2 (1.92)	4 (1.44)	162 (43.43)	421 (86.09)
occasional	0	5 (4.81)	14 (5.04)	129 (34.58)	66 (13.50)
none	36 (100.00)	97 (93.27)	260 (93.53)	82 (21.98)	2 (0.41)
Spleen size[*]					
size <3 cm	32 (88.89)	71 (68.27)	115 (41.37)	76 (20.38)	12 (2.45)
3-10 cm	4 (11.11)	32 (30.77)	143 (51.44)	130 (34.85)	153 (31.29)
>10 cm or splenectomy	0	1 (0.96)	20 (7.19)	167 (44.77)	324 (66.26)
Height development[*]					
<3rd percentide	3 (8.33)	17 (16.35)	27 (9.71)	78 (20.91)	220 (44.99)
Weight development[*]					
<3rd percentide	2 (5.56)	5 (4.81)	19 (6.83)	73 (19.57)	156 (31.90)

[*] Number of cases (%) [**] mean±SD

Table 1. Clinical and hematologic parameters among the different severity groups of β-thalassemia/HbE disease

α-Thalassemias	α-Globin genotype	Mild	Moderate	Severe	Total
		Number (%)	Number (%)	Number (%)	Number (%)
Normal	αα/αα	321	378	501	1200 (90.2)
Triplicated α-globin	αααanti3.7/αα	0 (0.0)	0 (0.0)	6 (0.5)	6 (0.5)
α-thalassemias all genotypes		113 (91.1)	11 (8.9)	0 (0.0)	124 (9.3)
Two α-globin genes defect					
α-thalassemia 1 heterozygote	--SEA/αα	7 (100.0)	0 (0.0)	0 (0.0)	7 (0.5)
α-thalassemia 2 homozygote	$-\alpha^{3.7}/-\alpha^{3.7}$	2 (100.0)	0 (0.0)	0 (0.0)	2 (0.2)
One α-globin gene defect					
α-thalassemia 2 (3.7 kb deletion) heterozygote	$-\alpha^{3.7}/\alpha\alpha$	73 (90.1)	8 (9.9)	0 (0.0)	81 (6.1)
α-thalassemia 2 (4.2 kb deletion) heterozygote	$-\alpha^{4.2}/\alpha\alpha$	6 (75.0)	2 (25.0)	0 (0.0)	8 (0.6)
HbCS heterozygote	$\alpha^{CS}\alpha/\alpha\alpha$	23 (95.8)	1 (4.2)	0 (0.0)	24 (1.8)
HbPS heterozygote	$\alpha^{PS}\alpha/\alpha\alpha$	2 (100.0)	0 (0.0)	0 (0.0)	2 (0.2)
Total		434 (32.6)	389 (29.3)	507 (38.1)	1330 (100.0)

Table 2. The effect of α-globin genotype on β-thalassemia/HbE disease phenotypes

Increased α-globin chains are also synthesized from the α-globin triplicated allele (Higgs et al., 1980). The excess α-globin chains lead to a greater globin chain imbalance in β-thalassemia, and hence, the clinical severity of patients is expected to be worsened. The effect of increased α-globin chains by two extra α-globin genes in homozygous triplicated α-globin genes (ααα/ααα) or heterozygous quadruplicated α-globin genes (αααα/αα) was clearly demonstrated in β-thalassemia heterozygotes, which resulted in thalassemia intermedia (Galanello et al., 1983; Thompson et al., 1989). However, the effect of one extra α-globin gene on heterozygous triplicated α-globin genes (ααα/αα) in heterozygous β-thalassemia is more variable and depends on the severity of the β-thalassemia allele (Camaschella et al., 1997; Traeger-Synodinos et al., 1996). Co-inheritance of triplicated α-globin genes (ααα/αα) resulting in severe anemia in β-thalassemia patients has been observed (Camaschella et al., 1995; Galanello et al., 1983; Sripichai et al., 2008a). In this β-thalassemia/HbE cohort, all patients carrying triplicated α-genes (0.5 % of patients) showed a severe clinical phenotype (Table 2). However, the triplicated and quadruplicated α-globin genes occur at a low frequency in most populations. The frequency of triplicated α-globin genes in Cambodian and Chinese cohorts was about 0.5% of patients (Carnley et al., 2006;

Ma et al., 2001). A higher frequency (1-3%) was observed in other countries such as Argentina and Mexico (Bragos et al., 2003; Nava et al., 2006). The quadruplicated α-globin genes were found at an even lower frequency than the triplicated α-globin genes. In Sri Lanka the triplicated and quadruplicated α-globin genes frequencies in the patients were 2.0% and 0.2 %, respectively (Fisher et al., 2003).

The HbF level, which is high at birth and decreases thereafter, is an extremely complex process and still poorly understood. However, the high production of HbF during the neonatal period protects the newborn from the clinical manifestations of β-thalassemia. The role of increased HbF as an ameliorating factor was shown in the group of homozygous β-thalassemia patients who are unable to produce any HbA but showed a mild disease with a reasonable level of HbF (Thein et al., 1988). Studies in β-thalassemia patients have shown that increased Hb F production can reduce the ratio of α- to non-α-globins and ameliorate the severity of the anemia (Rees et al., 1999). The absolute HbF level in mild patients who do not carry the two known modifying factors (β$^+$-thalassemia or α-thalassemia) was 3.28±1.20 g/dL. This level is significantly higher than that of severe patients, 1.50±0.81 g/dL or mild patients carrying β$^+$-thalassemia or α-thalassemia, 1.47±0.71 and 1.94±0.91 g/dL, respectively (Table 1).

The broad distribution of HbF levels in normal adults, in which HbF levels decrease steadily with age, and in which females have higher levels than males, suggests that more than one genetic factor may control HbF production. A twin study composed of 264 monozygotic and 511 dizygotic twins showed that approximately 90% of the variations in the level of HbF and F-cells (HbF containing erythrocytes) production in adult life is genetically controlled by some factor located near the γ-globin gene, while other factors are present on different chromosomes (Garner et al., 2000).

It is known that the genetic variant (C→T) at position -158 upstream of ^{G}γ-globin gene, XmnI ^{G}γ-globin polymorphism, is associated with high HbF production (Labie et al., 1985a; Thein et al., 1987). In addition, more than 50% of the genetic variances in levels of F-cells are caused by factors that are not linked to the β-globin gene cluster (Garner et al., 2000). Intensive linkage studies have mapped trans-acting quantitative trait loci (QTLs) controlling F-cell levels to three regions of the genome: chromosome 6q23, Xp22 and 8q11 (Craig et al., 1996; Dover et al., 1992; Garner et al., 2002). The genetic factors regulating HbF production are discussed in more detail below.

3.2.3 Tertiary modifying factors

Tertiary modifying factors, while not being involved in hemoglobin synthesis, cause variation in the progression of the disease. For example, the glucuronosyltransferase 1 (UGT1A) gene was found to be associated with the levels of bilirubin in response to hemolysis, ineffective erythropoiesis and the incidence of gallstones (Premawardhena et al., 2001). Similarly, the hemochromatosis (Venter et al.) gene has been identified as influencing the degree of iron loading (Longo et al., 1999; Rees et al., 1997) and the apolipoprotein E (APOE) ε4 allele is associated with organ damage and cardiac failure (Economou-Petersen et al., 1998). Variability of at least three different loci; vitamin D receptor (VDR), type 1 collagen (COLIA1) and transforming growth factor beta 1 (TGFB1), has the potential to modify the severity of the bone disease, which is particularly common in patients with severe β-thalassemia (Perrotta et al., 2000).

4. General genomic study

Completion of the human genome project (Frazer et al., 2004; Lander et al., 2001; Venter et al., 2001), dramatically accelerated biomedical research. In parallel, characterization of the inherited variation in human populations, focusing mainly on DNA variants that are common in the general population and that confer increases in diseases risk, has led to exploration of disease susceptibility.

4.1 Genomic variation

Genetic and environmental factors are the two keys that cause human phenotypic variation. Although more than 99% of human DNA sequences are the same across the population there is substantial variation in the sequence at many points throughout the genome. DNA sequence variations are described as mutations and polymorphisms. A mutation is defined as any change in a DNA sequence to a rare and abnormal variant in comparison to the normal allele that is prevalent in the population. In contrast, a polymorphism is a DNA sequence variation that is common in the population. The arbitrary cut-off point between a mutation and a polymorphism is 1% (Brookes, 1999). Genetic variations are responsible for individual phenotypic characteristics and impact on how humans respond to diseases, bacterias, viruses, toxins, chemicals, drugs and other therapies.

Since the early 1980s, humans were known to carry a heterozygous site roughly every 1,300 bases. Genetic maps containing a few thousand markers, which are adequate for rudimentary linkage mapping of Mendelian diseases, were constructed in the late 1980s and early 1990s (Lander, 2011; Lander et al., 2001). A map of 1.42 million single nucleotide polymorphisms (SNPs) distributed throughout the human genome was reported in a companion to the human genome project (Sachidanandam et al., 2001). Today, the vast majority of human variants with frequency >5% have been discovered and 95% of heterozygous SNPs in an individual are represented in current databases. The combination of marker alleles on a single chromosome is called a haplotype (*Haplo*id Geno*type*). Haplotype includes markers that tightly linked with each other and these markers often display statistical dependence, called linkage disequilibrium (LD). The International Haplotype Map Project defined the SNPs patterns across the entire genome by genotyping 3 million SNPs (Frazer et al., 2005).

The presence of a specific allele variation can be implicated as a causative factor in human genetic disorders and a genetic modifying factor in disease phenotypes. Therefore, screening for such an allele in an individual might enable detection of a genetic predisposition to disease or particular phenotype. The importance of finding genetic contribution to disease, therefore, has led to collection of DNA samples from a large number of patients with particular disorders. Two major approaches have been used to map genetic variants that influence disease or phenotype: linkage analysis and association studies.

4.2 Linkage studies

Linkage analysis (family-based studies) is based on the principle that a disease locus in a family will segregate as part of an undisturbed chromosomal region. Genetic markers that tag a chromosomal region that includes the disease gene will co-segregate with the disease. In practice, highly variable markers, such as microsatellites that can be distinguished between most mating couples, have been used to tag regions of the chromosomes (Hauser et al., 2004). Families in which sibling pairs are affected with the disorder are typed with genetic markers to find a polymorphism that is co-inherited with the disease. If the polymorphic allele is found in a large number of affected sibling pairs, the polymorphism is probably linked to a gene that confers susceptibility to that disease. The genetic markers and the disease allele must generally be inherited together within the one or two generations spanned by the family. To find polymorphisms that are linked to a specific disease requires the typing of 200–300 families with multiple affected relatives using a set of a few hundred or a few thousand markers, spaced millions of bases apart along the human genome. However, the linkages reported by one group have often not been replicated by others. Failure to replicate the linkages may result from a lack of statistical power or false positive results in the original study. Furthermore, there might also be different sets of susceptibility genes operating in different populations. Linkage analysis has been less successful for polygenic diseases and quantitative traits, perhaps in part because of a limited power to detect the effect of common alleles with modest effects on disease.

4.3 Association studies

Association studies rely on the retention of adjacent polymorphisms over several generations across the population. The prevalences of a particular genetic marker or a set of markers, in affected and unaffected individuals, are compared instead of analysis of large family pedigrees (population-based studies) (Cardon & Bell, 2001; Hirschhorn & Daly, 2005). The "common disease–common variant" hypothesis posited that common genetic variants could have a role in the etiology of common diseases (Reich & Lander, 2001). The vast majority of genetic variance in the population is due to common variants. The susceptibility alleles for a trait will include many common variants unless the alleles have had a large deleterious effect on reproductive fitness over long periods. For common diseases or traits, many susceptibility alleles may have been only mildly deleterious, neutral or even advantageous. By testing all common variants, one could pinpoint key genes and shed light on underlying mechanisms.

Genome-wide association studies (GWAS) are association studies that survey most of the genome for causal genetic variants. In GWAS, hundreds of thousand SNPs tested for association with a disease in hundreds or thousands of persons have revolutionized the search for genetic influences on complex traits (Manolio, 2010). Such conditions, in contrast with single-gene disorders, are caused by many genetic and environmental factors working together, each of which has a relatively small effect and few if any being absolutely required for the disease to occur. Rapid advances in technology and quality control now permit affordable, reliable genotyping of up to 1 million SNPs in a single scan of a person's DNA. In 2010, nearly 600 genome-wide association studies covering 150 distinct diseases and traits were published, with nearly 800 SNP–trait associations being reported as significant (P-$value$ <5×10^{-8}).

5. Genomic study in thalassemias

Even after exclusion of known genetic modifying factors, the phenotypic severity in the majority of β-thalassemia/HbE patients still can not be predicted. As mention above, family studies indicated that multiple genetic factors are involved in determining the clinical variability and additional genetic modifying factors remain to be discovered. In order to identify these variants, two GWAS were performed in Thai β-thalassemia/HbE patient cohorts, from which β- or α-globin mutations that are known to affect disease severity were excluded.

The first GWAS was carried out using a two-stage study design, which allowed cost effective identification of a targeted set of SNPs for individual genotyping. Initially pooled DNA of 197 mild and 198 severe cases was examined (Sherva et al., 2010). Then the SNPs with allele frequency differences between the pooled DNA (P-$value$ < 0.02) were further genotyped in individual samples of 198 mild and 305 severe cases. The assay panel corresponded to 119,811 gene-based SNPs with a median spacing of 10.4 kilobases, covering approximately 99% of all known and predicted human genes. The pooled genotyping was conducted using the MassARRAY platform (Sequenom, Inc., San Diego, CA, USA). The results showed that 50 SNPs were significantly associated with disease severity (P-$value$ < 0.05). Forty-one SNPs in a large linkage disequilibrium (LD) block within the β-globin gene cluster were associated with severe disease, of which the most significant was bthal_bg200 (odds ratio (OR) = 5.56, P-$value$ = 2.6×10^{-13}).

The second GWAS was conducted using the Illumina Human 610-Quad BeadChips array (Illumina, San Diego, CA, USA) with DNAs from 235 mild and 383 severe cases of Thai β⁰-thalassemia/HbE patients (Nuinoon et al., 2010). The result identified 27 SNPs located in three genes/regions, having P-$value$ of 1.00×10^{-7} or lower to be associated with the disease severity. The quantile–quantile plot of the observed P-$value$ for association to the disease severity and Manhattan plot are shown in Figure 1. The strongest SNPs associated with the disease severity were located in the β-globin gene cluster on chromosome 11p15.5 and olfactory receptor genes upstream of β-globin gene cluster. The 9 most significant disease severity associated SNPs (P-$value$ < 1.00×10^{-10}) were located in a large LD spanning over 62 kb containing the locus control region (LCR) of the β-globin gene cluster, 4 functional β-globin-like genes (ε-, Gγ-, Aγ- and δ-globin) and 1 pseudogene (ψβ-globin). The most significantly-associated SNP, rs2071348, was in the ψβ-globin gene (P-$value$ = 2.96×10^{-13}, OR = 4.33 with 95% CI; 2.74-6.84). The second most significant region was mapped to the *HBS1L-MYB* intergenic region on chromosome 6q23. Five SNPs of this region showed strong association with disease severity (P-$value$ < 1.00×10^{-7}) and rs9376092 revealed the most significant association with P-$value$ = 2.36×10^{-10} (OR = 3.07 with 95% CI; 2.16-4.38). The third significant gene is the *BCL11A* on chromosome 2p15. Four SNPs were significantly associated with the disease severity, with the most significant SNP rs766432 located in intron 2 (P-$value$ = 5.87×10^{-10}, OR = 3.06 with 95% CI; 2.15-4.37). In addition, 101 SNPs on 69 genes also showed association with disease severity with P-$values$ of 1.00×10^{-5} to 1.00×10^{-6}. These SNPs are located on several genes/regions and can be classified into various biological functions such as cell cycle, cell growth, structural proteins, enzymes, hormones, signaling molecules, genes involved in gene expression, protein degradation, inflammatory response and hypothetical proteins with unknown functions. These genes may have less effect on disease severity compared to the three regions. However, they may play some roles in modification of disease severity and need further investigation.

No SNPs in the *BCL11A* region were typed in the first GWAS, suggested that the pooled genotyping was done on a marker panel that was less dense than the second GWAS and did not have the same level of genome coverage as the high density SNP arrays. However, the low marker density can identify two of the three SNPs highly associated with disease severity identified by the second GWAS, the β-globin gene cluster and *HBS1L-MYB* region.

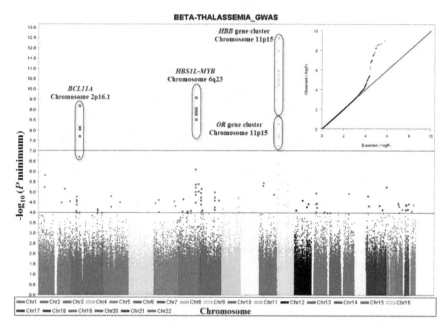

Fig. 1. Genome-wide association study scatter plots of *P-values* (analyzed with disease severity) with chromosome location. The red line denoted the significance threshold (*P-value* = 1.00 x 10^{-7}), and the blue line denoted the suggestive *P-value* (P = 1.00 x 10^{-4}). Inset shows the quantile–quantile plot of the *P-values* (allelic association) (Nuinoon et al., 2010). With kind permission from Springer Science+Business Media

Interestingly, the absolute HbF level among mild β^0-thalassemia/HbE patients without α-thalassemia co-inheritance was significantly higher than those of the mild cases who were β$^+$-thalassemia/HbE or having co-inheritance of α-thalassemia and the severe cases (Table 1). The three most significant regions associated with disease severity were also reported to be quantitative trait loci (QTLs) associated with HbF level in the previous genetic linkage and association studies.

6. HbF quantitative trait loci

It is clear from isolated family, linkage and GWAS studies that there are several QTLs for HbF and F-cells. Moreover, in many family studies, the high HbF phenotype segregates independently of the β-globin gene cluster, implicating the presence of *trans*-acting factors. The major QTLs for HbF and F-cells that have been extensively studied are located in three loci, one is *in-cis* with the β-globin gene cluster and two are *in-trans* with the β-globin gene cluster, the *HBS1L-MYB* intergenic region and *BCL11A* gene.

6.1 β-globin cluster

It has been recognized since the 1980s that the C→T single base substitution at position -158 in the promoter of the ^{G}γ-globin gene is associated with high HbF levels (Gilman &

Huisman, 1985; Labie et al., 1985a). Evidence for the influence of a genetic variant within the β-globin gene cluster came from families with β-thalassemia or sickle cell anemia which showed a tendency for co-segregation of higher or lower HbF levels with the disease mutation. The HbS mutation is found on four major β-globin cluster haplotypes (HbS-Senegal, -Benin, -Bantu, and –Arab/Indian). Carriers for the β^S gene on the HbS-Senegal or HbS-Arab/Indian β^S haplotype (including the T allele of $XmnI$ -158 $^G\gamma$-globin) have high HbF levels, and a mild clinical course, whereas carriers of the β^S gene on a HbS-Bantu haplotype (including the C allele of $XmnI$ -158 $^G\gamma$-globin) have low HbF levels (Labie et al., 1985b). Despite the long time since the identification of this locus as a major QTL for HbF expression, functional studies have been inconclusive. Identification of the pinpoint causative variant is still unknown, in part because the QTL is located in a large LD block spanning over 62 kb. A plausible explanation of the genetic variant in β-globin cluster and olfactory receptor genes upstream function is the regulation of globin genes expression and hemoglobin switching. In erythroblasts, the β-globin locus forms an erythroid-specific spatial structure called the active chromatin hub (ACH). The ACH composed of the HS sites of the LCR, active β-globin genes, remote 5' HS sites (HS-110 in human) and 3' HS-1 (Fang et al., 2007). A chromatin hub is formed by looping 3' HS-1, 5' HS-110, and the 5' part of the LCR together. The β-globin gene locus is surrounded by the genes encoding olfactory receptors that are expressed in olfactory epithelium, but not in erythroid cells (Bulger et al., 1999). The HS-110 and 3' HS-1 site are located in the olfactory receptor genes (ORGs) cluster. An RNA FISH study in erythroid cells indicated that intergenic transcription of the β-globin locus occurs over a region of more than 250 kb including several genes in the nearby olfactory receptor gene cluster (Miles et al., 2007).

6.2 *HBS1L-MYB* intergenic region

Extensive studies over the years of Thein and colleages showed that a quantitative trait locus (QTL) for HbF expression in adults is located in the *HBS1L-MYB* intergenic region, the so called HBS1L-MYB intergenic polymorphisms (HMIP). A genome-wide linkage analysis study covered seven generations of 210 family members of an Asian-Indian kindred with heterocellular HPFH, β-thalassemia and α-thalassemia identified QTLs for HbF expression on chromosome 6q23-q24 (Lod score = 12.4) (Craig et al., 1996; Garner et al., 1998). Fine mapping of the 1.5 Mb region of human chromosome 6q23 encompassing the area showed five genes, *ALDH8A1*, *HBS1L*, *MYB*, *AHI1* and *PDE7B* (Close et al., 2004). To narrow down the candidate region, a high-resolution association study was performed in twin pairs of North European origin. Three LD blocks within the 79 kb long *HBS1L-MYB* intergenic region showed very strong associations with F-cell levels ($P\text{-}value$= 10^{-75}), with the strongest effect in the second block (24 kb) (Thein et al., 2007). The HMIP accounts for about 19% of the North European population trait variance. In Thai β-thalassemia/HbE, a GWAS study also showed that the most significantly-associated SNP with the HbF level in the *HBS1L-MYB* region, rs9399137, is also located within the HMIP second block. The HbF expression QTL at HMIP is also reported in healthy individuals of African descent (Creary et al., 2009), sickle cell patients from Tanzania, Brazil, African American (Creary et al., 2009; Lettre et al., 2008; Makani et al., 2011), β-thalassemia heterozygotes (So et al., 2008) and β-thalassemia patients (Galanello et al., 2009; Nuinoon et al., 2010).

The HMIP has been reported to contain distal regulatory elements that generate a key part of the overall control of the *MYB* expression (Wahlberg et al., 2009). In *MYB* expressing primary human erythroid cells, the core *HBS1L-MYB* intergenic region harbors several potential cis-regulatory elements for GATA-1 signals that coincided with DNase I hypersensitive sites. HbF expression is linked to the kinetics of erythrocyte maturation and differentiation. *MYB* plays role in erythroid proliferation and differentiation, and in turn, the control of HbF levels (Jiang et al., 2006). The HMIP was associated not only with the HbF levels but also with the cell numbers of platelets and monocytes in the peripheral blood (Menzel et al., 2007). Recently, a 3-bp deletion, between 135,460,326 and 135,460,328 bp on chromosome 6q23 in HMIP was identified as the functional motif (Farrell et al., 2011).

6.3 BCL11A gene

The association of *BCL11A* and HbF expression was first identified by two GWAS studies (Menzel et al., 2007; Uda et al., 2008). The first GWAS with the F-cell trait was performed in a European twin cohort, targeting 179 individuals with contrasting extreme F-cell values. Association analysis identified not only the *Xmn*I -158 $^{G}\gamma$-globin and the chromosome 6 locus but also a new F-cell locus in intron 2 of the oncogene *BCL11A* on chromosome 2p15 (Menzel et al., 2007). The second GWAS based on HbF of 4,000 individuals from Sardinia also showed association to the same three loci, the β-globin locus, HMIP and *BCL11A*, which was the first replication of the *BCL11A* locus in patients with SCA and β-thalassemia (Uda et al., 2008). This locus was subsequently replicated in additional SCA patients from the USA and Brazil (Lettre et al., 2008; Sedgewick et al., 2008), and β-thalassemia heterozygotes from Hong Kong and the parents of β-thalassemia/HbE patients from Thailand (Nuinoon et al., 2010; Sedgewick et al., 2008).

The *BCL11A* gene encodes several isoforms of a zinc finger transcription factor, the shorter isoforms appeared to be restricted to primitive erythroblasts, and the full-length isoforms to adult-stage erythroblasts (Sankaran et al., 2008). Down-regulation of BCL11A expression in adult human erythroid precursors results in induction of HbF (Sankaran et al., 2008; Wilber et al., 2011). High-resolution chromatin immunoprecipitation (ChIP)–chip analysis and chromosome conformation capture (3C) assay showed that BCL11A binds the upstream locus control region (LCR), ε-globin and the intergenic regions between γ-globin and δ-globin genes cooperating with SOX6 that reconfigures the β-globin cluster by modulating chromosomal loop formation, which finally leads to transcriptional silencing of the γ-globin genes (Xu et al., 2010).

7. Conclusion

Thalassemias are the most common genetic disease in the world resulting from the defective globin chain synthesis. The main pathophysiologic feature of thalassemia is the accumulation of unpaired globin chains in erythrocyte precursors and red blood cells (β-globin in α-thalassemia and α-globin in β-thalassemia). The unmatched globin chains precipitated in the erythroid precursors in the bone marrow as well as in peripheral erythrocyte membranes contribute to ineffective erythropoiesis and shortened peripheral RBC survival resulting in chronic anemia in these patients. As a monogenic disorder, thalassemia is a very heterogeneous disorder. Patients with identical β-thalassemia genotypes show a remarkable variability in disease severity, ranging from nearly asymptomatic (mild disease) to transfusion-dependent anemia with additional complications (severe disease). Thus, thalassemias are good example of the Mendelian genetic disease that demonstrate phenotypic variations due to the result of multigene interactions. Understanding the roles played by genetic factors in diseases will revolutionize diagnosis, treatment, and prevention, in addition to increase understanding of the environmental contributions. Three levels of genetic modifiers which influence the severity of β-thalassemia have been classified into primary, secondary and tertiary modifiers. The primary modifying factor is described by expression of the β-globin alleles due to the heterogeneity of the molecular lesions of the underlying the β-thalassemia mutation itself. Secondary modifying factors are factors that can affect the degree of globin chain imbalance, which are α-globin genotype and variation in fetal hemoglobin production. Tertiary modifiers are candidate genes which may be involved in several pathological alterations in patients. Our recent GWAS in Thai β-thalassemia/HbE patient cohorts suggests that a number of additional genetic modifier genes may account for the variability in clinical expression. The three genes/regions that are most significant in β-thalassemia/HbE disease severity are also associated with HbF expression, namely the β-globin gene cluster and olfactory receptor genes upstream of β-globin gene cluster on chromosome 11p15.5, the HBS1L-MYB intergenic region on chromosome 6q23 and the BCL11A gene on chromosome 2p15. It is noteworthy that the HbF expression QTL in the β-globin cluster was discovered by family and population studies in the 1980s and subsequently validated by genetic studies. The second QTL, the HBS1L-MYB intergenic region, was discovered by linkage analysis in extensive kindred in 1990s, and subsequently validated by genetic association studies. The third QTL, the BCL11A, was discovered in 2000s by GWAS. This shows the significant development of genomic technologies and knowledge of the human genome. The rapid development of next-generation sequencing technologies seems likely to accelerate further genomic studies. The many less significant variants may be identified in near future. There are several less significant genes compared to the three above mentioned regions, which may play roles in modification of disease severity. More studies are also needed to address the effect of these modifying factors.

8. Acknowledgment

This study was supported in part by the Office of the Higher Education Commission and Mahidol University under the National Research University Initiative, Thailand Research Fund and National Science and Technology Development Agency, Thailand.

9. References

Bragos, I. M.; Noguera, N. I., et al. (2003). Triplication (/ααα$^{anti3.7}$) or deletion (-α$^{3.7}$/) association in Argentinian β-thalassemic carriers. *Ann Hematol,* Vol. 82, No. 11, (Nov), pp. 696-698, ISSN 0939-5555

Brookes, A. J. (1999). The essence of SNPs. *Gene,* Vol. 234, No. 2, (Jul 8), pp. 177-186, ISSN 0378-1119

Bulger, M.; van Doorninck, J. H., et al. (1999). Conservation of sequence and structure flanking the mouse and human β-globin loci: the β-globin genes are embedded within an array of odorant receptor genes. *Proc Natl Acad Sci USA,* Vol. 96, No. 9, (Apr 27), pp. 5129-5134, ISSN 0027-8424

Camaschella, C.; Kattamis, A. C., et al. (1997). Different hematological phenotypes caused by the interaction of triplicated α-globin genes and heterozygous β-thalassemia. *Am J Hematol*, Vol. 55, No. 2, (Jun), pp. 83-88, ISSN 0361-8609

Camaschella, C.; Mazza, U., et al. (1995). Genetic interactions in thalassemia intermedia: analysis of β-mutations, α-genotype, gamma-promoters, and β-LCR hypersensitive sites 2 and 4 in Italian patients. *Am J Hematol*, Vol. 48, No. 2, (Feb), pp. 82-87, ISSN 0361-8609

Cardon, L. R.&Bell, J. I. (2001). Association study designs for complex diseases. *Nat Rev Genet*, Vol. 2, No. 2, (Feb), pp. 91-99, ISSN 1061-4036

Carnley, B. P.; Prior, J. F., et al. (2006). The prevalence and molecular basis of hemoglobinopathies in Cambodia. *Hemoglobin*, Vol. 30, No. 4, pp. 463-470, ISSN 0363-0269

Close, J.; Game, L., et al. (2004). Genome annotation of a 1.5 Mb region of human chromosome 6q23 encompassing a quantitative trait locus for fetal hemoglobin expression in adults. *BMC Genomics*, Vol. 5, No. 1, (May 31), pp. 33, ISSN 1471-2164

Craig, J. E.; Rochette, J., et al. (1996). Dissecting the loci controlling fetal haemoglobin production on chromosomes 11p and 6q by the regressive approach. *Nat Genet*, Vol. 12, No. 1, (Jan), pp. 58-64, ISSN 1061-4036

Creary, L. E.; Ulug, P., et al. (2009). Genetic variation on chromosome 6 influences F cell levels in healthy individuals of African descent and HbF levels in sickle cell patients. *PLoS One*, Vol. 4, No. 1, pp. e4218, ISSN 1932-6203

Dover, G. J.; Smith, K. D., et al. (1992). Fetal hemoglobin levels in sickle cell disease and normal individuals are partially controlled by an X-linked gene located at Xp22.2. *Blood*, Vol. 80, No. 3, (Aug 1), pp. 816-824, ISSN 0006-4971

Economou-Petersen, E.; Aessopos, A., et al. (1998). Apolipoprotein E epsilon4 allele as a genetic risk factor for left ventricular failure in homozygous β-thalassemia. *Blood*, Vol. 92, No. 9, (Nov 1), pp. 3455-3459, ISSN 0006-4971

Fang, X.; Xiang, P., et al. (2007). Cooperativeness of the higher chromatin structure of the β-globin locus revealed by the deletion mutations of DNase I hypersensitive site 3 of the LCR. *J Mol Biol*, Vol. 365, No. 1, (Jan 5), pp. 31-37, ISSN 0946-2716

Farrell, J. J.; Sherva, R. M., et al. (2011). A 3-bp deletion in the HBS1L-MYB intergenic region on chromosome 6q23 is associated with HbF expression. *Blood*, Vol 117, No 18, (May 5), pp. 4935-4945, ISSN 0006-4971

Fisher, C. A.; Premawardhena, A., et al. (2003). The molecular basis for the thalassaemias in Sri Lanka. *Br J Haematol*, Vol. 121, No. 4, (May), pp. 662-671, ISSN 0007-1048

Frazer, K. A.; Ballinger, D. G., et al. (2004). Finishing the euchromatic sequence of the human genome, *Nature*, Vol 431, No 7011, (Oct 21), pp. 931-945, ISSN 0028-0836.

Frazer, K. A.; Ballinger, D. G., et al. (2005). A haplotype map of the human genome. *Nature*, Vol. 437, No. 7063, (Oct 27), pp. 1299-1320, ISSN 0028-0836

Fucharoen, S.&Winichagoon, P. (1997). Hemoglobinopathies in Southeast Asia: molecular biology and clinical medicine. *Hemoglobin*, Vol. 21, No. 4, (Jul), pp. 299-319, ISSN 0363-0269

Fucharoen, S.&Winichagoon, P. (2000). Clinical and hematologic aspects of hemoglobin E β-thalassemia. *Curr Opin Hematol*, Vol. 7, No. 2, (Mar), pp. 106-112, ISSN 1065-6251

Fucharoen, S.; Winichagoon, P., et al. (1984). Determination for different severity of anemia in thalassemia: concordance and discordance among sib pairs. *Am J Med Genet,* Vol. 19, No. 1, (Sep), pp. 39-44, ISSN 1552-4825

Fucharoen, S.; Winichagoon, P., et al. (1987). Variable severity of Southeast Asian β⁰-thalassemia/Hb E disease. *Birth Defects Orig Artic Ser,* Vol. 23, No. 5A, pp. 241-248, ISSN 1542-0752

Galanello, R.; Ruggeri, R., et al. (1983). A family with segregating triplicated α globin loci and β-thalassemia. *Blood,* Vol. 62, No. 5, (Nov), pp. 1035-1040, ISSN 0006-4971

Galanello, R.; Sanna, S., et al. (2009). Amelioration of Sardinian β⁰-thalassemia by genetic modifiers. *Blood,* Vol. 114, No. 18, (Oct 29), pp. 3935-3937, ISSN 0006-4971

Garner, C. P.; Tatu, T., et al. (2002). Evidence of genetic interaction between the β-globin complex and chromosome 8q in the expression of fetal hemoglobin. *Am J Hum Genet,* Vol. 70, No. 3, (Mar), pp. 793-799, ISSN 0002-9297

Garner, C.; Mitchell, J., et al. (1998). Haplotype mapping of a major quantitative-trait locus for fetal hemoglobin production, on chromosome 6q23. *Am J Hum Genet,* Vol. 62, No. 6, (Jun), pp. 1468-1474, ISSN 0002-9297

Garner, C.; Tatu, T., et al. (2000). Genetic influences on F cells and other hematologic variables: a twin heritability study. *Blood,* Vol. 95, No. 1, (Jan 1), pp. 342-346, ISSN 0006-4971

Gilman, J. G.&Huisman, T. H. (1985). DNA sequence variation associated with elevated fetal $^{G}\gamma$ globin production. *Blood,* Vol. 66, No. 4, (Oct), pp. 783-787, ISSN 0006-4971

Hardison, R. C.; Chui, D. H., et al. (1998). Access to a syllabus of human hemoglobin variants (1996) via the World Wide Web. *Hemoglobin,* Vol. 22, No. 2, (Mar), pp. 113-127, ISSN 0363-0269

Hauser, E. R.; Watanabe, R. M., et al. (2004). Ordered subset analysis in genetic linkage mapping of complex traits. *Genet Epidemiol,* Vol. 27, No. 1, (Jul), pp. 53-63, ISSN 0741-0395

Higgs, D. R.; Old, J. M., et al. (1980). A novel α-globin gene arrangement in man. *Nature,* Vol. 284, No. 5757, (Apr 17), pp. 632-635, ISSN 0028-0836

Hirschhorn, J. N.&Daly, M. J. (2005). Genome-wide association studies for common diseases and complex traits. *Nat Rev Genet,* Vol. 6, No. 2, (Feb), pp. 95-108, ISSN 1061-4036

Jiang, J.; Best, S., et al. (2006). cMYB is involved in the regulation of fetal hemoglobin production in adults. *Blood,* Vol. 108, No. 3, (Aug 1), pp. 1077-1083, ISSN 0006-4971

Labie, D.; Dunda-Belkhodja, O., et al. (1985a). The -158 site 5' to the $^{G}\gamma$ gene and $^{G}\gamma$ expression. *Blood,* Vol. 66, No. 6, (Dec), pp. 1463-1465, ISSN 0006-4971

Labie, D.; Pagnier, J., et al. (1985b). Common haplotype dependency of high Gγ-globin gene expression and high Hb F levels in β-thalassemia and sickle cell anemia patients. *Proc Natl Acad Sci USA,* Vol. 82, No. 7, (Apr), pp. 2111-2114, ISSN 0027-8424

Lander, E. S. (2011). Initial impact of the sequencing of the human genome. *Nature,* Vol. 470, No. 7333, (Feb 10), pp. 187-197, ISSN 0028-0836

Lander, E. S.; Linton, L. M., et al. (2001). Initial sequencing and analysis of the human genome. *Nature,* Vol. 409, No. 6822, (Feb 15), pp. 860-921, ISSN 0028-0836

Lettre, G.; Sankaran, V. G., et al. (2008). DNA polymorphisms at the BCL11A, HBS1L-MYB, and β-globin loci associate with fetal hemoglobin levels and pain crises in sickle cell disease. *Proc Natl Acad Sci U S A,* Vol. 105, No. 33, (Aug 19), pp. 11869-11874, ISSN 0027-8424

Longo, F.; Zecchina, G., et al. (1999). The influence of hemochromatosis mutations on iron overload of thalassemia major. *Haematologica*, Vol. 84, No. 9, (Sep), pp. 799-803, ISSN 0390-6078

Ma, S. K.; Au, W. Y., et al. (2001). Clinical phenotype of triplicated α-globin genes and heterozygosity for β^0-thalassemia in Chinese subjects. *Int J Mol Med*, Vol. 8, No. 2, (Aug), pp. 171-175, ISSN 1107-3756

Makani, J.; Menzel, S., et al. (2011). Genetics of fetal hemoglobin in Tanzanian and British patients with sickle cell anemia. *Blood*, Vol. 117, No. 4, (Jan 27), pp. 1390-1392, ISSN 0006-4971

Manolio, T. A. (2010). Genomewide association studies and assessment of the risk of disease. *N Engl J Med*, Vol. 363, No. 2, (Jul 8), pp. 166-176, ISSN 0028-4793

Menzel, S.; Jiang, J., et al. (2007). The HBS1L-MYB intergenic region on chromosome 6q23.3 influences erythrocyte, platelet, and monocyte counts in humans. *Blood*, Vol. 110, No. 10, (Nov 15), pp. 3624-3626, ISSN 0006-4971

Miles, J.; Mitchell, J. A., et al. (2007). Intergenic transcription, cell-cycle and the developmentally regulated epigenetic profile of the human β-globin locus. *PLoS One*, Vol. 2, No. 7, pp. e630, ISSN 1932-6203

Modell, B.&Darlison, M. (2008). Global epidemiology of haemoglobin disorders and derived service indicators. *Bull World Health Organ*, Vol. 86, No. 6, (Jun), pp. 480-487,

Nava, M. P.; Ibarra, B., et al. (2006). Prevalence of $-\alpha^{(3.7)}$ and $\alpha\alpha\alpha^{(anti3.7)}$ alleles in sickle cell trait and β-thalassemia patients in Mexico. *Blood Cells Mol Dis*, Vol. 36, No. 2, (Mar-Apr), pp. 255-258, ISSN 1079-9796

Nuinoon, M.; Makarasara, W., et al. (2010). A genome-wide association identified the common genetic variants influence disease severity in β^0-thalassemia/hemoglobin E. *Hum Genet*, Vol. 127, No. 3, (Mar), pp. 303-314, ISSN 0340-6717

Orkin, S. H.; Kazazian, H. H., Jr., et al. (1982). Abnormal RNA processing due to the exon mutation of β^E-globin gene. *Nature*, Vol. 300, No. 5894, (Dec 23), pp. 768-769, ISSN 0028-0836

Perrotta, S.; Cappellini, M. D., et al. (2000). Osteoporosis in β-thalassaemia major patients: analysis of the genetic background. *Br J Haematol*, Vol. 111, No. 2, (Nov), pp. 461-466, ISSN 0007-1048

Premawardhena, A.; Fisher, C. A., et al. (2001). Genetic determinants of jaundice and gallstones in haemoglobin E β-thalassaemia. *Lancet*, Vol. 357, No. 9272, (Jun 16), pp. 1945-1946, ISSN 0140-6736

Rees, D. C.; Luo, L. Y., et al. (1997). Nontransfusional iron overload in thalassemia: association with hereditary hemochromatosis. *Blood*, Vol. 90, No. 8, (Oct 15), pp. 3234-3236, ISSN 0006-4971

Rees, D. C.; Porter, J. B., et al. (1999). Why are hemoglobin F levels increased in HbE/β thalassemia? *Blood*, Vol. 94, No. 9, (Nov 1), pp. 3199-3204, ISSN 0006-4971

Reich, D. E.&Lander, E. S. (2001). On the allelic spectrum of human disease. *Trends Genet*, Vol. 17, No. 9, (Sep), pp. 502-510, ISSN 0168-9525

Rund, D.&Rachmilewitz, E. (2005). β-Thalassemia. *N Engl J Med*, Vol. 353, No. 11, (Sep 15), pp. 1135-1146, ISSN 0028-4793

Sachidanandam, R.; Weissman, D., et al. (2001). A map of human genome sequence variation containing 1.42 million single nucleotide polymorphisms. *Nature*, Vol. 409, No. 6822, (Feb 15), pp. 928-933, ISSN 0028-0836

Sankaran, V. G.; Menne, T. F., et al. (2008). Human fetal hemoglobin expression is regulated by the developmental stage-specific repressor BCL11A. *Science*, Vol. 322, No. 5909, (Dec 19), pp. 1839-1842, ISSN 0036-8075

Sedgewick, A. E.; Timofeev, N., et al. (2008). BCL11A is a major HbF quantitative trait locus in three different populations with β-hemoglobinopathies. *Blood Cells Mol Dis*, Vol. 41, No. 3, (Nov-Dec), pp. 255-258, ISSN 1079-9796

Sherva, R.; Sripichai, O., et al. (2010). Genetic modifiers of Hb E/β⁰-thalassemia identified by a two-stage genome-wide association study. *BMC Med Genet*, Vol. 11, No. pp. 51, ISSN 1471-2350

So, C. C.; Song, Y. Q., et al. (2008). The HBS1L-MYB intergenic region on chromosome 6q23 is a quantitative trait locus controlling fetal haemoglobin level in carriers of β-thalassaemia. *J Med Genet*, Vol. 45, No. 11, (Nov), pp. 745-751, ISSN 0022-2593

Sripichai, O.; Makarasara, W., et al. (2008a). A scoring system for the classification of β-thalassemia/Hb E disease severity. *Am J Hematol*, Vol. 83, No. 6, (Jun), pp. 482-484, ISSN 0361-8609

Sripichai, O.; Munkongdee, T., et al. (2008b). Coinheritance of the different copy numbers of α-globin gene modifies severity of β-thalassemia/HbE disease. *Ann Hematol*, Vol. 87, No. 5, (May), pp. 375-379, ISSN 0939-5555

Thein, S. L. (2008). Genetic modifiers of the β-haemoglobinopathies. *Br J Haematol*, Vol. 141, No. 3, (May), pp. 357-366, ISSN 0007-1048

Thein, S. L.; Hesketh, C., et al. (1988). The molecular basis of thalassaemia major and thalassaemia intermedia in Asian Indians: application to prenatal diagnosis. *Br J Haematol*, Vol. 70, No. 2, (Oct), pp. 225-231, ISSN 0007-1048

Thein, S. L.; Menzel, S., et al. (2007). Intergenic variants of HBS1L-MYB are responsible for a major quantitative trait locus on chromosome 6q23 influencing fetal hemoglobin levels in adults. *Proc Natl Acad Sci U S A*, Vol. 104, No. 27, (Jul 3), pp. 11346-11351, ISSN 0027-8424

Thein, S. L.; Wainscoat, J. S., et al. (1987). Association of thalassaemia intermedia with a β-globin gene haplotype. *Br J Haematol*, Vol. 65, No. 3, (Mar), pp. 367-373, ISSN 0007-1048

Thompson, C. C.; Ali, M. A., et al. (1989). The interaction of anti 3.7 type quadruplicated α-globin genes and heterozygous β-thalassemia. *Hemoglobin*, Vol. 13, No. 2, pp. 125-135, ISSN 0363-0269

Traeger-Synodinos, J.; Kanavakis, E., et al. (1996). The triplicated α-globin gene locus in β-thalassaemia heterozygotes: clinical, haematological, biosynthetic and molecular studies. *Br J Haematol*, Vol. 95, No. 3, (Dec), pp. 467-471, ISSN 0007-1048

Tubsuwan, A.; Munkongdee, T., et al. (2011) Molecular analysis of globin genes expression in different thalassaemia disorders individual variation of β^E pre-mRNA splicing determine disease severity. *Br J Haematol*. Vol. 154, No. 5, (Sep), pp. 635-643, ISSN 0007-1048

Uda, M.; Galanello, R., et al. (2008). Genome-wide association study shows BCL11A associated with persistent fetal hemoglobin and amelioration of the phenotype of β-thalassemia. *Proc Natl Acad Sci U S A*, Vol. 105, No. 5, (Feb 5), pp. 1620-1625, ISSN 0027-8424

Venter, J. C.; Adams, M. D., et al. (2001). The sequence of the human genome. *Science*, Vol. 291, No. 5507, (Feb 16), pp. 1304-1351, ISSN 0036-8075

Wahlberg, K.; Jiang, J., et al. (2009). The HBS1L-MYB intergenic interval associated with elevated HbF levels shows characteristics of a distal regulatory region in erythroid cells. *Blood,* Vol. 114, No. 6, (Aug 6), pp. 1254-1262, ISSN 0006-4971

Wainscoat, J. S.; Kanavakis, E., et al. (1983). Thalassaemia intermedia in Cyprus: the interaction of α and β thalassaemia. *Br J Haematol,* Vol. 53, No. 3, (Mar), pp. 411-416, ISSN 0007-1048

Weatherall, D. J.; Clegg, J. B., et al. (1965). Globin synthesis in thalassaemia: an in vitro study. *Nature,* Vol. 208, No. 5015, (Dec 11), pp. 1061-1065, ISSN 0028-0836

Wilber, A.; Hargrove, P. W., et al. (2011). Therapeutic levels of fetal hemoglobin in erythroid progeny of β-thalassemic CD34+ cells after lentiviral vector-mediated gene transfer. *Blood,* Vol. 117, No. 10, (Mar 10), pp. 2817-2826, ISSN 0006-4971

Winichagoon, P.; Fucharoen, S., et al. (1995). Role of alternatively spliced β^E-globin mRNA on clinical severity of β-thalassemia/hemoglobin E disease. *Southeast Asian J Trop Med Public Health,* Vol. 26 Suppl 1, No. pp. 241-245,

Xu, J.; Sankaran, V. G., et al. (2010). Transcriptional silencing of γ-globin by BCL11A involves long-range interactions and cooperation with SOX6. *Genes Dev,* Vol. 24, No. 8, (Apr 15), pp. 783-798, ISSN 0890-9369

2

HMG–CoA Lyase Deficiency

Beatriz Puisac, María Arnedo, Mª Concepción Gil-Rodríguez,
Esperanza Teresa, Angeles Pié, Gloria Bueno, Feliciano J. Ramos,
Paulino Goméz-Puertas and Juan Pié
Unit of Clinical Genetics and Functional Genomics
School of Medicine, University of Zaragoza
Spain

1. Introduction

The HMG-CoA lyase (HL) deficiency or 3-hydroxy-3-methylglutaric aciduria (MIM 246450) is an inborn error of intermediary metabolism that was first described in 1976 by Faull et al (Faull et al., 1976). Because its clinical manifestations, it has been included within the Sudden Infant Death Syndrome (Wilson et al., 1984). At present, it is considered a rare disease (<1/100,000 live neonates) that should be diagnosed at early age because there is a simple and effective treatment (Watson et al., 2006).

HL is a mitochondrial enzyme that catalyzes the cleavage of HMG-CoA to acetyl-CoA and acetoacetate, which is the common final step of ketogenesis and leucine catabolism (Figure 1). Patients with this disease suffer on the one hand, the absence of ketone bodies as alternative energy source of glucose and on the other hand, the accumulation of toxic metabolites of leucine catabolism. The most frequently affected organs are the liver and the brain, but the pancreas and the heart can also be involved. This chapter discusses a recent study of differential expression of human HL in liver, pancreas, testis, heart, skeletal muscle and brain that can help us to understand the consequences of this deficiency (Puisac et al., 2010).

It is an autosomal recessive disease caused by mutations in the *HMGCL* gene. The study of these mutations and patients´ origin helps to draw a map of incidence in which three countries stand out for their high frequency: Saudi Arabia (Ozand et al., 1992), Spain and Portugal (Menao et al., 2009).

At present, the functional study of missense mutations is possible thanks to the knowledge of the structure (Fu et al., 2006) and mechanism of the enzyme (Fu et al., 2010) and also by the development of a method of simple and efficient expression of the protein (Menao et al., 2009). Finally, despite the current knowledge of the disease, genotype-phenotype correlations are difficult to establish.

2. HL enzyme

HL is a 325-aminoacid enzyme that has been purified from a variety of organisms and tissues, including pig heart (Bachawat et al., 1955), chicken liver (Kramer et al., 1980) and *Pseudomonas mevalonii* (Scher et al., 1989). In addition to the isoform located in the mitochondrial matrix, it has been described another in peroxisomes (Ashmarina et al., 1994). The native mitochondrial isoform contains a leader peptide of 27 aminoacids at the N-terminal end, which guides HL towards the mitochondrial matrix, where the leader peptide is removed. This final isoform has a molecular mass of 31.5 kDa and an isoelectric point of 6.2.

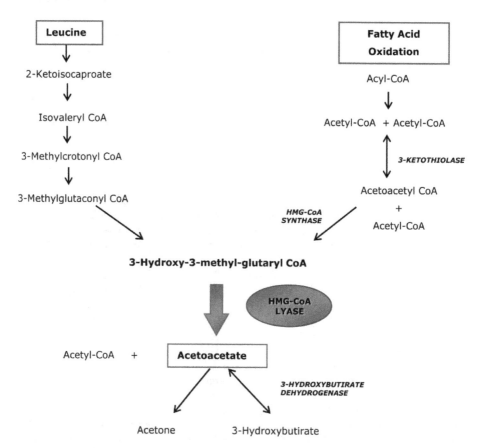

Fig. 1. Metabolic interrelationships of HL

Human HL has 87% simmilarity with its mouse homologue, 82% with its chicken homologue, and 52% with *P. mevalonii*, and the sequence has been highly conserved throughout evolution (Pié et al., 2007). The cathalytic active form is a homodimer of two identical monomers bound by a disulphide bridge (Roberts, 1994). The human enzyme is very sensitive to oxidation, showing higher activity in reductive conditions. It is also sensitive to the conditions of pH, showing an optimum activity at alkaline pH (pH=9). HL activity requires the presence of a divalent cation, such as Mg^{+2} or Mn^{+2}. The Mg^{+2} ion has an octahedral coordination with two water molecules, the imidazole nitrogens of catalitic residues His[233] and His[235], the carboxylate group of Asp[42] and the amide oxygen of Asn[275]. Other catalytic residues in the vicinity include Arg[41] and Cys[266].

2.1 Protein structure

The first attempt to build a 3D structural model of human 3-hydroxy-3-methylglutaryl-CoA lyase was based on a threading procedure using the crystallized structure of the TIM-barrel hisA gene from *Thermotoga maritima* as a template (Casals et al., 2003). The proposed model correspond to a $(\alpha\beta)_8$ barrel with short loops on the NH$_2$ terminal face and, in contrast, long and probably non-structured loops on the COOH-terminal face of the β-barrel. This model showed, for the first time, the structural proximity of the residues involved in the cathalytic activity of the protein: Arg[41], Asp[42], Glu[72], His[233] and His[235], located near the cavity opened in the COOH-terminal face of the protein model (Figure 2).

This model was confirmed when the cristal structure of human HL was obtained (Fu et al., 2006). In addition to the basic TIM barrel structure, the monomer of human HL includes an additional polypeptide region made of residues 290-323 containing β-strand 9, and α-helices 11 and 12. The active site is accessible only from the C-terminal side of the TIM barrel and the N-terminal barrel end is occluded. Crystal structures of the wild-type enzyme complex and inhibitor hydroxyglutaryl-CoA has demostrated the interaction of Arg[41] and acyl-CoA´s C1 carbonyl oxygen of sustrate and explains why Arg[41] mutations cause drastic enzyme deficiency (Fu et al., 2010).

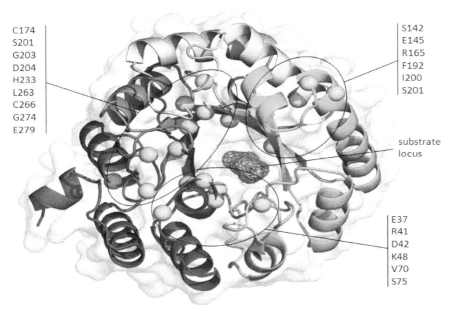

Fig. 2. Structural location of missense mutations in human HL. Blue spheres represent mutated residues

The native enzyme is a dimer in solution (Tuinstra et al., 2002) that was confirmed when the protein was crystallized. The area of contact between monomers is formed by additional secondary elements that are not part of the core TIM barrel structure, β-strand 9, and α-helices 11 and 12. Recently it was suggested that multiple cysteine residues influence covalent adduct formation in HMG-CoA lyase as well as the dependence of enzyme activity on reducing agent (Montgomery & Miziorko, 2011).

2.2 Enzymatic reaction

The cleavage of HMG-CoA, catalyzed by the HL enzyme is the final step of ketogenesis, in which acetyl-CoA, mainly from the β-oxidation of fatty acids, is converted to acetoacetate, β-hydroxybutyrate and acetone (Figure 1). From a chemical point of view, the enzyme reaction is a retro-Claisen condensation, which requires an acid and a base for catalysis (Roberts et al., 1996). The base abstracts a proton from the C3 hydroxyl of HMG-CoA, which leads to the formation of a ketone (acetoacetate) and C2–C3 bond cleavage (Figure 3). In addition, a transient carbanion form of acetyl-CoA, is regenerated by the acid proton. However, the exact identity of molecules or residues that act as base or as acid was not precised. Recently a water molecule, positioned between D42 and the C3 hydroxyl of bound sustrate has been proposed as a proton shuttle (Fu et al., 2010).

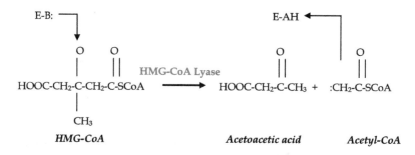

Fig. 3. Chemical reaction catalyzed by the enzyme HMG-CoA lyase. E-B: base, E-AH acid

2.3 Enzyme expression

HL is widely expressed in most tissues (Clikenbeard et al., 1975) mainly because it is necessary not only in tissues that synthesize ketone bodies, but for the catabolism of leucine as well. Activity levels of this enzyme have been reported in different eucaryotes organism tissues: pig heart (Bachawat et al., 1955), bovine liver (Stegink & Coon, 1968) and chicken liver, kidney, heart, brain, ileum and muscle (Clikenbeard et al., 1975). However, its distribution and activity in human tissues have been limited to enzyme assay in fibroblast (Wanders et al., 1988b) lymphoblast (Wysocki et al, 1976b) liver biopsy (Robinson et al,1980) amniocytes and chorionic villi (Wanders et al., 1988b) or pancreatic islets (MacDonald et al., 2007).

Recently, it has been reported the first study of mRNA levels, protein expression and enzyme activity of human HMG-CoA lyase in kidney, pancreas, testis, heart, skeletal muscle and brain (Puisac et al., 2010). The highest HL activity was found in liver and pancreas was the second with more activity (Figure 4c). This finding indicates that the pancreas has a high ketogenic capacity and suggests that if ketone bodies regulate the release of insulin (Biden & Taylor, 1983; Malaisse et al., 1990; Rhodes et al., 1985) some of them could be produced in the pancreas. HL activity in kidney was high and moderately high in testis and skeletal muscle. Surprisingly in muscle, although the mRNA levels were very low (Figure 4a), moderate HL activity was measured. Similar cases are reported in the literature (Lewin et al., 2001), which suggests that certain tissues may have a lower turnover of the HL protein versus an unstable mRNA. In testis, the low activity levels of HL compared with the high enzyme expression (Figure 4b), suggest that HL activity could be regulated after translation in this tissue. However, very little HL is found in heart tissue and it is not present in the mitochondria from human brain.

2.4 Isoforms
Two different protein isoforms of HL have been found, which are codified by a single gene located in chromosome 1. While most HL is found in mitochondria, about 16-20% is located in peroxisomes (Ashmarina et al., 1999). To date, no satisfactory explanation has been found to explain this distribution. The protein found in peroxisomes is guided by the signal CKL tripeptide in the C-terminal end and it has 325 aminoacids, a molecular mass of 34.1 kDa and an isoelectric point of 7.6, which is much more basic than the mitochondrial protein (Ashmarina et al., 1994). As the mitochondrial isoform, it is a dimeric form and has lyase activity; however its role inside peroxisomes is still unknown. Probably, this is related to cholesterol synthesis or long chain fat acids degradation (Krisans et al., 1996).

3. HL deficiency

HMG-CoA lyase deficiency or 3-Hydroxy-3-methylglutaric aciduria (OMIM 246450) is a rare autosomal recessive genetic disorder that affects ketogenesis and L-leucine catabolism. For this reason, it is included within alterations of fatty acid metabolism and also within organic acidemias. This deficiency was first described by Faull et al in 1976 in a 7 month-old male with acidosis and hypoglycemia (Faull et al., 1976). Later, Wysocki et al showed that HL activity in the leukocytes of this patient was null (Wysocky et al., 1976). The gene knock-out in mice results in embryonic lethality (Wang et al., 1998) reflecting the physiological importance of this enzyme.

3.1 Clinical features
3-Hydroxy-3-methylglutaric aciduria is a severe condition in children, in fasting or in high glucose consumption, when ketone bodies are essential as alternative energy substrate. In approximately 30% of the cases the first symptoms appear between the second and fifth days of life or between 3 and 11 months. However, four patients with late onset (puberty and adult) have been reported (Sweetman et al., 1995; Vargas et al., 2007; Bischof et al., 2004; Reimao et al., 2009).

3.1.1 Acute crisis
Acute crises tend to occur when there is no exogenous intake of glucose (starving cases) or when there is an excessive glucose metabolization (conditions of metabolic stress, febrile stress and exercise). Initial symptoms may include poor feeding, vomiting, diarrhea, followed by further complication as hypotonia, hypothermia, lethargy, cyanosis and apnea. (Schutgens et al., 1979; Gibson et al., 1988a; Gibson et al., 1988b). In some cases the progresive lowered state of consciousness leads to coma and subsequent death (Wysocki et al., 1986). Laboratory data that stand out are the metabolic acidosis and non-ketotic hypoglycemia (Table 1). Hypoglycemia can be explained by fasting or other intercurrent illness, while the hipoketonemia shows the inability of patients to synthesize ketone bodies. Metabolic acidosis and aciduria can be explained by the accumulation of acids metabolites from leucine catabolism: 3-hydroxy-isovaleric acid, 3-methylglutaconic acid, 3-methylglutaric acid and 3-hydroxy-3-methylglutaric acid. Occasionally, patients present with increased

bilirubin, liver transaminases and prothrombin time. It is also reported the appearance of hyperammonemia associated with increased proteolysis by deficiency of ketone bodies.

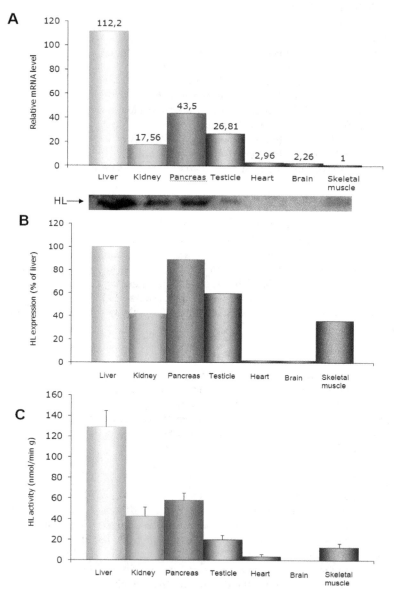

Fig. 4. Comparative analysis of mRNA levels, protein expression and enzymatic activity of HMG-CoA lyase in different human tissues. (A) Relative levels of mRNA HL expression in human tissues (B) HL protein expression measured in mitochondrial fraction from human tissues (C) HL activity was measured in the mitochondrial fraction of human tissues spectrophotometrically. Data are presented as mean ±SEM

Clinical manifestations in acute clinical episodes	
Vomiting	
Diarrhea	
Hipotonia	Frequent all of them if the clinical picture worsens
Hypothermia	
Lethargy	
Apnea	
Coma	

Laboratory test

General biochemistry	
Metabolic acidosis	Always present
Hypoglycemia	Always present
Hypoketonemia	Always present
Ketonuria	Absent
Hyperammonemia	Elevated frequently
Hepatic transaminases	Elevated frequently
Bilirrubin	Elevated in some cases
Prothrombin time	Elevated in some cases
Organic acids	
3-hydroxy-3-methylglutaric	Elevated very frequently
3-methylglutaric	Elevated frequently
3-methylglutaconic	Elevated sometimes
3-hydroxyisovaleric	Elevated sometimes
HL enzyme activity	Less than 5%

Affected organs	
Brain	Macro o Microcephaly (infrequent)
	Alterations of the white matter (frequent)
	Epilepsy (infrequent)
	Cerebral infarction (infrequent)
Pancreas	Acute pancreatitis (infrequent)
Liver	Hepatomegaly (very frequent)
Heart	Dilated cardiomyopathy with arrythmia (infrequent)

Table 1. Clinical and laboratory findings of the HMG-CoA lyase deficiency

3.1.2 Chronic complications

Chronic complications are uncommon but include: hepatomegalia, macrocephalia (Gibson et al., 1988b; Stacey et al., 1985) microcephalia (Lisson et al., 1981) and delayed development (Gibson et al., 1994). It has been reported that organs such as the brain, the liver and occasionally the pancreas and the heart are affected (Gibson et al., 1994; Leung et al., 2009; Muroi et al., 2000a; Urganci et al., 2001; Wilson et al., 1984; Zafeiriou et al., 2007; Zoghbi et al., 1986). Recently, a study of mRNA levels, protein expression and enzyme activity of human HMG-CoA lyase in kidney, pancreas, testis, heart, skeletal muscle and brain has contributed to better understanding of the enzyme function and of the involvement of these organs in 3-hydroxy-3-methylglutaric aciduria (Puisac et al., 2010).

The liver is the organ most frequently affected in this deficiency, although involvement is usually mild, with elevated transaminases and hepatomegaly (Urganci et al., 2001; Wysocki & Hahnel, 1986). Ketogenesis is more active in the liver and the blockage of this pathway could result in an accumulation of toxic intermediate metabolites.

Pancreatitis is a potential complication in patients with organic acidemias, (Kahler et al., 1994) and some cases have been reported in 3-hydroxy-3-methylglutaric aciduria (Muroi et al., 2000a; Wilson et al., 1984). The finding of higher enzymatic activity in pancreas (Puisac et al., 2010) indicates that it may be more susceptible to toxic accumulation of metabolites. Among the brain abnormalities in these patients, cerebral white matter involment is the most common reported finding (Lisson et al., 1981; Yalcinkaya et al., 1999; Zafeiriou et al., 2007) and also one case of prominent corticospinal tract and pontine involvement has also been reported (Yylmaz et al., 2006). HL is not found at different levels of mRNA, protein and enzymatic activity, in the mitochondria from human brain (Puisac et al., 2010). This suggests that the neurological alterations frequently associated with this deficiency, are related to hypoglycaemia and to the absence of the only alternative substrate to glucose for the brain, ketone bodies. Concomitantly, the organic acids would not be produced in situ, although they could cross the blood-brain barrier of an immature brain (Wajner et al., 2004) and cause damage.

Dilated cardiomyopathy has been described in two patients with 3-hydroxy-3-methylglutaric aciduria, one young male (Gibson et al., 1994) and one adult (Leung et al., 2009). In this last case, the authors suggest that the cardiomyopathy results from impaired ketogenesis, intracellular fatty acid accumulation and a secondary carnitine deficiency. However, very little HL was found in heart tissue (Puisac et al., 2010). This result does not support the hypothesis of local accumulation of organic acids or regulation the entry of fatty acids to the heart and thus prevent their accumulation as a cause of the cardiomyopathy. In HL deficiency heart disease could be caused by the lack of an alternative energy substrate. The heart is a continuously active muscle which uses various energy substrates depending on their availability (Kodde et al., 2007). Although ketone bodies are not an indispensable substrate, the added L-carnitine deficiency, which is caused by the HL deficiency, could alter the transport of fatty acids to the mitochondria for oxidation and the coupling between glycolysis and glucose oxidation (Allard et al., 2006).

3.2 Diagnosis

This deficiency should be suspected in children with hypoglycaemia, hipoketonemia and metabolic acidosis. A preliminary diagnosis is made from a characteristic pattern of organic acids in urine, with high levels of 3-hydroxy-3-methylglutaric acid, 3-hydroxy-isovaleric acid, 3-methylglutaric acid and 3-methylglutaconic acid (Table 1). The characteristic metabolite of this disease is the 3-hydroxy-3-methylglutaric acid, but can also occur in the deficiency of carbamyl phosphate synthetase or Leigh-like disease (Faull et al., 1976). The confirmation of HL deficiency requires direct assay of the enzyme activity in leukocytes (Wysocki et al., 1976a) fibroblasts (Wysocki et al., 1976b; Wanders et al., 1988a) or liver biopsy (Schutgens et al., 1979). In prenatal diagnosis the pattern of organic acids in amniotic liquid (Chalmers et al., 1979), in maternal urine (Duran et al., 1979) and measurements of HL activity in cultured amniocytes or chorionic villi (Mitchell et al., 1995; Chalmers et al., 1979) could be used as diagnostic tools. The molecular characterization of mutations in the gene *HMGCL*, including alterations in the mRNA, helps to complete the diagnosis.

3.3 Treatment

During acute episodes, treatment is based on symptoms and consists of intravenous administration of glucose to control hypoglycemia, and bicarbonate to correct acidosis. Maintenance therapy is based on restrictive protein and fat diet, whose aim is to reduce the formation of toxic metabolites. However, the most important concern is to avoid metabolic stress such as intercurrent illnesses and starvation. Carnitine treatment has been proposed to improve the patient´s general state by facilitating urinary excretion of toxic metabolites (Dasouki et al., 1979). Moreover, L-carnitine, can be essential to prevent the development of cardiomyopathy (Puisac et al., 2010).

3.4 Prognosis

Despite this disease belongs to a group of 29 genetic conditions for which effective treatment is currently available (Watson et al., 2006), HMG-CoA lyase deficiency is fatal in approximately 20% of the cases. Nevertheless, early and careful treatment may result in a good prognosis with normal growth and development. Besides, in absence of complications, illness tends to improve with time and adults are usually free of symptoms.

4. *HMGCL* gene

The *HMGCL* gene (Gen Bank NM_000191.2) located in the short arm of chromosome 1 (1p36.1-p35), between *FUCA1* and *TCEB3* encodes human HL. It has 9 exons and 8 introns (Figure 5) and a total of 24,336 base pairs. Its 5'-untranslated region bears the characteristic elements of a housekeeping gene, as well as a CpG island that contains binding sites for SP1. There is no evidence of the existence neither of a TATA box nor a CAAT box (Wang et al., 1996). Exons size varies between 64 and 527 base pairs (bp) and the introns range between 600 and 3400 bp. Exon 1 and part of exon 2 codify a 27 aminoacids array that forms the signal peptide for mitochondrial entering. Exon 9 codifies for 33 codons at the C-terminal ending and also has 406 bp from the 3'untranslated region (Mitchell et al., 1993). The polyadenylation signal in humans and mouse is ATTAAA. This gene is present in both eukaryotes and prokaryotes and it has been cloned and studied in a variety of organisms, including humans (Mitchell et al., 1993), chicken (Mitchell et al., 1993), mouse (Wang et al., 1993), the *Rhodospilirrum rubrum* (Baltscheffsky et al., 1997) and bacterial strains such as *Pseudomonas mevalonii* (Anderson et al., 1989), *Brucella mellitensis* and *Bacillus subtillus* (Forouhar et al., 2006).

The mRNA transcribed from *HMGCL* human gene has a size of 1.6 Kb and it has been found in all tissues studied albeit in widely differing amounts (Puisac et al., 2010) (Figure 4a) Tissues with the highest expression are liver 112.2 arbitrary units (100%) pancreas 43.5 (39%), kidney 17.56 (16%), testis 26.81 (24%), heart 2.96 (2,6%) brain 2.26 (2%) and skeletal muscle 1 (0.89%).

This gene presents a physiological splicing with three variants, one with all exons encoding the active protein and two with deletion of exons 5 and 6 and deletion of exons 5, 6 and 7 that encode inactive proteins (Muroi et al., 2000; Beatriz Puisac PhD thesis). These last two transcripts appear in tissues such as heart, brain and skeletal muscle which have little or no ketogenic potential.

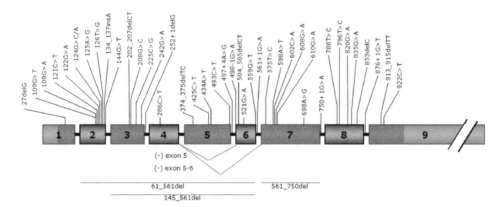

Fig. 5. Scheme of mutations located in the human *HMGCL* gene

4.1 Mutational update

To date 50 variant alleles in the *HMGCL* gene (48 mutations and 2 SNPs) in more than 100 patiens have been reported (Table 2). The missense mutations are the most frequent (25) followed by intronic mutations (7), frameshift deletions (6), nonsense mutations (6), large deletions (3) and insertions (1). The mutations are uniformly distributed along the gene sequences, although some clustering is observed in exon 2 and exon 7, suggesting that they could be hot spots for mutations (Figure 5).

Three mutations are more common than the rest: one is the c.122G>A (81 alleles, 43 patients: 38 homozygous, 5 heterozygous with an allele unknown), prevalent in Saudi Arabia, where 40 patients carry it (Mitchell et al., 1998; Al-Sayed et al., 2006) and that has also been found in a patient in Italy, another in Turkey (Mitchell et al., 1998) and one in the Tcheck Republic suggesting that this mutation may have arisen independently more than once (Pospisilova et al., 2003).

Allelic variant	Exon/ Intron	Aminoacid change/ Predicted effect	Patients	Mutant Aleles	Origin	References
Missense mutations						
c.109G>A	E2	E37K	2	4	2 Pakistani	Menao 2009 Al-Sayed 2006;
c.122G>A	E2	R41Q	43	81	1 Czech, 1 Italian (ht), 40 Saudi (4 ht), 1 Turkish	Mitchell 1998; Pospisilova 2003
c.124G>A	E2	D42N	1	1	1 Brazilian (ht)	Vargas 2007
c.124G>C	E2	D42H	1	1	1 Cajun (ht)	Mitchell 1998
c.125A>G	E2	D42G	2	4	1 German, 1 Palestinian	Menao 2009; Mitchell 1998
c.126T>G	E2	D42E	1	2	1 Austrian	Mitchell 1998

Allelic variant	Exon/ Intron	Aminoacid change/ Predicted effect	Patients	Mutant Aleles	Origin	References
c.144G>T	E2	K48N	1	1	1 Spanish	Carrasco 2007
c.208G>C	E3	V70L	1	1	1 French-Canadian (ht)	Mitchell 1992
c.225C>G	E3	S75R	1	2	1 German	Casals 2003
c.425C>T	E5	S142F	1	1	1 Spanish (ht)	Menao 2009
c.434A>T	E5	E145V	1	1	1 Japanese (ht)	Muroi 2000
c.493C>T	E5	R165W	1	2	1 Turkish	Koling 2000
c.494G>A	E5	R165Q	1	1	1 French? (ht)	Pierron 2009
c.494G>T	E5	R165Q	1	1	1Tawianese (ht)	Lin 2009
c.521G>A	E6	C174Y	1	2	1 Palestinian	Menao 2009
c.575T>C	E7	F192S	1	2	1 Spanish	Menao 2009
c.598A>T	E7	I200F	1	2	1 French	Menao 2009
c.602C>A	E7	S201Y	1	2	1 English	Casals 2003
c.608G>A	E7	G203E	1	2	1 Italian	Mir 2006
c.610G>A	E7	D204N	2	3	1 Argentinean ,1 Portuguese (ht)	Casals 2003; Cardoso 2004
c.698A>G	E7	H233R	4	5	2 Czech (1ht), 1 French (ht), 1 English (ht)	Menao 2009; Pospisilova 2003; Roberts 1996; Zapater 1998
c.788T>C	E8	L263P	1	1	1 French (ht)	Zapater 1998
c.796T>C	E8	C266R	1	1	1 Greek (ht)	Zafeiriou 2007
c.820G>A	E8	G274R	1	1	1 French? (ht)	Pierron 2009
c.835G>A	E8	E279K	2	3	2 Japanese (1 ht)	Muroi 2000

Nonsense mutations

Allelic variant	Exon/ Intron	Aminoacid change/ Predicted effect	Patients	Mutant Aleles	Origin	References
c.109G>T	E2	E37X; Exon 2 skipping	31	55	1 Argentinian, 2 Moroccan, 13 Portuguese (4ht) , 11 Spanish (1ht), 1 Turkish, 3 portuguese-brazilian (2ht)	Cardoso 2004; Casale 1998; Menao 2009; Pié 1997; Puisac 2005
c.121C>T	E2	R41X	1	1	1 English/German (ht)	Mitchell 1998
c. 242G>A	E3	W81X	1	2	1 Ecuatorian	Menao 2009
c.286C>T	E4	Q96X	1	2	1 Italian	Funghini 2001
c.559G>T	E6	E187X	1	1	1 Spanish (ht)	Menao 2009
c.922C>T	E9	Q308X	1	2	1 Japanese	Muroi 2000

Allelic variant	Exon/ Intron	Aminoacid change/ Predicted effect	Patients	Mutant Aleles	Origin	References
Deletions/ insertions						
c.27delG	E1	P9P/ frameshift: stop codon 33	1	1	1 Czech (ht)	Pospisilova 2003
c.134-137insA	E2	N46K/frameshift: stop codon 47	2	4	2 Italian	Mitchell 1995
c.61-561del	E2,E3,E4,E5, E6	Deletes V21-E187 in frame	1	1	1 English	Wang 1996
c.202-207delCT	E3	S69C/ frameshift: stop codon 79	3	6	2 Acadian French-Canadian, 1 Spanish	Mitchell 1993
c.145-561del	E3,E4,E5, E6	Deletes E49-E187 in frame	1	1	1 Turkish	Wang 1996
c.374-375delTC	E5	V125D/frameshift: stop codon 150	1	1	1 Greek (ht)	Zafeiriou 2007
c.504-505delCT	E6	V168V/frameshift: stop codon 176; Exon 5 and 6, 6 skipping	10	11	3 Portuguese-brazilian (3ht), 2 Portuguese (2ht), 5 Spanish (4 ht)	Cardoso 2004; Casals 1997; Menao 2009; Vargas 2007
c.561-750del	E7	Deletes E187-Q250 in frame	1	2	1 Japanese	Muroi 2000
c.853delC	E8	Frameshift: stop codon 258	1	1	1 English (ht)	Menao 2009
c.913-915delTT	E9	F305Y/ frameshift: stop codon 314	3	6	3 Saudi	Al-Sayed 2006; Mitchell 1998
Intronic mutations						
IVS3+1Gdel	I3	Exon 3 deletion	1	2	1 Japanese	Muroi 2000
IVS3+1G>A	I3	Exon 3 deletion	1	1	1 Tawianese (ht)	Lin 2009
IVS5+4A>G	I5	Exon 5 deletion/ exon 5-6 deletion	1	1	1 English (ht)	Menao 2009
IVS6-1G>A	I5		1	1	1 Taiwanese (ht)	Lin 2009
IVS6+1G>A	I6		1	2	1 Saudi	Al-Sayed 2006
IVS7+1G>A	I7	r.slp	2	2	2 Spanish (2 ht)	Menao 2009
IVS8+1G>T	I8	Exon 8 deletion	1	2	1 Turkish	Buesa 1996

Allelic variant	Exon/ Intron	Aminoacid change/ Predicted effect	Patients	Mutant Aleles	Origin	References
Polimorfism						
c.252+34C>T	I3		1	1	1 Palestinian (ht)	Menao 2009
c.654A>G	E7	L218L	1	-	1 Spanish	Pié 1997
c.727A>G	E7	T243A	4	8	1 Moroccan, 1 Portuguese, 2 Spanish	Pié 1997

Table 2. Mutations and polymorphisms in the *HMGCL* gene. Position refers to the numbering of the HL cDNA sequence in Mitchell et al., 1993. ht, heterozygous

The second most frequent mutation is the c.109G>T (Mediterranean mutation) (55 alleles, 31 patients: 24 homozygous, 6 double heterozygous, 1 heterozygous with an allele unknown), found mostly in the Iberian Peninsula (13 patients in Portugal, 11 in Spain and 3 in brazilian-portugueses). It has also been described two cases in Morocco and another in Turkey (Pié et al., 1997; Casale et al., 1998; Cardoso et al., 2004; Puisac et al., 2005; Menao et al., 2009). It has been hypothesized that in Portugal and Spain the genetic hit was introduced during the Arabian invasions of the Iberian Peninsula in the eighth century. Further studies should be necessary to dillucidate if the mutation origin is the Iberian Peninsula itself or the Magreb (Pié et al., 2007).

The third most frequent mutation is c.504_505delCT (11 alleles, 10 patients: 1 homozygous, 9 double heterozygous), although its incidente is much lower than the first two. It seems to be exclusively located in the Iberian Peninsula, where 15% of Portuguese (2 cases) (Cardoso et al., 2004) and 27% of Spanish patients have it (Menao et al., 2009). This mutation is also present in 3 of the 4 molecularly diagnosed Brazilians patients, though they were of Portuguese origin (Vargas et al., 2007).

In most of the remaining countries, only a few patients are reported, with a high level of allelic heterogeneity. In Japan 4 mutations have been reported in 5 unrelated patients (Muroi et al., 2000b), in Taiwan 3 mutations in 2 patients (Lin et al., 2009) in Italy, 5 mutations in 5 patients (Mitchell et al., 1995; Mitchell et al., 1998; Funghini et al., 2001) in Turkey 4 mutations in 4 patients (Wang et al., 1996; Buesa et al., 1996; Pié et al., 1997; Mitchell et al., 1998) . In the United Kingdom 6 mutations in 5 patients, though one of them was of German origin (c.121C>T) (Wang et al., 1996; Mitchell et al., 1998; Casals et al., 2003; Menao et al., 2009), 3 mutations in 3 patients in the Tcheck Republic (Pospisilova et al., 2003) and in Germany 2 mutations in 2 patients (Mitchell et al., 1998; Casals et al., 2003). The French group, the Acadians (descendents of the 17th-century French colonists), the Cajuns (Acadians settled in Louisiana) and the French-Canadians, despite of their common origin, present a great allelic heterogenicity: 6 mutations in 6 patients (Mitchell et al., 1992; Mitchell et al., 1993; Zapater et al., 1998; Mitchell et al., 1998; Menao et al., 2009).

4.2 Genotype-phenotype correlations

The genotype-phenotype correlation is difficult to establish because the progress of the disease seems to be more related to the causes that produce hypoglycaemia (fasting or acute illness) than to a specific genotype. For example, patients carrying the same mutation, for instance the so-called Mediterranean mutation (c.109G>T) may have from moderate to severe crises of lethal consequences. This is why in clinical practice it is fundamental to avoid situations that may cause hypoglycemia in these patients (Pié et al., 2007).

Several studies agree that studied missense mutations cause a loss of enzyme activity greater than 95% although these mutations often produce mild phenotypes (Mitchell et al., 1998; Carrasco et al., 2007; Menao et al., 2009). This suggests that the illness appears only in very severe genotypes, and that partial disruption of the enzyme is probably compatible with normal function. This adds more difficulties to establish genotype-phenotype correlations because we only see the effects of very severe genotypes.

5. Conclusion

Although 3-hydroxy-3-methylglutaric aciduria is a very rare disease, given the availability of an effective treatment, we recommend the screening of this disease in any child with hypoglycemia and metabolic acidosis. Moreover, in countries with a greater number of diagnosed cases (Saudi Arabia, Portugal and Spain), we also recommend to screen for the following mutations: c.122G>A, c.109G>T and c.504_505delCT. The high percentage of splicing mutations justifies including the measurement of the mRNA.

6. Acknowledgment

This study was supported by Spanish grants from: Diputación General de Aragón (Ref.# Grupo Consolidado B20) and University of Zaragoza (Ref.# PIF-UZ_2009-BIO-02). We also thank to "Biomol-Informatics SL -www.bioinfo.es-" for bioinformatic support.

7. References

Allard, ML., Jeejeebhoy, KN., & Sole, MJ. (2006). The management of conditioned nutritional requirements in heart failure. *Heart Failure Reviews,* Vol. 11, No. 1, (March 2006), pp. 75-82, ISSN 1382-4147

Al-Sayed, M., Imtiaz, F., Alsmadi, OA., Rashed, MS., & Meyer, BF. (2006). Mutations underlying 3-hydroxy-3-methylglutaryl CoA lyase deficiency in the Saudi population. *BMC Medical Genetics,* Vol. 16, No. 7, (December 2006), ISSN 1471-2350

Anderson, DH., & Rodwell, VW. (1989). Nucleotide sequence and expression in Escherichia coli of the 3-hydroxy-3-methylglutaryl coenzyme A lyase gene of Pseudomonas mevalonii. *Journal of Bacteriology,* Vol. 171, No. 12, (December 1989), pp. 6468-6472, ISSN 0021-9193

Ashmaina, LI., Rusnak, N., Miziorko, HM., & Mitchell, GA. (1994). 3-Hydroxy-3-methylglutaryl-CoA lyase is present in mouse and human liver peroxisomes. *The Journal of Biological Chemistry,* Vol. 269, No. 50 (December 1994), pp. 31929-31932, ISSN 0752-7399

Ashmarina, LI., Pshezhetsky, AV., Branda, SS., Isaya, G., & Mitchell, GA. (1999). 3-Hydroxy-3-methylglutaryl coenzyme A lyase: targeting and processing in peroxisomes and mitochondria. *Journal of Lipid Research,* Vol. 40, No. 1, (January 1999), pp. 70-75, ISSN 0022-2275

Bachhawat, BK., Robinson, WG., & Coon, MJ. (1955). The enzymatic cleavage of beta-hydroxy-beta-methylglutaryl coenzyme A to acetoacetate and acetyl coenzyme A. *Journal of Biological Chemistry,* Vol. 216, (August 1955), pp. 727-736, ISSN 0021-9258

Baltscheffsky, M., Brosché, M., Hultman, T., Lundvik, L., Nyrén, P., Sakai-Nore, Y., Severin, A., & Strid, A. (1997). A 3-hydroxy-3-methylglutaryl-CoA lyase gene in the photosynthetic bacterium Rhodospirillum rubrum. *Biochimica Biophysica Acta*, Vol. 1337, No. 1, (January 1997), pp. 113-122, ISNN 0005-2736

Biden, TJ., & Taylor, KW. (1983). Effects of ketone bodies on insulin release and islet-cell metabolism in the rat. *Biochemical Journal*, Vol. 212, No. 2, (May 1983), pp. 371-377, ISSN 0264-6021

Bischof, F., Nagele, T., Wanders, RJ., Trefz, FK., & Melms, A. (2004). 3-Hydroxy-3-methylglutaryl-coenzyme A lyase deficiency in an adult with leukoencephalopathy. *Annals of Neurology*, Vol. 56, No. 5, (November 2004), pp. 727-730. ISNN 0364-5134

Buesa, C., Pié, J., Barceló, A., Casals, N., Mascaró, C., Casale, CH., Haro, D., Duran, M., Smeitink, JA., Hegardt, FG. (1996). Aberrantly spliced mRNAs of the 3-hydroxy-3-methylglutaryl coenzyme A lyase (HL) gene with a donor splice-site point mutation produce hereditary HL deficiency. *Journal of Lipid Research*, Vol. 37, No.11, (November 1996), pp. 2420-2432, ISSN 0022-2275

Cardoso, ML., Rodrigues, MR., Leão, E., Martins, E., Diogo, L., Rodrigues, E., Garcia, P., Rolland, MO., & Vilarinho, L. (2004). The E37X is a common HMGCL mutation in Portuguese patients with 3-hydroxy-3-methylglutaric CoA lyase deficiency. *Molecular Genetics and Metabolism*, Vol. 82, No. 4, (August 2004), pp. 334-338, ISSN 1096-7192

Carrasco, P., Menao, S., López-Viñas, E., Santpere, G., Clotet, J., Sierra, AY., Gratacós, E., Puisac, B., Gómez-Puertas, P., Hegardt, FG., Pie, J., & Casals, N. (2007). C-terminal end and aminoacid Lys48 in HMG-CoA lyase are involved in substrate binding and enzyme activity. *Molecular Genetics and Metabolism*, Vol. 91, No. 2, (June 2007), pp. 120-127, ISSN 1096-7192

Casale, CH., Casals, N., Pié, J., Zapater, N., Pérez-Cerdá, C., Merinero, B., Martínez-Pardo, M., García-Peñas, JJ., García-Gonzalez, JM., Lama, R., Poll-The, BT., Smeitink, JA., Wanders, RJ., Ugarte, M., & Hegardt, FG. (1998). A nonsense mutation in the exon 2 of the 3-hydroxy-3-methylglutaryl coenzyme A lyase (HL) gene producing three mature mRNAs is the main cause of 3-hydroxy-3-methylglutaric aciduria in European Mediterranean patients. *Archives of Biochemistry and Biophysics*, Vol. 349, No.1, (January 2001), pp. 129-137, ISSN 0003-9861

Casals, N., Gomez-Puertas, P., Pie, J., Mir, C., Roca, R., Puisac, B., Aledo, R., Clotet, J., Menao, S., Serra, D., Asins, G., Till, J., Elias-Jones, AC., Cresto, JC., Chamoles, NA., Abdenur, JE., Mayatepek, E., Besley, G., Valencia, A., & Hegardt, FG. (2003). Structural (betaalpha)$_8$ TIM barrel model of 3-hydroxy-3-methylglutaryl-coenzyme A lyase. *Journal of Biological Chemistry*, Vol. 278, No. 31, (May 2003), pp. 29061-29023, ISSN 0021-9258

Chalmers, RA., Tracey, BM., Mistry, J., Stacey, TE., & McFadyen, IR. (1989). Prenatal diagnosis of 3-hydroxy-3-methylglutaric aciduria by GC-MS and enzymology on cultured amniocytes and chorionic villi. *Journal of Inherited Metabolic Disease*, Vol. 12, No. 3, pp. 286-292, ISSN 0141-8955

Clinkenbeard, KD., Reed, WD., Mooney, RA. (1975). Intracellular localization of the 3-hydroxy-3-methylglutaryl coenzyme A cycle enzymes in liver. Separate cytoplasmic and mitochondrial 3-hydroxy-3-methylglutaryl coenzyme A generating systems for cholesterogenesis and ketogenesis. *Journal of Biological Chemistry*, Vol. 250, No. 8, (April 1975), pp. 3108-3116, ISSN 0021-9258

Dasouki, M., Buchanan, D., Mercer, N., Gibson, KM., & Thoene, J. (1987). 3-Hydroxy-3-methylglutaric aciduria: response to carnitine therapy and fat and leucine restriction. *Journal of Inherited Metabolic Disease*, Vol. 10, No. 2, (1987), pp. 142-146, ISSN 0141-8955

Duran, M., Ketting, D., Wadman, SK., Jakobs, C., Schutgens, RB., & Veder, HA. (1978). Organic acid excretion in a patient with 3-hydroxy-3-methylglutaryl-CoA lyase deficiency: facts and artefacts. *Clinica Chimica Acta*, Vol. 90, No. 2, (December 1978), pp. 187-193, ISSN 0009-8981

Faull, KF., Bolton, PD., Halpern, B., Hammond, J., Danks, DM., Hähnel, R., Wilkinson, SP., Wysocki, SJ., & Masters, PL. (1976). Letter: Patient with defect in leucine metabolism. *New England Journal of Medicine*, Vol. 294, No. 18, (April 1976), pp. 1013, ISSN 0028-4793.

Forouhar, F., Hussain, M., Farid, R., Benach, J., Abashidze, M., Edstrom, WC., Vorobiev, SM., Xiao, R., Acton, TB., Fu, Z., Kim, JJ., Miziorko, HM., Montelione, GT., & Hunt, JF. (2006). Cristal structures of two bacterial 3-hydroxy-3-methylglutaryl-CoA lyases suggest a common catalytic mechanism among a family of TIM barrel metalloenzymes cleaving carbon-carbon bonds. *Journal of Biological Chemistry*, Vol. 281, No. 11, (March 2006), pp. 7533-7545, ISSN 0021-9258

Fu, Z., Runquist, JA., Forouhar, F., Hussain, M., Hunt, JF., Miziorko, HM., & Kim, JJ. (2006). Crystal structure of human 3-hydroxy-3-methylglutaryl-CoA Lyase: insights into catalysis and the molecular basis for hydroxymethylglutaric aciduria. *Journal of Biological Chemistry*, Vol. 281, No. 11, (March 2006), pp. 7526-7532, ISSN 0021-9258.

Fu, Z., Runquist, JA., Montgomery, C., Miziorko, HM., & Kim, JJ. (2010). Functional insights into human HMG-CoA lyase from structures of Acyl-CoA-containing ternary complexes. *Journal of Biological Chemistry*, Vol. 285, No. 34, (August 2010), pp. 26341-26349, ISSN 0021-9258

Funghini, S., Pasquini, E., Cappellini, M., Donati, MA., Morrone, A., Fonda, C., & Zammarchi, E. (2001). 3-Hydroxy-3-methylglutaric aciduria in an Italian patient is caused by a new nonsense mutation in the HMGCL gene. *Molecular Genetics and Metabolism*, Vol. 73, No. 3, (July 2004), pp. 268-275, ISSN 1096-7192

Gibson, KM., Breuer, J., & Nyhan, WL. (1988a). 3-Hydroxy-3-methylglutaryl-coenzyme A lyase deficiency: review of 18 reported patients. *European Journal of Pediatrics*, Vol. 148, No. 3, (December 1988), pp. 180-186, ISSN 0340-6199

Gibson, KM., Breuer, J., Kaiser, K., Nyhan, WL., McCoy, EE., Ferreira, P., Greene, CL., Blitzer, MG., Shapira, E., & Reverte, F. (1988b). 3-Hydroxy-3-methylglutaryl-coenzyme A lyase deficiency: report of five new patients. *Journal of Inherited Metabolic Disease*, Vol. 11, No. 1, pp. 76-87, ISNN 0141-8955

Gibson, KM., Cassidy, SB., Seaver, LH., Wanders, RJ., Kennaway, NG., Mitchell, GA., & Spark, RP. (1994). Fatal cardiomyopathy associated with 3-hydroxy-3-methylglutaryl-CoA lyase deficiency. *Journal of Inherited Metabolic Disease*, Vol. 17, No. 3, pp. 291-294, ISNN 0141-8955

Kahler, SG., Sherwood, WG., Woolf, D., Lawless, ST., Zaritsky, A., Bonham, J., Taylor, CJ., Clarke, JT., Durie, P., & Leonard, JV. (1994). Pancreatitis in patients with organic acidemias. *The Journal of Pediatrics*, Vol. 124, No. 2, (February 1994), pp. 239-243, ISSN 0022-3476

Kodde, IF., van der Stok, J., Smolenski, RT., & de Jong, JW. (2007). Metabolic and genetic regulation of cardiac energy substrate preference. *Comparative Biochemistry and Physiology*, Vol. 146, No. 1, (January 2007), pp. 26-39, ISSN 1095-6433

Kramer, PR., & Miziorko, HM. (1980). Purification and characterization of avian liver 3-hydroxy-3-methylglutaryl coenzyme A lyase. *Journal of Biological Chemistry*, Vol. 255, No. 22, (November 1980), pp. 11023-11028, ISSN 0021-9258

Krisans, SK. (1996). Cell compartmentalization of cholesterol biosynthesis. *Annals of the New York Academy of Sciences*, Vol. 804, (December 1999), pp. 142-164, ISSN 0077-8923

Leung, AA., Chan, AK., Ezekowitz, JA. & Leung, AK. (2009). A Case of Dilated Cardiomyopathy Associated with 3-Hydroxy-3-Methylglutaryl-Coenzyme A (HMG CoA) Lyase Deficiency. *Case Report in Medicine*, Vol. 2009, (2009), pp.1-3 ISSN 1687-9627

Lewin, TM., Granger, DA., & Kim, JH. (2001). Regulation of mitochondrial sn-glycerol-3-phosphate acyltransferase activity: response to feeding status is unique in various rat tissues and is discordant with protein expression. *Archives of Biochemistry and Biophysics*, Vol. 396, No. 1, (December 2001), pp. 119-127, ISSN 0003-9861

Lin, WD., Wang, CH., Lai, CC., Tsai, Y., Wu, JY., Chen, CP., & Tsai , FJ. (2009). Molecular analysis of Taiwanese patients with 3-hydroxy-3-methylglutaryl CoA lyase deficiency. *Clinica Chimica Acta*, Vol. 401, No. 1-2, (March 2009), pp. 33-36, ISNN 0009-8981

Lisson, G., Leupold, D., Bechinger, D., & Wallesch, C. (1981). CT findings in a case of deficiency of 3-hydroxy-3-methylglutaryl-CoA-lyase. *Neuroradiology*, Vol. 22, No.2, pp.99-101, ISSN 0028-3940

MacDonald, MJ., Smith, AD., & Hasan, NM. (2007). Feasibility of pathways for transfer of acyl groups from mitochondria to the cytosol to form short chain acyl-CoAs in the pancreatic beta cell. *Journal of Biological Chemistry*, Vol. 282, No. 42, (October 2007), pp. 30596-30606, ISSN 0021-9258

Malaisse, WJ., Lebrun, P., & Rasschaert, J. (1990). Ketone bodies and islet function: 86Rb handling and metabolic data. *American Journal of Physiology*, Vol. 259, (January 1990), pp. E123-E130, ISSN 0363-6135

Menao, S., López-Viñas, E., Mir, C., Puisac, B., Gratacós, E., Arnedo, M., Carrasco, P., Moreno, S., Ramos, M., Gil, MC., Pié, A., Ribes, A., Pérez-Cerda, C., Ugarte, M., Clayton, PT., Korman, SH., Serra, D., Asins, G., Ramos, FJ., Gómez-Puertas, P., Hegardt, FG., Casals, N., & Pié, J. (2009). Ten novel HMGCL mutations in 24 patients of different origin with 3-hydroxy-3-methyl-glutaric aciduria. *Human Mutation*, Vol. 30, No. 3, (March 2009), pp.E520-529, ISSN 1098-1004

Mitchell, GA., Robert, MF., Fontaine, G., Wang, S., Lambert, M., Cole, D., Lee, C., Gibson, M., & Miziorko, MH. (1992). HMG CoA lyase (HL) deficiency: detection of a causal mutation in an affected French-Canadian sibship. *American Journal of Human Genetics*, Vol.51, A173, ISSN 0002-9297

Mitchell, GA., Robert, MF., Hruz, PW., Wang, SP., Fontaine, G., Behnke, CE., Mende-Mueller, LM., Schappert, K., Lee, C., Gibson, KM., & Miziorko, HM. (1993). 3-Hydroxy-3-methylglutaryl coenzyme A lyase (HL). Cloning of human and chicken liver HL cDNAs and characterization of a mutation causing human HL deficiency. *Journal of Biological Chemistry*, Vol. 268, No. 6, (February 1993), pp. 4376-4381, ISSN 0021-9258

Mitchell, GA., Jakobs, C., Gibson, KM., Robert, MF., Burlina, A., Dionisi-Vici, C., & Dallaire, L. (1995). Molecular prenatal diagnosis of 3-hydroxy-3-methylglutaryl CoA lyase deficiency. *Prenatal Diagnosis*, Vol. 15, No. 8, (August 1995), pp. 725-729, ISSN 0197-3851

Mitchell, GA., Ozand, PT., Robert, MF., Ashmarina, L., Roberts, J., Gibson, KM., Wanders, RJ., Wang, S., Chevalier, I., Plöchl, E., & Miziorko, H. (1998). HMG CoA lyase deficiency: identification of five causal point mutations in codons 41 and 42, including a frequent Saudi Arabian mutation, R41Q. *American Journal of Human Genetics*, Vol. 62, No .2, (February 1998), pp. 295-300, ISSN 0002-9297

Montgomery, C., & Miziorko, HM. (2011). Influence of multiple cysteines on human 3-hydroxy-3-methylglutaryl-CoA lyase activity and formation of inter-subunit adducts. *Archives of Biochemistry and Biophysics*, Vol.511, No. 1-2, (April 2011), pp.48-55, ISSN 0003-9861.

Muroi, J., Yorifuji, T., Uematsu, A., & Nakahata, T. (2000a). Cerebral infarction and pancreatitis: possible complications of patients with 3-hydroxy-3-methylglutaryl-CoA lyase deficiency. *Journal of Inherited Metabolic Disease*, Vol. 23, No. 6, (September 2000), pp. 636-637, ISSN 0141-8955

Muroi, J., Yorifuji, T., Uematsu, A., Shigematsu, Y., Onigata, K., Maruyama, H., Nobutoki, T., Kitamura, A., & Nakahata, T. (2000b). Molecular and clinical analysis of Japanese patients with 3-hydroxy-3-methylglutaryl CoA lyase (HL) deficiency. *Human Genetics*, Vol. 107, No. 4, (October 2000), pp. 320-326, ISSN 0340-6717

Ozand, PT., Devol, EB., & Gascon, GG. (1992). Neurometabolic diseases at a national referral center: five years experience at the King Faisal Specialist Hospital and Research Centre. *Journal of Child Neurology*, Suppl. 7, (April 1992), pp.S4-S11, ISSN 0883-0738.

Pié, J., Casals, N., Casale, CH., Buesa, C., Mascaró, C., Barceló, A., Rolland, MO., Zabot, T., Haro, D., Eyskens, F., Divry, P., & Hegardt, FG. (1997). A nonsense mutation in the 3-hydroxy-3-methylglutaryl-CoA lyase gene produces exon skipping in two patients of different origin with 3-hydroxy-3-methylglutaryl-CoA lyase deficiency. *Biochemical Journal*, Vol. 323, No. 2, (April 1997), pp. 329-335, ISSN 0264-6021

Pié, J., López-Viñas, E., Puisac, B., Menao, S., Pié, A., Casale, C., Ramos, FJ., Hegardt, FG., Gómez-Puertas, P., & Casals, N. (2007). Molecular genetics of HMG-CoA lyase deficiency. *Molecular Genetics and Metabolism*, Vol. 92, No. 3, (November 2007), pp. 198-209, ISSN 1096-7192

Pospísilová, E., Mrázová, L., Hrdá, J., Martincová, O., & Zeman, J. (2003). Biochemical and molecular analyses in three patients with 3-hydroxy-3-methylglutaric aciduria. *Journal of Inherited Metabolic Disease*, Vol. 26, No. 5, (2003), pp. 433-441, ISSN 0141-8955

Puisac, B. (2004). Splicing variants and three-dimensional structure of human HMG-CoA lyase. Molecular and functional characterization of four new allelic variants. *PhD thesis. University of Zaragoza, Department of Pharmacology and Physiology* (September 2004).

Puisac, B., López-Viñas, E., Moreno, S., Mir, C., Pérez-Cerdá, C., Menao, S., Lluch, D., Pié, A., Gómez-Puertas, P., Casals, N., Ugarte, M., Hegardt, F., & Pié, J. (2005). Skipping of exon 2 and exons 2 plus 3 of HMG-CoA lyase (HL) gene produces the loss of beta sheets 1 and 2 in the recently proposed (beta-alpha) 8 TIM barrel model of HL. *Biophysical Chemistry*, Vol. 115, No. 2-3, (April 2005), pp. 241-245, ISSN 0301-4622

Puisac, B., Arnedo, M., Casale, CH., Ribate, MP., Castiella, T., Ramos, FJ., Ribes, A., Pérez-Cerdá, C., Casals, N., Hegardt, FG., & Pié, J. (2010). Differential HMG-CoA lyase expression in human tissues provides clues about 3-hydroxy-3-methylglutaric aciduria. *Journal of Inherited Metabolic Disease*, Vol. 33, No. 4, (August 2010), pp. 405-410, ISSN 1573-2665

Reimão, S., Morgado, C., Almeida, IT., Silva, M., Real, HC., & Campos, J. (2009). 3-Hydroxy-3-methylglutaryl-coenzyme A lyase deficiency: Initial presentation in a young adult. *Journal of Inherited Metabolic Disease*, (February 2009), ISSN 0141-8955

Rhodes, CJ., Campbell, IL., & Szopa, TM. (1985). Effects of glucose and D-3-hydroxybutyrate on human pancreatic islet cell function. *Clinical Science*, Vol. 68, No.5, (May 1985), pp. 567-572, ISSN 0143-5221

Roberts, JR., Narasimhan, C., Hruz, PW., Mitchell, GA., & Miziorko, HM. (1994). 3-Hydroxy-3-methylglutaryl coenzyme A lyase: Expression and isolation of the recombinant human enzyme and investigation of a mechanism for regulation of enzyme activity. *Journal of Biological Chemistry*, Vol. 269, No. 27, (July 1994), pp.17841-17846, ISSN 0021-9258

Roberts, JR., Narasimhan, C., & Miziorko, HM. (1995). Evaluation of cysteine 266 of human 3-hydroxy-3-methylglutaryl coenzyme A lyase as a catalytic residue. *Journal of Biological Chemistry*, Vol. 270, No. 31, (July 1995), pp. 17311-17316, ISSN 0021-9258

Roberts, JR., Mitchell, GA., & Miziorko, HM. (1996). Modeling of a mutation responsible for human 3-hydroxy-3-methylglutaryl-CoA lyase deficiency implicates histidine 233 as an active site residue. *Journal of Biological Chemistry*, Vol. 271, No. 40, (October 1996), pp. 24604-24609, ISSN 0021-9258

Robinson, AM., & Williamson, DH. (1980). Physiological roles of ketone bodies as substrates and signals in mammalian tissues. *Physiological Reviews*, Vol. 60, No. 1, (January 1980), pp. 143-187, ISSN 0031-9333

Scher, DS., & Rodwell, VW. (1989). 3-Hydroxy-3-methylglutaryl coenzyme A lyase from Pseudomonas mevalonii. *Biochimica and Biophysica Acta*, Vol. 1003, No. 3, (June 1989) pp. 321-326, ISSN 0304-4165

Schutgens, RB., Heymans, H., Ketel, A., Veder, HA., Duran, M., Ketting, D., & Wadman, SK. (1986). Lethal hypoglycemia in a child with a deficiency of 3-hydroxy-3-methylglutarylcoenzyme A lyase. *The Journal of Pediatrics*, Vol. 94, No. 1 (January 1979), pp. 89-91, ISSN 0022-3476

Stacey, TE., de Sousa, C., Tracey, BM., Whitelaw, A., Mistry, J., Timbrell, P., & Chalmers, RA. (1985). Dizygotic twins with 3-hydroxy-3-methylglutaric aciduria; unusual presentation, family studies and dietary management. *European Journal of Pediatrics*, Vol. 144, No. 2, (July 1985), pp. 177-181, ISSN 0340-6199

Sweetman, L., & William, JC. (1995). In: *The Metabolic and Molecular Basis of Inherited Disease*, C.R. Schreiver, A.L. Beaudet, W.S. Sly, D. Valle (Eds.), pp.1400-1402, McGraw-Hill, New York

Tuinstra, RL., Burgner, JW., & Miziorko, HM. (2002). Investigation of the oligomeric status of the peroxisomal isoform of human 3-hydroxy-3-methylglutaryl-CoA lyase. *Archives of Biochemistry and Biophysics*, Vol. 408, No. 2, (December 2001), pp. 286-294, ISSN 0003-9861

Urgançi, N., Arapoğlu, M., Evrüke, M., & Aydin, A. (2001). A rare cause of hepatomegaly: 3-hydroxy-3-methylglutaryl coenzyme-a lyase deficiency. *Journal of Pediatrics Gastroenterol & Nutrition*, Vol. 33, No. 3, (September 2001), pp. 339-41, ISSN 0277-2116

Vargas, CR., Sitta, A., Schmitt, G., Ferreira, GC., Cardoso, ML., Coelho, D., Gibson, KM., & Wajner, M. (2007). Incidence of 3-hydroxy-3-methylglutaryl-coenzyme A lyase (HL) deficiency in Brazil, South America. *Journal of Inherited Metabolic Disease*, (December 2007), ISSN 0141-8955

Wajner, M., Latini, A., Wyse, AT., & Dutra-Filho, CS. (2004). The role of oxidative damage in the neuropathology of organic acidurias: insights from animal studies. *Journal of Inherited Metabolic Disease*, Vol. 27, No. 4, (2004), pp. 427-448, ISSN 0141-8955

Wanders, RJ., Schutgens, RB., & Zoeters, PH. (1988a). 3-Hydroxy-3-methylglutaryl-CoA lyase in human skin fibroblasts: study of its properties and deficient activity in 3-hydroxy-3-methylglutaric aciduria patients using a simple spectrophotometric method. *Clinica Chimica Acta*, Vol. 171, No. 1, (January 1988), pp. 95-101, ISSN 0009-8981

Wanders, RJ., Schutgens, RB., & Zoeters, BH. (1988b). Prenatal diagnosis of 3-hydroxy-3-methylglutaric aciduria via enzyme activity measurements in chorionic villi, chorionic villous fibroblasts or amniocytes using a simple spectrophotometric method. *Journal of Inherited Metabolic Disease*, Vol. 11, No. 4, (1988), pp. 430, ISSN 0141-8955

Wang, SP., Robert, MF., Gibson, KM., Wanders, RJ., & Mitchell, GA. (1996). 3-Hydroxy-3-methylglutaryl CoA lyase (HL): mouse and human HL gene (*HMGCL*) cloning and detection of large gene deletions in two unrelated HL-deficient patients. *Genomics*, Vol. 33, No. 1, (April 1996), pp. 99-104, ISSN: 0888-7543

Wang, SP., Marth, JD., Oligny, LL., Vachon, M., Robert, MF., Ashmarina, L., & Mitchell, GA. (1998). 3-Hydroxy-3-methylglutaryl-CoA lyase (HL): gene targeting causes prenatal lethality in HL-deficient mice. *Human Molecular Genetics*, Vol. 7, No.13, (December 1998) pp. 2057-2062, ISSN 0964-6906

Watson, MS., Mann, MY., Lloyd-Puryear, MA., & Rinaldo, M. (2006). Newborn screening: toward a uniform screening panel and system. *Genetics in Medicine*, 8 Suppl 1: 1S-252S, ISSN 1098-3600

Wilson, WG., Cass, MB., Søvik, O., Gibson, KM., & Sweetman, L. (1984). A child with acute pancreatitis and recurrent hypoglycemia due to 3-hydroxy-3-methylglutaryl-CoA lyase deficiency. *European Journal of Pediatrics*, Vol. 142, No. 4, (September 1984), pp. 289-291, ISSN 0340-6199

Wysocki, SJ., & Hahnel, R. (1976a). 3-Hydroxy-3-methylglutaric aciduria: deficiency of 3-hydroxy-3-methylglutaryl coenzyme A lyase. *Clinica Chimica Acta*, Vol. 71, No. 2, (September 1976), pp.349-351, ISSN 0009-8981

Wysocki, SJ., & Hahnel. R. (1976b). 3-Hydroxy-3-methylglutaric aciduria: 3-hydroxy-3-methylglutaryl-coenzyme A lyase levels in leucocytes. *Clinica Chimica Acta*, Vol. 73, No. 2, (December 1976), pp. 373-375, ISSN 0009-8981

Wysocki, SJ., & Hähnel, R. (1986). 3-Hydroxy-3-methylglutaryl-coenzyme a lyase deficiency: a review. *Journal of Inherited Metabolic Disease*, Vol. 9, No. 3, (1986), pp. 225-233, ISSN 0141-8955

Yalçinkaya, C., Dinçer, A., Gündüz, E., Fiçicioğlu, C., Koçer, N., & Aydin, A. (2007). MRI and MRS in HMG-CoA lyase deficiency. *Pediatrics Neurology*, Vol. 20, No. 5, (May 2007), pp. 375-380, ISSN 0887-8994

Yýlmaz, Y., Ozdemir, N., Ekinci, G., Baykal, T., & Kocaman, C. (2006). Corticospinal tract involvement in a patient with 3-HMG coenzyme A lyase deficiency. *Pediatrics Neurology*, Vol. 35, No. 2, (August 2006), pp. 139-141, ISSN 0887-8994

Zafeiriou, DI., Vargiami, E., Mayapetek, E., Augoustidou-Savvopoulou, P., & Mitchell, GA. (2007). 3-Hydroxy-3-methylglutaryl coenzyme a lyase deficiency with reversible white matter changes after treatment. *Pediatrics Neurology*, Vol. 37, No.1, (July 2007), pp. 47-50, ISSN 0887-8994

Zapater, N., Pié, J., Lloberas, J., Rolland, MO., Leroux, B., Vidailhet, M., Divry, P., Hegardt, FG., & Casals, N. (2001). Two missense point mutations in different alleles in the 3-hydroxy-3-methylglutaryl coenzyme A lyase gene produce 3-hydroxy-3-methylglutaric aciduria in a French patient. *Archives of Biochemistry and Biophysics*, Vol. 358, No. 2, (October 1998), pp. 197-203, ISSN 0003-9861

Zoghbi, HY., Spence, JE., Beaudet, AL., O'Brien, WE., Goodman, CJ., & Gibson, KM. (1986). Atypical presentation and neuropathological studies in 3-hydroxy-3-methylglutaryl-CoA lyase deficiency. *Annals of Neurology*, Vol. 20, No. 3, (September 1986), pp. 367-369, ISSN 0364-5134.

3

Mitochondrial HMG–CoA Synthase Deficiency

María Arnedo, Mónica Ramos, Beatriz Puisac,
Mª Concepción Gil-Rodríguez, Esperanza Teresa, Ángeles Pié,
Gloria Bueno, Feliciano J. Ramos, Paulino Gómez-Puertas and Juan Pié
Unit of Clinical Genetics and Functional Genomics, School of Medicine,
University of Zaragoza
Spain

1. Introduction

The mitochondrial 3-hydroxy-3-methylglutaryl-CoA (HMG-CoA) synthase deficiency (MIM 600234) is an autosomic recessive inborn error of metabolism, hard to characterize and probably underdiagnosed (Thompson et al., 1997). The enzyme failure is caused by mutations in the gene *HMGCS2,* located in chromosome 1. The illness was first diagnosed in 1997 (Thompson et al., 1997), in a six-year old boy, who presented a semicomatose state after three days with gastroenteritis and diet (Bouchard et al., 2001). Up to date, only eight patients have been reported with an estimated incidence of <1/1,000,000, although it could be higher because some patients probably have been misdiagnosed as Reye syndrome.

The mitochondrial HMG-CoA synthase enzyme (mHS, EC 4.1.3.5) has a main role in the synthesis of the ketone bodies and in the HMG-CoA formation. Ketone bodies act as an alternative glucose fuel in a number of tissues as heart, muscle and brain, and have a critical role during metabolic stress and starving, situations where the symptoms of the disease appear.

2. Ketogenesis

The ketogenesis is a metabolic process that takes place inside the mitochondria. The acetyl-CoA, originated during the fatty acids β-oxidation, is converted to acetoacetate, β-hidroxybutyrate and acetone. These metabolites are known as ketone bodies and act as a glucose alternative fuel in many tissues as heart, skeletal muscle and brain. In brain, ketone bodies play an essential role in situations of hypoglycemia (Edmond, 1992; Zammit & Moir, 1994). Besides their alternative fuel role, ketone bodies are lipogenic precursors too. They play a role during the myelinating process in the neonates' brain (Nehlig & Pereira de Vasconcelos, 1993), and in a minor degree in the mammary gland during suckling (Zammit, 1981). Moreover, they seem to have some functions in metabolism regulation (Robinson & Williamson, 1980).

The main tissue where ketogenesis takes place is the liver (Zammit & Moir, 1994). However, it has been also found in kidney, adipose tissue (Thumelin et al., 1993), and intestine of suckling rats (Hahn & Taller, 1987) and, in a minor degree, in cortical astrocytes of newborn rats (Cullingford et al., 1998; Blázquez et al., 1998).

Ketone bodies can be elevated in physiological situations as: fasting, prolonged exercise, high-fat diet or pregnancy (Felig & Lynch, 1970), in the neonate (Hawkins et al., 1971); and in pathologic situations as: diabetes (Bates et al., 1968), obesity and disease of the glucose or glycogen metabolism (Mitchell et al., 1997).

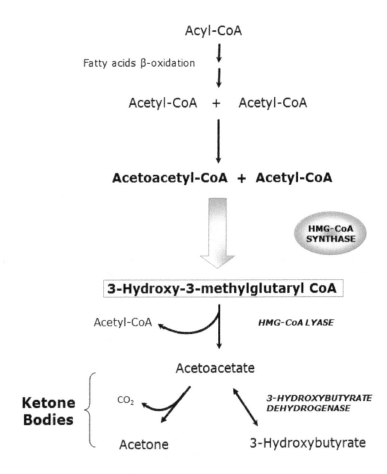

Fig. 1. Ketone bodies synthesis pathway

The main pathway of ketone bodies from acetyl-CoA includes the following reactions (Figure 1):

- In the first reaction, two acetyl-CoA molecules join to form acetoacetyl-CoA. This reaction is catalyzed by the acetoacetyl-CoA thiolase enzyme.
- Then, acetoacetyl-CoA reacts with another acetyl-CoA to produce the HMG-CoA. This is a condensation reaction where the mHS enzyme is involved, and whose failure is responsible of the disease.

- In the third reaction, the HMG-CoA is cleaved into acetoacetate, the first ketone body produced, and acetyl-CoA. This step is catalyzed by the HMG-CoA lyase (HL).
- Finally, in the last reaction, the acetoacetate is reduced to β-hydroxybutyrate, the second ketone body generated. The enzyme involved in this reaction is the β-hydroxybutyrate dehydrogenase. Acetone is formed by the spontaneous decarboxylation of acetoacetate.

There is an alternative ketogenic pathway different from the previously described, which takes place with substrates of aminoacids catabolism. Both pathways converge in the mitochondrial HL enzyme.

3. mHS enzyme

The mHS catalyzes the second reaction of the main pathway of the synthesis of ketone bodies and it is considered as the key enzyme of pathway regulation.

3.1 Enzymatic reaction

The mHS enzyme catalyzes the condensation of acetyl-CoA and acetoacetyl-CoA into HMG-CoA. The HMG-CoA, produced inside the mitochondria, drives towards the formation of ketone bodies. The mHS catalyzed reaction follows a Bi Bi Ping-Pong substitution mechanism (Cleland, 1963; Miziorko et al., 1975). This reaction has three steps (Miziorko et al., 1977) (Figure 2):

- Firstly, acetyl-CoA reacts with the thiol group of the catalytic Cys[166] in order to produce a covalent intermediate form of the acetyl-enzyme. This is the limiting reaction step (Miziorko et al., 1977).
- Then, acetoacetyl-CoA (second substrate) condenses with the intermediate product to give HMG-CoA, which will be attached to the enzyme by a covalent bond.
- In the final step, HMG-CoA is released from the enzyme by hydrolysis.

High concentrations of acetoacetyl-CoA inhibit the first reaction step, because it competes with acetyl-CoA for the active site of the enzyme (Page & Tubbs, 1978). Magnesium can act as an inhibitor of the reaction too.

3.2 Protein structure

Human mHS has 508 amino acids and its structure is a homodimer formed by two identical monomers linked by a salt bridge (Figure 3). At the N-terminal end is the leader peptide, with 37 aa, which drives the protein to the mitochondria.

In 1985, the catalytic sequence of the enzyme was identified in a purified protein from chicken liver (Miziorko & Behnke, 1985). This sequence has 21 aa and a 100% homology with HMG-CoA synthases from other mammals. The catalytic aminoacid Cys[129], whose human homolog is the Cys[166], is located inside this region (Misra et al., 1995). The protein analysis shows three regions rich in proline, glutamine, serine and threonine, which could be PEST sequences (Pro-Glu-Ser-Thr) (Rogers et al., 1986). These regions are characterized by a quick turnover of proteins (Boukaftane et al., 1994; Ayté et al., 1990).

Recently, the human enzyme has been crystallized and its alpha/beta structure, with 17 beta sheets and 19 alpha helices, has been well characterized. The tunnel of substrate entry and product exit is located outside of the molecule, at the opposite side of the interaction between the two monomers (Shafqat et al., 2010).

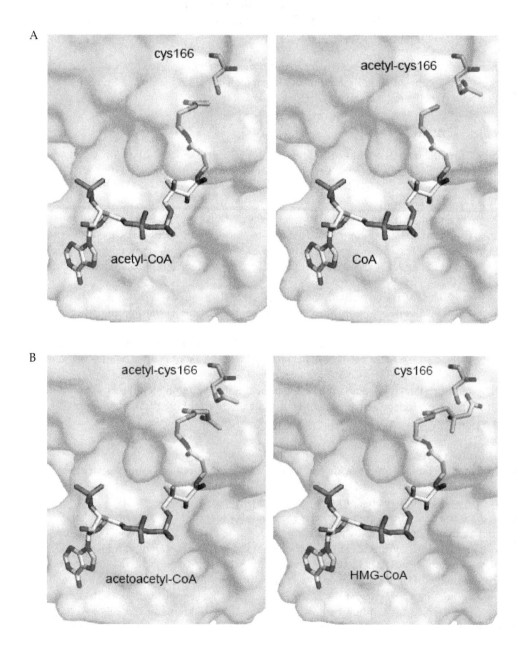

Fig. 2. A. Acetyl-enzyme intermediate formation. B. HMG-CoA formation

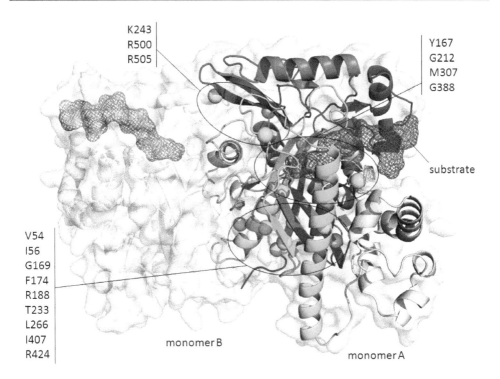

Fig. 3. Structural location of missense mutations in human mHS, represented as blue spheres

3.3 Enzyme expression

Studies of gene expression in human tissues in basal conditions showed a tissue-specific expression. High mRNA levels are detected in the liver, the organ with the highest ketogenic capacity. Expression is also high in colon, which is related to the fermentative processes that take place in it (Mascaró et al., 1995). A minor level of mRNA expression has been observed in heart, skeletal muscle, gonads, kidney and pancreas (Mascaró et al., 1995; Royo et al., 1993). Studies in rats have found mRNA expression in cortical astrocytes from newborns (Cullingford et al., 1998; Blazquez et al., 1998), and in the intestine of suckling animals (Bekesi & Williamson, 1990; Thumelin et al., 1993; Serra et al., 1993).

Changes in the level of gene expression have been reported during development. In suckling rats, the highest levels of expression were detected at the third day of life, decreasing progressively until weaning, when mRNA levels are similar to those of adult well fed rats (Serra et al., 1993).

3.4 Enzyme regulation

Production of ketone bodies in hepatic mitochondria is a complex and highly regulated process (Guzmán & Geelen, 1993; Zammit & Moir, 1994). Their synthesis increases in starving situations and in high fat intake, while it decreases after feeding or insulin administration and in the suckling-weaning transition (Williamson & Whitelaw, 1978; McGarry & Foster, 1980; Robinson et al., 1980).

Initially, the acyl-CoA input to the mitochondria was considered the principal check-point of ketogenesis (Guzman & Geelen, 1993; McGarry & Brown, 1997). However, later studies showed that the mHS enzyme can regulate ketogenesis (Williamson et al., 1968). Therefore, metabolic conditions that imply an increase of ketone bodies are linked to an increase of the levels of *HMGCS2* gene expression (Casals et al., 1992) and of the mHS enzyme (Serrá et al., 1993). Meanwhile, conditions that cause a decrease of the synthesis of ketone bodies are related to a decrease in the mRNA levels of the *HMGCS2* gene (Casals et al., 1992) and of the mHS enzyme (Serrá et al., 1993).

Currently, two check-points are recognized in the control of the synthesis of ketone bodies, one at the same step that of the Carnitine Palmitoyl Transferase 1 reaction, which provides the substrate acetyl-CoA, and another in the ketogenic pathway, at the step of the mHS enzyme (Williamson et al., 1968; Dashti & Ontko, 1979). Regulation of mHS is the most important step and depends on two mechanisms: a long term regulation of the transcription of the *HMGCS2* gene (Casals et al., 1992; Hegardt, 1999), and a short term regulation of the protein. This one depends on succinyl and desuccinyl enzymes reactions (Lowe & Tubbs, 1985; Quant et al., 1990). All of these mechanisms are influenced by nutritional and hormonal factors.

3.5 Isoenzymes

Two HMG-CoA synthase isoenzymes which catalyze the same reaction are known, however, they are located in different structures inside the cell. The mHS (Clinkenbeard et al., 1975) is involved in the synthesis of ketone bodies in the mitochondria, while the cytosolic HMG-CoA synthase (cHS) is critical for the synthesis of cholesterol (Clinkenbeard et al., 1975; Reed et al., 1975).

Expression pattern of cHS is different from the one described for mHS. The cytosolic enzyme is expressed in most of the tissues, and its gene is considered a house-keeping gene. High mRNA levels are observed in liver followed by heart, placenta and pancreas (Mascaró et al., 1995). Their transcriptional regulation is different from the mHS and it is negatively regulated by cholesterol and other isoprenoids (Hua et al., 1993).

The activity measures of the HMG-CoA synthase in a liver crude extract is divided between a 20-40% for the cHS and a 60-80% for the mHS (Clinkenbeard et al., 1975). Surprisingly, there is not reported any case with cHS deficiency.

4. mHS deficiency

Deficiency of mHS is an inborn error of metabolism that affects the synthesis of ketone bodies. It is a very rare autosomal recessive disorder reported in 1997 (Thompson et al., 1997), in a six year old boy. The patient had hypoglycemia, hypoketonemia and semicomatous state, after three days with gastroenteritis and dieting. Symptoms quickly reversed after intravenous administration of glucose. Liver biopsy showed a decrease in the activity of mHS. Molecular study of the gene confirmed the diagnosis (Bouchard et al., 2001). Generally, the disease shows unspecific clinical symptoms and metabolites excretion profile, sometimes attributed to a fatty acid β-oxidation enzyme defect and that makes it to be underdiagnosed. Some authors pointed out that it can be misdiagnosed as Reye syndrome and be associated with the sudden infant death syndrome (Thompson et al., 1997). Symptoms usually appear after situations of starving and/or high energy expenditure (fever, stress, exercise). In normal conditions, metabolic pathways that provide alternative glucose sources, as the synthesis of ketone bodies, are activated. A defect of ketogenesis can trigger a coma in the individual with low glucose availability.

4.1 Clinical features

In all the cases reported, clinical symptoms have appeared in childhood, specially during the first year of life; however, two of the 8 cases were diagnosed at the age of four and six years, respectively.

Clinical features of mHS deficiency are unspecific (Table 1), which makes it hard to diagnose. Initial symptoms include vomiting and lethargy that can progress to coma. In most cases these symptoms are accompanied with hepatomegaly (Thompson et al., 1997) and in some cases with respiratory disease and encephalopathy. These symptoms quickly improve after glucose administration. Up to date, all the reported cases have had a favorable outcome, despite severe acute episodes. All the reported patients with mHS deficiency are still alive.

4.2 Diagnosis
4.2.1 Biochemical data

Hypoglycemia is the main biochemical anomaly detected during an acute episode. Increase of the levels of plasmatic free fatty acids and urine dicarboxylic acids is also found. Plasma levels of acylcarnitines, lactate and ammonium are within normal limits (Morris et al., 1998). In some cases, metabolic acidosis has been reported (Table 1).

This disease, as opposite to the HL deficiency, does not show a characteristic organic acids pattern in urine. The mHS substrate does not accumulate because it can be metabolized to acetyl-CoA during the β-oxidation.

4.2.2 Enzyme activity

An enzymatic assay in liver biopsy is needed to confirm the mHS deficiency, because liver is the tissue with the highest enzyme expression. This method has several limitations, being the main one that in liver homogenate we cannot distinguish between mHS and cHS enzyme activity. This problem impairs the interpretation of the results and explains that the assay has only been carried out in two patients (Thompson et al., 1997; Morris et al., 1998). The possibility to use other tissues or alternative cells as lymphocytes or fibroblasts has been proposed, but the low expression levels in these tissues did not allow investigators to obtain valid measurable levels (Thompson et al., 1997).

4.2.3 Molecular diagnosis

Molecular analysis is the method of choice to confirm the clinical diagnosis. It is done from genomic DNA of the patient, by PCR amplification and sequencing of the *HMGCS2* gene.

4.2.4 Differential diagnosis with HMG-CoA lyase deficiency

The HL is the immediately posterior to mHS enzyme in the pathway of the ketone bodies synthesis. HL deficiency (3-hydroxy-3-methylglutaric aciduria) has very similar clinical manifestations to mHS deficiency, although there are significant differences that the clinicians should know in order to differentiate them.

	Signs and laboratory data	mHS deficiency	HL deficiency
SIGNS	Encephalopathy	+/-	+/-
	Hypotonia	-	+/-
	Lethargy	+/-	+/-
	Abnormal Breathing	+/-	+/-
	Coma	+/-	+/-
	Hepatomegaly	+	+/-
	Normal development	+	+/-
	Death	-	+/-
BIOCHEMICAL DATA	Hypoglycaemia	+	+
	Hypoketonemia	+	+
	Hyperammonemia	-	+/-
	Transaminase	+/-	+/-
	Metabolic acidosis	+/-	+
	High urine dicarboxylic acid	+	-
	High 3-hydroxy-3-methylglutaric, 3-hydroxyisovaleric, 3-methylglutaconic and 3-methylglutaric acids	-	+
	Normal level of carnitine	+	+/-

+Always; -Never; +/- Sometimes.

Table 1. Signs and Biochemical data of mHS and HL deficiency

Patients with HL deficiency may present acute crisis as well, during the neonatal or early infancy periods. Both diseases appear when exogenous supply of glucose fails (fasting periods), or when excessive glucose consumption exists (stress, fever or exercise). In the majority of patients with mHS deficiency, the acute crisis begins with hepatomegaly and superficial coma. However, in HL deficiency, or other β-oxidation enzymes, symptoms of the deficiency usually involve several tissues (Thompson et al., 1997). In the latter, most of the patients show muscular weakness and myopathy (Ribes et al., 2003). In the HL deficiency symptoms as dehydration, hypotonia, hypothermia, tachypnea, lethargy, coma and even death, have been reported (Wysocki & Hahnel, 1986; Menao et al., 2009). Up to date, no patient with mHS deficiency has died due to this disease.

Complications of 3-hydroxy-3-methylglutaric aciduria include, macrocephaly (Stacey et al., 1985), development delay and dilated cardiomyopathy with arrhythmia (Gibson et al., 1994). Microcephaly has been reported in one patient (Lisson et al., 1981). Up to date, no complications have been reported in patients with mHS deficiency.

The most important difference between both diseases is found in the urine profile of the organic acids, which is characteristic only in HL deficiency. Metabolites that accumulate in urine are the 3-hydroxy-isovaleric acid, the 3-methylcrotonyl glycine, the 3-methylglutaric acid, the 3-methylglutaconic acid and the 3-hydroxy-3-methylglutaric acid. Neither of these metabolites is increased in mHS deficiency. Clinical and biochemical data of both deficiencies are included in Table 1.

4.3 Treatment
Treatment is symptomatic during acute episodes and consists of intravenous administration of glucose to correct hypoglycemia. Long-term maintenance therapy includes low-fat diet and avoidance of fasting periods of more than 12 hours. It is also important to avoid situations of metabolic stress, mainly produced by recurrent illness that can be prevented by extra caloric intake (Morris et al., 1998).

5. *HMGCS2* gene

Although mHS is codified by a gene (Ayte et al., 1990) different from the cHS gene (Gil et al., 1986), their high homology suggests a common origin about 500 millions years ago, when vertebrates appeared (Boukaftane et al., 1994).
Human *HMGCS2* gene is located in chromosome 1 (1p12-p13), between the markers WI-7519 and D1S514. It has 10 exons and 9 introns, with a total size of 21,708 bp (Figure 4). Exons length oscillates between 107 and 846 bp, and the intron's size varies between 0.4 and 4.1 kDa. cDNA has a total size of 2,082 bp.
So far, no splice variants of the gene have been experimentally confirmed, although the current Expressed Sequence Tag database includes a variant with a deletion of exon 4.

5.1 Mutation update
Up to date, 8 patients have been diagnosed by molecular analysis. Among them nine allelic variants have been identified: seven missense variants, one nonsense and one intronic mutation (Figures 3 and 4). One of these variants, the Y167C, affects to a closed Cys[166] amino acid, which is considered the catabolic site of the enzyme (Hegard, 1999). The nonsense variant R424X (Bouchard et al., 2001; Morris et al., 1998), produced a truncated protein of 424 amino acids that probably cannot be incorporated into the active protein dimer. The intronic mutation is located in the first nucleotide of the intron 5 (c.1016+1G>A). In general, this type of mutations produces the deletion of the affected exon (exon 5 in this case), although in this disease the mechanism has not been confirmed (Zschocke et al., 2002).
In order to prove the effect of the mutation in the enzyme activity, protein over-expression has been tried with recombinant DNA techniques although with no success (Bouchard et al., 2001).

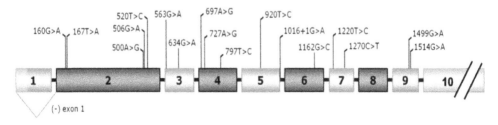

Fig. 4. Scheme of the mutations located in the human gene *HMGCS2*

Patient	Disease debut	Genotype	Symptoms and signs	Organic acids	Acylcarnitine	Reference
Patient 1	6 years	F174L/F174L	Gastroenteritis, hypoglycemia, hipoketonemia, superficial coma	Normal	Normal	Bouchard 2001; Thompson 1997
Patient 2	1 year and 4 months	R424X/unknown	Diarrhea, vomiting, hepatomegaly, hypoglycemia, hipoketonemia, coma	Dicarboxylic aciduria	Normal	Bouchard 2001; Morris 1998
Patient 3	11 months	G212R/R500H	Gastroenteritis, vomiting, hepatomegaly, hypoglycemia, hipoketonemia, coma	Dicarboxylic aciduria	Normal	Aledo 2001
Patient 4	9 months	G212R/IVS5+1G>A	Gastroenteritis, diarrhea, vomiting, hepatomegaly, hypoglycemia, hipoketonemia, coma	Dicarboxylic aciduria	Normal	Zschocke 2002
Patient 5	4 years and 6 months	V54M/Y167C	Gastroenteritis, diarrhea, vomiting, hypoglycemia, hipoketonemia, coma	Dicarboxylic aciduria	Normal	Wolf 2003
Patient 6	1 year and 7 months	V54M/Y167C	Hepatomegaly, normal hepatic function	Dicarboxylic aciduria	Normal	Wolf 2003
Patient 7	7 months	M307T/R188H	Vomiting, hepatomegaly, hipoglycemia hipoketonemia, encephalopathy.	Dicarboxylic aciduria	Normal	Aledo 2006
Patient 8	1 year	M307T/R188H	Vomiting, lethargy	Normal	Normal	Aledo 2006

Mutations G169D, T233A, K243E, L266S, I407T, R505Q, R84X and exon 1 deletion were reported by Pitt et al., at the 11th International Congress on Inborn Errors of Metabolism, San Diego CA and by Shafqat et al., 2010.
Mutations I56N, T233A, K243E and R84X were reported by Shafqat et al., 2010.
No clinical data were available from the patients who carried these mutations.

Table 2. Clinical findings and biochemical data from patients with mHS deficiency

Another approach consisted in studying, with an indirect method, the mutation effect in MEV-1 cell cultures (Aledo et al., 2001). These studies were based in the cell mevalonate auxotrophy correction when they are transfected with cDNA of the *HMGCS2* gene. The expression of the mHS gene gives to MEV-1 cells the capacity to synthesize HMG-CoA inside the mitochondria, which is transformed in mevalonate and cholesterol (Ortiz et al., 1994). As expected, the mutated mHS cDNA transfection does not correct the MEV-1 cells auxotrophy, which proves the deficiency of HMG-CoA synthesis.

Recently, new mutations in mHS deficiency patients have been reported, but no clinical information was given. There are 8 missense mutations and one nonsense (Shafqat et al., 2010).

In Table 2 an updated list of mutations reported in the *HMGCS2* gene is displayed, together with the patients´ clinical data.

6. Genotype-phenotype correlations

With the current knowledge available, it is difficult to establish strong genotype-phenotype correlations, among other reasons, for instance, because we ignore relevant information such as the levels of enzyme activity in affected patients. The seriousness of the disease may be more related to the agent that triggered hypoglycemia and to the time without treatment than with the mutation itself.

7. Conclusion

Although mHS deficiency is an extremely rare disease, it is likely underdiagnosed and its prevalence is higher than estimated. Pediatricians may suspect this disorder in infants with vomiting, mild hepatomegaly, hypoglycemia, metabolic acidosis, increased levels of plasmatic free fatty acids and dicarboxylic aciduria, specially if symptoms appeared after a situation of metabolic stress, usually due to dieting in a gastroenteritis or during an infection process. Currently, the only reliable diagnostic –confirmatory- test is the molecular analysis of the gene, since measurements of the levels of enzymatic activity are masked by the activity of isoenzyme cHS.

8. Acknowledgment

This study was supported by Spanish grants from: Diputación General de Aragón (Ref.# Grupo Consolidado B20) and University of Zaragoza (Ref.# PIF-UZ_2009-BIO-02). We also thank to "Biomol-Informatics SL -www.bioinfo.es-" for bioinformatic support.

9. References

Aledo, R., Zschocke, J., Pie, J., Mir, C., Fiesel, S., Mayatepek, E., Hoffmann, GF., Casals, N., & Hegardt, FG. (2001). Genetic basis of mitochondrial HMG-CoA synthase deficiency. *Human Genetics*, Vol. 1, No. 109, (July 2001), pp. 19-23, ISSN 11479731

Ayte, J., Gil-Gomez, G., Haro, D., Marrero, PF., & Hegardt, FG. (1990). Rat mitochondrial and cytosolic 3-hydroxy-3-methylglutaryl-CoA synthases are encoded by two different genes. *Proceedings of the National Academy of Sciences of the United States of America*, Vol. 10, No. 87, (May 1990), pp. 3874-3878, ISSN 1971108

Bates, MW., Krebs, HA., & Williamson, DH. (1968). Turnover rates of ketone bodies in normal, starved and alloxan-diabetic rats. *Biochemical Journal*, Vol. 110, No. 4, (December 1968), pp. 655-661, ISSN 5704813

Békési, A., & Williamson, DH. (1990). An explanation for ketogenesis by the intestine of the suckling rat: the presence of an active hydroxymethylglutaryl-coenzyme A pathway. *Biology of the Neonate*, Vol. 58, No. 3, (1990), pp. 160-165, ISSN 2279051

Blázquez, C., Sanchez, C., Velasco, G., & Guzman, M. (1998). Role of carnitine palmitoyltransferase I in the control of ketogenesis in primary cultures of rat astrocytes. *Journal of Neurochemistry*, Vol. 4, No. 71, (October 1998), pp. 1597-1606, ISSN 9751193

Bouchard, L., Robert, MF., Vinarov, D., Stanley, CA., Thompson, GN., Morris, A., Leonard, JV., Quant, P., Hsu, BY., Boneh, A., Boukaftane, Y., Ashmarina, L., Wang, S., Miziorko, H., & Mitchell, GA. (2001). Mitochondrial 3-hydroxy-3-methylglutaryl-CoA synthase deficiency: clinical course and description of causal mutations in two patients. *Pediatric Research*, Vol. 3, No. 49, (March 2001), pp. 326-331, ISSN 11228257

Boukaftane, Y., Duncan, A., Wang, S., Labuda, D., Robert, MF., Sarrazin, J., Schappert, K., & Mitchell, GA. (1994). Human mitochondrial HMG CoA synthase: liver cDNA and partial genomic cloning, chromosome mapping to 1p12-p13, and possible role in vertebrate evolution. *Genomics*, Vol. 3, No. 23, (October 1994), pp. 552-559, ISSN 7851882

Casals, N., Roca, N., Guerrero, M., Gil-Gómez, G., Ayté, J., Ciudad, CJ., & Hegardt, FG. (1992). Regulation of the expression of the mitochondrial 3-hydroxy-3-methylglutaryl-CoA synthase gene. Its role in the control of ketogenesis. *The Biochemical Journal*, Vol. 1, No. 283, (April 1992), pp. 261-264, ISSN 1348927

Cleland, WW. (1963). The kinetics of enzyme-catalyzed reactions with two or more substrates or products. I. Nomenclature and rate equations. *Biochimica et Biophysica Acta*, Vol. 67 (January 1968), pp. 104-137, ISSN 1402166

Clinkenbeard, KD., Reed, WD., Mooney, RA., & Lane, MD. (1975). Intracellular localization of the 3-hydroxy-3-methylglutaryl coenzyme A cycle enzymes in liver. Separate cytoplasmic and mitochondrial 3-hydroxy-3-methylglutaryl coenzyme A generating systems for cholesterogenesis and ketogenesis. *The Journal of Biological Chemistry*, Vol. 8, No. 250, (April 1975), pp. 3108-3116, ISSN 164460

Cullingford, TE., Bhakoo, KK., & Clark, JB. (1998). Hormonal regulation of the mRNA encoding the ketogenic enzyme mitochondrial 3-hydroxy-3-methylglutaryl-CoA synthase in neonatal primary cultures of cortical astrocytes and meningeal fibroblasts. *Journal of Neurochemistry*, Vol. 5, No. 71, (November 1998), pp. 1804-1812, ISSN 9798904

Dashti, N., & Ontko, JA. (1979). Rate-limiting function of 3-hydroxy-3-methylglutaryl-coenzyme A synthase in ketogenesis. *Biochemical Medicine*, Vol. 3, No. 22, (December 1979), pp. 365-374, ISSN 93966

Edmond J. (1992). Energy metabolism in developing brain cells. *Canadian Journal of Physiology and Pharmacoogyl*, Vol. 70, No. S1 (May 1992), pp. S118-S129, ISSN 1295662

Felig, P., & Lynch, V. (1970). Starvation in human pregnancy: hypoglycemia, hypoinsulinemia, and hyperketonemia. *Science*, Vol. 170, No. 961, (November 1970), pp.990-992, ISSN 5529067

Gibson, KM., Cassidy, SB., Seaver, LH., Wanders, RJ., Kennaway, NG., Mitchell, GA., & Spark, RP. (1994). Fatal cardiomyopathy associated with 3-hydroxy-3-methylglutaryl-CoA lyase deficiency. *Journal of Inherited Metabolic Disease*, Vol. 3, No. 17 (1994), pp. 291-294, ISSN 7807935

Gil, G., Goldstein, JL., Slaughter, CA., & Brown, MS. (1986). Cytoplasmic 3-hydroxy-3-methylglutaryl coenzyme A synthase from the hamster. I. Isolation and sequencing of a full-length cDNA. *The Journal of Biology Chemistry*, Vol. 261, No. 8, (March 1986), pp. 3710-3716, ISSN 286903

Guzmán, M., & Geelen, MJ. (1993). Regulation of fatty acid oxidation in mammalian liver. *Biochimical et Biophysucal Acta* Vol. 1167, No. 3 (April 1993), pp. 227-241, ISSN 8097

Hahn, P., & Taller, M. (1987). Ketone formation in the intestinal mucosa of infant rats. *Life Science*, Vol. 12, No. 41, (September 1987), pp. 1525-1528, ISSN 3626770

Hawkins, RA., Williamson, DH., & Krebs, HA. (1971). Ketone-body utilization by adult and suckling rat brain in vivo. *Biochemical Journal*, Vol. 122, No. 1, (March 1971), pp. 13-18, ISSN 5124783

Hegardt, FG. (1999). Mitochondrial 3-hydroxy-3-methylglutaryl-CoA synthase: a control enzyme in ketogenesis. *The Biochemical Journal*, Vol. 3, No. 338, (March 1999), pp. 569-582, ISSN 10051425

Hua, X., Yokoyama, C., Wu, J., Briggs, MR., Brown, MS., Goldstein, JL., & Wang, X. (1993). SREBP-2, a second basic-helix-loop-helix-leucine zipper protein that stimulates transcription by binding to a sterol regulatory element. *Proceedings of the National Academy of Sciences USA*, Vol. 90, No.24, (December 1993), pp. 11603-11607, ISSN 790345

Lisson, G., Leupold, D., Bechinger, D., & Wallesch, C. (1981). CT findings in a case of deficiency of 3-hydroxy-3-methylglutaryl-CoA-lyase. *Neuroradiology*, Vol. 22, No. 2, (1981), pp. 99-101, ISSN 6170906

Lowe, DM., & Tubbs, PK. (1985). Succinylation and inactivation of 3-hydroxy-3-methylglutaryl-CoA synthase by succinyl-CoA and its possible relevance to the control of ketogenesis. *The Biochemical Journal*, Vol. 1, No. 232, (November 1985), pp. 37-42, ISSN 2867762

Mascaró, C., Buesa, C., Ortiz, JA., Haro, D., & Hegardt, FG. (1995). Molecular cloning and tissue expression of human mitochondrial 3-hydroxy-3-methylglutaryl-CoA synthase. *Archives of Biochemistry and Biophysics*, Vol. 2, No. 317, (March 1995), pp. 385-390, ISSN 7893153

McGarry, JD., & Brown, NF. (1997). The mitochondrial carnitine palmitoyltransferase system. From concept to molecular analysis. *European Journal of Biochemistry*, Vol. 244, No. 1 (February 1997), pp. 1-14, ISSN 9063439

McGarry, JD., & Foster, DW. (1980). Regulation of hepatic fatty acid oxidation and ketone body production. *Annual Review of Biochemistry*, No. 49, (1980), pp. 395-420, ISSN 6157353

Menao, S., Lopez-Viñas, E., Mir, C., Puisac, B., Gratacós, E., Arnedo, M., Carrasco, P., Moreno, S., Ramos, M., Gil, MC., Pié, A., Ribes, A., Pérez-Cerda, C., Ugarte, M., Clayton, PT., Korman, SH., Serra, D., Asins, G., Ramos, FJ., Gómez-Puertas, P., Hegardt, FG., Casals, N., & Pié, J. (2009). Ten novel *HMGCL* mutations in 24 patients of different origin with 3-hydroxy-3-methyl-glutaric aciduria. *Human Mutation*, Vol. 3, No. 30, (March 2009), pp. E520-529, ISSN 19177531

Misra, I., Charlier, HA Jr., & Miziorko, HM. (1995). Avian cytosolic 3-hydroxy-3-methylglutaryl-CoA synthase: evaluation of the role of cysteines in reaction chemistry. *Biochemica et Biophysical Acta*, Vol. 1247, No. 2 (March 1995), pp. 253-259, ISSN 7696316

Mitchell, JB., DiLauro, PC., Pizza, FX., & Cavender, DL. (1997). The effect of preexercise carbohydrate status on resistance exercise performance. *International Journal of Sport Nutrition*, Vol. 7, No. 3, (1997), pp. 185-196, ISSN 9286742

Miziorko, HM., Clinkenbeard, KD., Reed, WD., & Lane, MD. (1975). 3-Hydroxy-3-methylglutaryl coenzyme A synthase. Evidence for an acetyl-S-enzyme intermediate and identification of a cysteinyl sulfhydryl as the site of acetylation. *The Journal of Biological Chemistry*, Vol. 250, No. 10 (August 1975), pp. 5768-5573, ISSN 238985

Miziorko, HM. & Behnke, CE. (1985). Active-site-directed inhibition of 3-hydroxy-3-methylglutaryl coenzyme A synthase by 3-chloropropionyl coenzyme A. *Biochemistry*, Vol. 13, No. 24, (June 1985), pp. 3174-3179, ISSN 2862911

Miziorko, HM., & Lane, MD. (1977). 3-Hydroxy-3-methylgutaryl-CoA synthase. Participation of acetyl-S-enzyme and enzyme-S-hydroxymethylgutaryl-SCoA intermediates in the reaction. *The Journal of Biological Chemistry*, Vol. 252, No. 4, (February 1977), pp. 1414-1420, ISSN 14151

Morris, AA., Lascelles, CV., Olpin, SE., Lake, BD., Leonard, JV., & Quant, PA. (1998). Hepatic mitochondrial 3-hydroxy-3-methylglutaryl-coenzyme a synthase deficiency. *Pediatric Research*, Vol. 3, No. 44, (September 1998), pp. 392-396, ISSN 9727719

Nehlig, A., & Pereira de Vasconcelos, A. (1993). Glucose and ketone body utilization by the brain of neonatal rats. *Progress in Neurobiology*, Vol. 40, No. 2 (February 1993), pp. 163-221, ISSN 8430212

Ortiz, JA., Gil-Gómez, G., Casaroli-Marano, RP., Vilaró, S., Hegardt, FG., & Haro, D. (1994). Transfection of the ketogenic mitochondrial 3-hydroxy-3-methylglutaryl-coenzyme A synthase cDNA into Mev-1 cells corrects their auxotrophy for mevalonate. *The Journal of Biological Chemistry*, Vol. 269, No. 46 (November 1994), pp.28523-28526 ISSN 7961793

Page, MA., & Tubbs, PK. (1978). Some properties of 3-hydroxy-3-methylglutaryl-coenzyme A synthase from ox liver. *Biochemical Journal*, Vol 173, No. 3, (September 1978), pp. 925-928, ISSN 39450

Quant, PA., Tubbs, PK., & Brand, MD. (1990). Glucagon activates mitochondrial 3-hydroxy-3-methylglutaryl-CoA synthase in vivo by decreasing the extent of succinylation of the enzyme. *European Journal of Biochemistry / FEBS*, Vol. 1, No. 187, (January 1990), pp. 169-174, ISSN 1967579

Reed, WD., Clinkenbeard, D., & Lane, MD. (1975). Molecular and catalytic properties of mitochondrial (ketogenic) 3-hydroxy-3-methylglutaryl coenzyme A synthase of liver. *The Journal of Biological Chemistry*, Vol. 8, No. 250, (April 1975), pp. 3117-3123, ISSN 804485

Ribes, A., Rodes, M., Gregersen, N., & Divry, P. (2003). Transtornos de la β-oxidación mitocondrial de los ácidos grasos. *Patología Molecular*, González-Sastre, F., Guinovart, JJ. pp. 333-359, Elseveir-Masson, ISBN 9788445812532

Robinson, AM., & Williamson, DH. (1980). Physiological roles of ketone bodies as substrates and signals in mammalian tissues. *Physiological Reviews,* Vol. 60, No. 1 (Janurary 1980), pp. 143-187, ISSN 6986618

Robinson, BH., Oei, J., Sherwood, WG., Slyper, AH., Heininger, J., & Mamer, OA. (1980). Hydroxymethylglutaryl CoA lyase deficiency: features resembling Reye syndrome. *Neurology,* Vol. 7 Pt 1, No. 30, (July 1980), pp. 714-718, ISSN 6156427

Rogers, S., Wells, R., & Rechsteiner, M. (1986). Amino acid sequences common to rapidly degraded proteins: the PEST hypothesis. *Science,* Vol 234, No. 4774 (October 1986), pp.364-368, ISSN 287651

Royo, T., Pedragosa, MJ., Ayte, J., Gil-Gómez, G., Vilaró, S., & Hegardt, FG. (1993). Testis and ovary express the gene for the ketogenic mitochondrial 3-hydroxy-3-methylglutaryl-CoA synthase. *Journal of Lipid Research,* Vol. 9, No. 34, (September 1993), pp. 867-874, ISSN 8102635

Serra, D., Casals, N., Asins, G., Royo, T., Ciudad, CJ., & Hegardt, FG. (1993). Regulation of mitochondrial 3-hydroxy-3-methylglutaryl-coenzyme A synthase protein by starvation, fat feeding, and diabetes. *Archives of Biochemistry and Biophysics,* Vol. 1, No. 307, (September 1993), pp. 40-45, ISSN 7902069

Shafqat, N., Turnbull, A., Zschocke, J., Oppermann, U., & Yue, WW. (2010). Crystal structures of human HMG-CoA synthase isoforms provide insights into inherited ketogenesis disorders and inhibitor design. *Journal of Molecular Biology,* Vol. 4, No. 398, (May 2010), pp.497-506, ISSN 20346956

Stacey, TE., de Sousa, C., Tracey, BM., Whitelaw, A., Mistry, J., Timbrell, P., & Chalmers, RA. (1985). Dizygotic twins with 3-hydroxy-3-methylglutaric aciduria; unusual presentation, family studies and dietary management. *European Journal of Pediatrics,* Vol. 2, No. 144, (July 1985), pp. 177-181, ISSN 2412823

Thompson, GN., Hsu, BY., Purr, JJ., Treacy, E., & Stanley, CA. (1997). Fasting hypoketotic coma in a child with deficiency of mitochondrial 3-hydroxy-3-methylglutaryc-CoA synthase. *The New England Journal of Medicine,* Vol.17, No.337, (October 1997), pp.1203-1207, ISSN 9337379

Thumelin, S., Forestier, M., Girard, J., & Pegorier, JP. (1993). Develpmental changes in mitochondrial 3-hydroxy-3-methylglutaryc-CoA synthase gene expression in rat liver, intestine and kidney. *The Biochemical Journal,* Vol.2 No. 192, (June 1993), pp.493-496, ISSN 8099282

Williamson, DH., & Whitelaw., E. (1978). Physiological aspects of the regulation of ketogenesis. *Biochemical Society symposium,* No. 43, (1978); pp.137-161, ISSN 571280

Williamson, DH., Bates, MW., & Krebs, HA. (1968). Activity and intracellular distribution of enzymes of ketone-body metabolism in rat liver. *The Biochemical Journal,* Vol. 3, No. 108, (July 1968), pp.353-361, ISSN 5667251

Wysocki, SJ., & Hahnel, R. (1986). 3-Hydroxy-3-methylglutaryc-coenzyme a lyase deficiency: a review. *Journal of Inherited Metabolic Disease,* Vol. 3, No. 9, (1986), pp. 225-233, ISSN 3099065

Zammit VA. (1981). Regulation of hepatic fatty acid metabolism. The activities of mitochondrial and microsomal acyl-CoA:sn-glycerol 3-phosphate O-acyltransferase and the concentrations of malonyl-CoA, non-esterified and esterified carnitine, glycerol 3-phosphate, ketone bodies and long-chain acyl-CoA esters in livers of fed or starved pregnant, lactating and weaned rats. *Biochemical Journal*, Vol. 198, No. 1 (July 1981), pp. 75-83 ISSN 7326003

Zammit, VA., & Moir, AM. (1994). Monitoring the partitioning of hepatic fatty acids in vivo: keeping track of control. *Trends of Biochemistry Science*, Vol. 19, No.8, (August 1994), pp.313-317, ISSN 7940674

Zschocke, J., Penzien, JM., Bielen, R., Casals, N., Aledo, R., Pié, J., Hoffmann, GF., Hegardt, FG., & Mayatepek, E. (2002). The diganosis of mitochondrial HMG-CoA synthase deficiency. *The Journal of Pediatrics*, Vol. 6, No. 140, (June 2002); pp.778-780, ISSN 12072887

4

Tangier Disease

Yoshinari Uehara[1], Bo Zhang[2] and Keijiro Saku[1]
[1]Department of Cardiology, Fukuoka University Faculty of Medicine,
Nanakuma, Jonan-ku, Fukuoka
[2]Department of Biochemistry, Fukuoka University Faculty of Medicine,
Nanakuma, Jonan-ku, Fukuoka
Japan

1. Introduction

Various clinical and epidemiological studies have demonstrated an inverse association between high-density lipoprotein (HDL) cholesterol and the risk of coronary events (von Eckardstein et al., 2001). However, it remains controversial whether this relationship is causal or only an epiphenomenon of a more general atherogenic disorder. HDL exerts various potential anti-atherogenic properties. For example, HDL particles transport cholesterol from cells of the arterial wall to the liver and steroidogenic organs, in which cholesterol is used for the synthesis of bile acids, lipoproteins, vitamin D, and steroid hormones (von Eckardstein et al., 2001). In contrast, low HDL cholesterol is frequently identified as a component of metabolic syndrome in many populations, i.e., together with overweight or obesity, glucose intolerance or overt diabetes mellitus, hypertriglyceridemia, and hypertension, which by themselves contribute to the pathogenesis of atherosclerosis (Despres and Marette, 1994). The most severe form of familial HDL deficiency is Tangier disease (TD), which is caused by a genetic disorder.

2. HDL metabolism and functions

HDL, isolated by ultracentrifugation, is a lipoprotein with a density in the range 1.063–1.21 g/ml (HDL_2, 1.063–1.125 g/ml; HDL_3, 1.125–1.21 g/ml) (Havel et al., 1955). However, HDL constitutes a heterogeneous group of particles differing in size, density, lipid composition, apolipoprotein content, and electrophoretic mobility. HDL can be separated into two main subfractions based on electrophoretic mobility, namely the major subfraction has the same mobility as alpha HDL, whereas the other subfractions migrate similar to pre-beta HDL. Most HDL particles in human plasma are alpha HDL, and pre-beta HDL represents only 2–14% of all apolipoprotein A-I (apoA-I) (Ishida et al., 1987; Kunitake et al., 1985).

HDL has a very complex metabolism associated with several HDL-related genes and is synthesized via a complex pathway. Although the underlying genetic defects in many cases of primary low HDL cholesterolemia are not clearly understood, mutations in three pivotal genes, namely apoA-I, lecithin:cholesterol acyltransferase, and ATP-binding cassette transporter A1 (ABCA1) are associated with low plasma HDL cholesterol levels (Miller et al., 2003). Some mutations of these genes are also associated with an increased risk of premature coronary artery disease (CAD).

3. Characters of TD

3.1 Clinical manifestations of TD

The most severe form of HDL deficiency is TD, first described by Fredrickson et al. (Fredrickson et al., 1961). The plasma lipid profiles in a typical TD patient (TD case 1) with peripheral neuropathy (Uehara et al., 2008a) and those of her younger brother are shown in Table 1. The biological hallmark of plasma in patients with TD is a deficiency of HDL cholesterol, low levels of low-density lipoprotein (LDL) cholesterol, and moderate hypertriglyceridemia. The concentration of apoA-I in plasma of patients with TD is 3% less than that in healthy subjects. TD is a rare autosomal recessive disorder characterized by the absence or extremely low levels of HDL cholesterol and apoA-I in plasma. Furthermore, cholesteryl esters accumulate in many macrophage-rich tissues including the tonsils, liver, spleen, peripheral nerves, lymph nodes, thymus, and arterial walls. Clinical symptoms in homozygotes include hyperplastic orange-yellow tonsils (Fig. 1), hepatosplenomegaly, corneal opacification, and premature CAD in 50% of cases, as well as relapsing peripheral neuropathy due to cholesteryl ester deposition in macrophages and Schwann cells (Assman et al., 1995; Fredrickson et al., 1961; Hobbs and Rader, 1999).

		Standard value	Tangier disease (Case)	Younger brother of case
Age, gender			50, Female	48, Male
Mutation with ABCA1 gene			homozygote, T940M	homozygote, T940M
Total Cholesterol	(mg/dl)	150-219	66	61
Triglyceride	(mg/dl)	50-149	204	191
HDL Choletserol	(mg/dl)	40-86	< 5	< 5
LDL Cholesterol	(mg/dl)	70-139	27	33
Apolipoprotein A-I	(mg/dl)	119-155	< 5	< 5
Apolipoprotein A-II	(mg/dl)	25.9-35.7	1.9	2
Apolipoprotein B	(mg/dl)	73-109	93	76
Apolipoprotein C-II	(mg/dl)	1.8-4.6	4.3	0.5
Apolipoprotein C-III	(mg/dl)	5.8-10.0	5.9	3.5
Apolipoprotein E	(mg/dl)	2.7-4.3	3.9	2.9
RLP cholesterol	(mg/dl)	< 7.5	3.4	5.5
Phospholipids	(mg/dl)	160-260	85	90
Total Bile Acids	(μmol/L)	< 10.0	38.8	22.0

Table 1. Serum lipid profiles in patient with Tangier disease

3.2 ABCA1 and TD

In 1999, TD was determined to be caused by a defect in the ABCA1 gene (formerly known as ABC1) (Brooks-Wilson et al., 1999; Rust et al., 1999; von Eckardstein et al., 2001) that is located on chromosome 9q31 and is composed of 50 exons spanning a region of approximately 149 kb (Remaley et al., 1999; Santamarina-Fojo et al., 2000). ABCA1 has been identified as a pivotal gene in the regulation of plasma levels of HDL cholesterol and cellular cholesterol homeostasis, which is defective in patients with TD. In these patients and their heterozygous relatives, ABCA1 gene mutations cause gene dose-dependent decreases in plasma levels of HDL cholesterol and in the capacity of skin fibroblasts and monocyte-derived macrophages to release cholesterol in the extracellular presence of apolipoproteins (Bodzioch et al., 1999; Brooks-Wilson et al., 1999; Lawn et al., 1999; Rust et al., 1999; von Eckardstein et al., 2001).

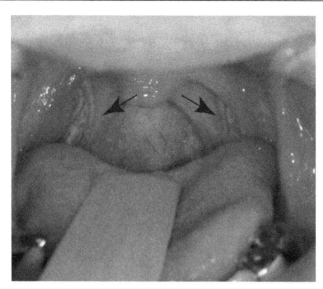

Fig. 1. Photograph of the oral cavity in a patient with Tangier disease reveals swollen orange colored tonsils with yellow lines (arrows). In a genetic sequence analysis, a homozygous missense point mutation was identified at nucleotide 2819 (mRNA position, AB055982) with a C to T mutation in exon 19. Thr940 was substituted by Met940 on the ATP-binding cassette transporter A1 (ABCA1) protein, which was found in the Walker-A motif, as the first nucleotide binding fold of the ABCA1 gene

ABC transporters are transmembrane proteins that facilitate the transport of specific substrates across the membrane in an ATP-dependent manner. ABCA1 is a member of the ABC transporter superfamily, which comprises 48 human transporters; the superfamily is divided into seven subfamilies, including full- or half-transporters, designated ABC A–G. ABC transporters are integral membrane proteins that transport various substrates such as lipids, peptides, amino acids, carbohydrates, vitamins, ions, glucuronides, glutathione conjugates, and xenobiotics to different cellular compartments (Dean and Annilo, 2005; Klein et al., 1999). ABC transporters are defined by the presence of nucleotide binding domains (NBD) that interact with ATP. These domains have two conserved peptide motifs, known as Walker-A and Walker-B, which are present in many proteins that utilize ATP (Walker et al., 1982). The ABC transporters also have a unique amino acid signature between the two Walker motifs that define ABC superfamilies (Klein et al., 1999).

Human ABCA1 belongs to the ABCA subfamily, which is composed of 12 full-transporters denoted ABCA1–13 (with the absence of a functional ABCA11) (Dean et al., 2001). All ABCA transporters are full-size transporters with 1543–5058 amino acids. Structurally, ABCA1 is a 2261 amino acid membrane transporter that is integrated into the membrane via transmembrane domains composed of six transmembrane helices. In addition, ABCA1 has two transmembrane domains and two nucleotide binding domains and is predicted to have an N-terminus oriented to the cytosol with two large extracellular loops (Fig. 2). ABCA1 is expressed in several human organs, with the highest expression levels occurring in the placenta, liver, lung, adrenal glands, and fetal tissues (Langmann et al., 1999).

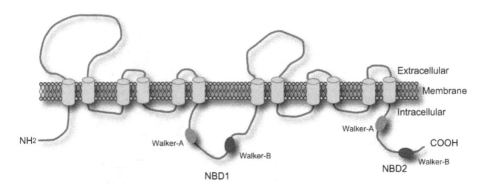

Fig. 2. Structure of the ATP-binding cassette transporter A1 (ABCA1) transporter. The ABCA1 protein consists of 2201 amino acids with two transmembrane domains composed of six transmembrane helices and two nucleotide binding domains (NBD-1 and NBD-2) containing two conserved peptide motifs known as Walker-A and Walker-B. It is predicted to have an N-terminus oriented into the cytosol and two large extracellular loops

4. Roles of ABC transporters in HDL metabolism

4.1 Functions of ABCA1 and its relationship to HDL metabolism

ABCA1 proteins transport cholesterol or phospholipids (PLs) from the membranous inner leaflet to the outer leaflet, and lipid-free or lipid-poor apoA-I subsequently takes up the transported cholesterol and PLs to form nascent HDL (Oram and Lawn, 2001). ABCA1 localizes to the plasma membrane and intracellular compartments, where it could potentially facilitate transport of lipids to either cell surface-bound (Neufeld et al., 2001) or internalized apolipoproteins (von Eckardstein and Rohrer, 2009). HDL metabolism has at least three steps. First, lipid-free or lipid-poor apoA-I removes free cholesterol from peripheral cells via ABCA1 to form nascent HDL. Second, nascent HDL is lipidated to mature HDL. Third, mature HDL interacts with other apoB containing triglyceride-rich lipoproteins (TRLs) such as very low density lipoprotein (VLDL) and intermediate-density lipoprotein (IDL). Therefore, ABCA1 is necessary to form nascent HDL and is an important key molecule in the initial step of the reverse cholesterol transport (RCT) pathway. Cultivated monocyte-derived macrophages from a normolipidemic healthy subject showed an approximately 125% increase in cholesterol efflux of lipid-free apoA-I, whereas macrophages derived from patients with TD did not respond to apoA-I during cholesterol efflux (Fig. 3A). Although cultivated monocyte-derived macrophages showed an increase in cholesterol efflux by lipid-free apoA-I in healthy subjects, the macrophages from patients with TD did not change apoA-I-mediated cholesterol efflux. These results demonstrate that apoA-I-mediated cholesterol efflux depends on ABCA1 in macrophages. Furthermore, ABCA1 plays a pivotal role in mediating PL and cholesterol efflux by lipid-free apoA-I, and thereby, in the formation of discoidal HDL precursors. However, ABCA1 interacts poorly with HDL_2 and HDL_3. Due to a genetic defect in ABCA1, patients with TD have an extremely low level of HDL and cannot form nascent HDL particles.

Disruption of the ABCA1 gene in mice results in an HDL deficiency and impaired cholesterol transport (McNeish et al., 2000; Orso et al., 2000), and overexpression of ABCA1 leads to increased apoA-I-mediated cholesterol efflux in transgenic mice (Singaraja et al., 2001; Vaisman et al., 2001). These results indicate that ABCA1 is a pivotal gene in the regulation of plasma HDL cholesterol and cellular cholesterol homeostasis.

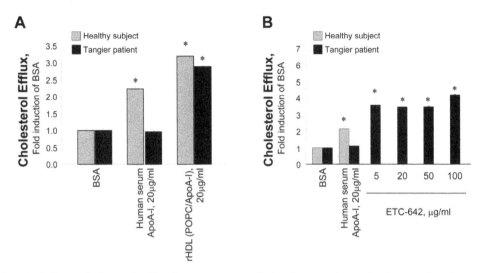

Fig. 3. Cellular cholesterol efflux from monocyte-derived macrophages in the peripheral blood of a patient with Tangier disease (TD). The human monocyte-derived macrophages from a healthy subject and a patient with TD were radiolabeled with ^{3}H-cholesterol. The cells were then equilibrated with 30 µg/ml cholesterol. Cholesterol efflux was induced by 4-h incubation with 20 µg/ml apolipoprotein A-I (apoA-I) and rHDL (POPC/apoA-I disc) (A) or ETC-642 (phospholipid (PL)/apoA-I mimetics) (B) using a previously modified method (Uehara et al.: *Diabetes* 2002;51:2922–8, Uehara et al.: *Atherosclerosis* 2008;197(1):283–9). rHDL, reconstituted HDL (POPC/apoA-I disc); ETC-642, synthetic peptide of 22 amino acids with 1,2-dipalmitoyl-sn-glycero-3-phosphocholine. n = 3–7; *P < 0.001 vs. BSA

4.2 Mechanisms of ABCA1 gene regulation

Cellular cholesterol efflux and ABCA1 expression are upregulated by cholesterol (Langmann et al., 1999; Lawn et al., 1999), oxysterols (Costet et al., 2000), rexinoids (Repa et al., 2000), and cAMP analogs (Bortnick et al., 2000; Lawn et al., 1999). The ABCA1 gene promoter has been analyzed (Costet et al., 2000; Santamarina-Fojo et al., 2000). Ligands of the nuclear transcription factor liver-X-receptors (LXRα and LXRβ) and retinoid-X-receptor alpha (RXRα), i.e., oxysterols and retinoids, respectively, have been identified as enhancers of ABCA1 gene expression (Costet et al., 2000; Oram et al., 2000; Repa et al., 2000; Venkateswaran et al., 2000). LXR and RXR form obligate heterodimers that preferentially bind to response elements within the ABCA1 gene promoter (Santamarina-Fojo et al., 2000; Wang et al., 2001). LXRα/β and RXRα bind to the response element direct repeat 4 (DR4) — two direct hexameric repeats separated by four nucleotides on the ABCA1 promoter that are activated by oxysterols and retinoic acid (Bungert et al., 2001; Willy et al., 1995). Binding of either one or both ligands activates ABCA1 transcription. Treating cells with either an oxysterol or 9-*cis*-retinoic acid induces ABCA1 expression, and their combined treatment has a marked synergistic effect (Schwartz et al., 2000). The activator of peroxisome proliferator activating receptor (PPAR)-α or -γ also enhances ABCA1 transcription in cultivated cells, but this stimulated ABCA1 transcription depends on an indirect effect by PPARs via upregulation of LXR expression. By contrast, the zinc finger protein ZNF202 transcription factor is a major repressor of ABCA1 transcription. Besides these regulatory factors, unsaturated fatty acids, but not saturated fatty acids, markedly inhibit ABCA1-mediated cholesterol efflux from macrophages because they act as antagonists during oxysterol binding to LXR (Uehara et al., 2002; Uehara et al., 2007). In addition to ZNF202 and unsaturated fatty acids, several potent transcription factors such as USF1, USF2, Fra2, and Sp3 are repressors of ABCA1 transcription (Yang et al., 2002).

4.3 Other ABC cholesterol transport proteins
ABCG1 (formerly known as ABC8), another member of the ABC transporter superfamily, has been mapped to chromosome 21q22.3 (Chen et al., 1996; Croop et al., 1997; Dean et al., 2001; Klucken et al., 2000; Savary et al., 1996; Walker et al., 1982). In contrast to ABCA1, ABCG1 is a half-transporter containing only one NBD and a transmembrane domain (Dean et al., 2001; Walker et al., 1982). Therefore, it is thought that ABCG1 requires a dimeric partner to become active. Wang et al. recently reported that ABCG1 and ABCG4 contribute to HDL$_2$- and HDL$_3$-dependent cellular cholesterol efflux (Wang et al., 2004) and appear to have an important function related to HDL lipidation (Smith, 2006; Uehara et al., 2008b; Wang et al., 2004).

Administering a high-fat high-cholesterol diet to ABCG1-deficient mice results in massive accumulation of lipids in tissue macrophages, whereas overexpression of human ABCG1 protects murine tissues from dietary fat-induced lipid accumulation (Kennedy et al., 2005). Furthermore, Mauldin et al. have shown that reduced ABCG1 function facilitates foam cell formation in type 2 diabetic mice (Mauldin et al., 2006). Transplantation of ABCG1-deficient (ABCG1$^{-/-}$) bone marrow into LDL receptor-deficient mice produces contrasting effects on atherosclerotic formation (Baldan et al., 2006; Out et al., 2006; Ranalletta et al., 2006). In contrast, a decrease in lesion formation and size has been observed in the absence of macrophage ABCG1 in mice (Baldan et al., 2006; Ranalletta et al., 2006). Total body expression of ABCG1 protects against the development of early atherosclerotic lesions (Out et al., 2007). However, the physiological roles of ABCG1 and its contribution to the progression of atherosclerosis in humans remain unclear. In addition to the nonspecific and passive pathway, mature-HDL particles, which are spherical and transport almost all HDL cholesterol, appear to induce cholesterol efflux via other ABC transporters, such as ABCG1 and ABCG4, rather than ABCA1 (Uehara et al., 2008b; Wang et al., 2004).

5. Lipoprotein profiles in TD measured by capillary isotachophoresis (cITP)
cITP is a newly established technique for characterizing plasma lipoprotein subfractions according to their electric charges. We have previously shown that plasma lipoproteins can be separated into eight fractions consisting of three HDL fractions with fast (fHDL), intermediate (iHDL), and slow (sHDL) electromobility, a fast VLDL fraction (fVLDL), a slow VLDL/IDL fraction (sVLDL),two LDL fractions with fast (fLDL) and slow (sLDL) electromobility, and a minor LDL fraction (mLDL) (Zhang et al., 2005) in normolipidemic (NL) subjects. Figure 4 shows the plasma lipoprotein profiles as characterized by cITP analysis in healthy NL subjects (Fig. 4A) and in two patients with TD (Fig. 4B and C). The

plasma lipoprotein profiles have a characteristic lipoprotein pattern in patients with TD, namely their fasting plasma shows an extremely low signal in the three HDL fractions (peaks 1, 2, and 3) (Fig. 4B-a, B-d, C-a, and C-d). Moreover, while the sLDL fraction corresponding to native LDL (peak 7) was extremely reduced, the sVLDL and fLDL fractions corresponding to electronegative LDL (some oxidized LDL, βVLDL, small dense LDL, or modified LDL) were significantly enhanced. Interestingly, peaks 4 and 5, TRLs, were identified in the LDL subfraction of plasma from patients with TD, which is usually detected only in the VLDL/IDL subfraction but not in LDL in NL plasma. These findings indicate that patients with TD not only have a deficiency in HDL particles but also have a characteristic lipid composition for other lipoproteins such as triglyceride-rich LDL.

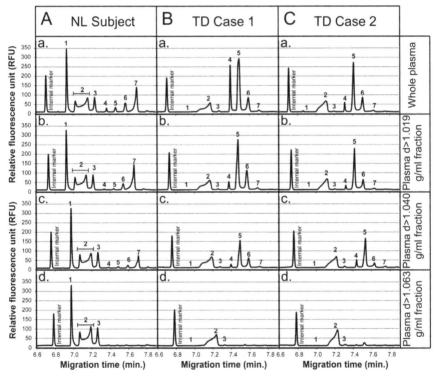

Fig. 4. Lipoprotein subfractions in whole plasma (a) and plasma density (d) > 1.019 g/ml (b), d > 1.040 g/ml (c), and d > 1.063 g/ml (d) fractions by ultracentrifugation in a normolipidemic (NL) subject (A) and two patients with Tangier disease (TD): Case 1, Thr940Met (B) and Case 2, Lys913X (C), as analyzed by capillary isotachophoresis. HDL peaks were not detected in whole plasma (a) or the HDL fraction (d) in patients with TD. Interestingly, peaks 4 and 5, triglyceride-rich lipoproteins (TRLs), were identified in the LDL subfraction of plasma from patients with TD, which was only detected in the VLDL/IDL subfraction but not in LDL in NL plasma. Peaks 1–3: fast-, intermediate-, and slow-migrating HDL; peaks 4 and 5 in a: fast- (fTRL) and slow-migrating (sTRL), respectively; peaks 4 and 5 in b, c: very-very-fast- and very-fast-migrating LDL (vvfLDL and vfLDL), respectively; peaks 6 and 7: fast- and slow-migrating LDL (fLDL and sLDL), respectively

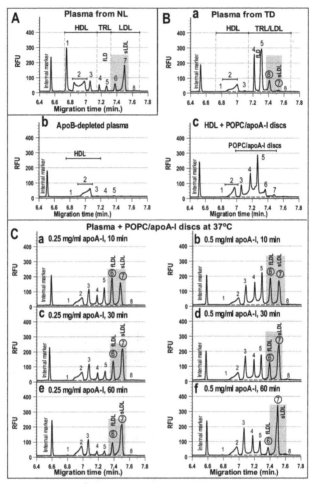

Fig. 5. Effects of 1-palmitoyl-2-oleoylphosphatidylcholine (POPC)/apolipoprotein A-I
(apoA-I) discs on lipoprotein profiles in plasma from normolipidemic (NL) subjects (A) and
a patient with Tangier disease (TD) (B) as characterized by capillary isotachophoresis (cITP).
cITP lipoprotein profiles in apoB-depleted plasma from a patient with TD (B-b). Direct
effects of discoidal reconstituted-HDL (rHDL) and the POPC/apoA-I disc (500 µg/ml) on
the cITP lipoprotein profile in apoB-depleted plasma from a patient with TD (B-c). Time-
dependent effects of rHDL and the POPC/apoA-I disc on the lipoprotein profiles by cITP
(C). Lipoprotein profiles in plasma from a patient with TD in the presence (C-a–C-f) of
POPC/apoA-I discs as characterized by cITP. Two doses (250 and 500 µg/ml) of
POPC/apoA-I discs were incubated *in vitro* with whole plasma at 37°C from a patient with
TD. The POPC/apoA-I discs were incubated with plasma for 10 min (C-a and C-b), 30 min
(C-c and C-d), or 60 min (C-e and C-f), respectively.
Peaks 1–3, fast (fHDL), intermediate (iHDL), and slow (sHDL) fractions; peaks 4, 5, fast
VLDL (fVLDL) and VLDL/IDL (sVLDL) fractions; peaks 6–8, fast (fLDL), slow (sLDL), and
minor LDL (mLDL) fractions. TRL, triglyceride-rich lipoprotein

6. Therapeutic approach for HDL deficiency and TD

Although the inhibition of cholesteryl ester transfer protein, PL transfer protein, or scavenger receptor BI and activation of apoA-I or ABCA1 increase HDL cholesterol, the effects of such interventions on atherosclerosis are uncertain in light of studies on animal models and inborn errors of human HDL metabolism. However, no small molecule has been found that strongly stimulates apoA-I production. An LXR agonist is a candidate for increasing HDL cholesterol by increasing ABCA1 expression and HDL cholesterol levels, and RCT also induces hypertriglycemia as a result of the induction of hepatic VLDL production. Substituting or mimicking apoA-I and other potentially anti-atherogenic HDL components has been attempted. Intravenous infusion of an apoA-I variant called apoA-I Milano rapidly decreases atherosclerotic plaque volumes (Nissen et al., 2003). Because TD is a rare genetic disorder, the basic treatment for the disease is still unknown. The development of neuropathy or atherosclerosis in patients with TD is based on a disorder of cellular cholesterol excretion as the initial step of RCT. If the process is able to performed in vitro, it leads to the generation of HDL particle, which can take up the excessive cholesterol from peripheral cell, and it acts as a new therapeutic target without using gene therapy in patients with TD. Reconstituted HDL (rHDL), which is a complex of apoA-I or apoA-I mimetics with PL, must be disc shaped and may be a candidate medication for patients with TD. ApoA-I-mediated cholesterol efflux depends on ABCA1 in macrophages, and ABCA1 plays a pivotal role in mediating PL and cholesterol efflux to lipid-free apoA-I, and thereby, in the formation of discoidal HDL precursors. Mature HDL particles, which are spherical and transport almost all HDL cholesterol, appear to induce cholesterol efflux via other ABC transporters, such as ABCG1 and ABCG4, rather than ABCA1 (Wang et al., 2004). Therefore, we prepared a discoidal reconstituted HDL, which is a complex with apoA-I that contains 1-palmitoyl-2-oleoylphosphatidylcholine (POPC) (Rye et al., 1997). Interestingly, the apoA-I complex with POPC/apoA-I discs was able to take up cholesterol from macrophages in patients with TD and normal subjects (Fig. 3A). Moreover, ETC-642, a newly developed PL/apoA-I mimetic, is a synthetic peptide of 22 amino acids that contains 1, 2-dipalmitoyl-sn-glycero-3-phosphocholine and also works on cholesterol efflux in macrophages of patients with TD as well as the POPC/apoA-I disc (Fig. 3B).

rHDL and the POPC/apoA-I discs not only have a beneficial action on cholesterol efflux in macrophages but are also involved in lipoprotein–lipoprotein interactions in circulating plasma. To clarify the direct effects of the POPC/apoA-I discs in plasma from patients with TD, 250 and 500 μg/ml discs (final concentrations) were incubated with plasma at 37°C (Fig. 5C). After incubation, peaks 4 and 5 comprised TRLs, such as VLDL, and time dependently decreased in addition to an increase in peak 3 as sHDL. The POPC/apoA-I discs did not affect the native-LDL subfraction; however, surprisingly, the native-LDL subfraction was time dependently generated in plasma from patients with TD by incubating it with POPC/apoA-I discs at 37°C. von Eckardstein et al. have shown that lipid-poor HDL precursors are converted into mature, lipid-rich HDL by acquiring PLs and unesterified cholesterol from either cells or apoB-containing lipoproteins or through association with additional lipoprotein (von Eckardstein et al., 1998b). In contrast to normal subjects, the plasma of patients with TD does not convert preβ-HDL into α-HDL, which is believed to be related to the absence of a lipid transfer factor in the cells and plasma of patients with TD (Huang et al., 1995; von Eckardstein et al., 1998a). Thus, a deficiency in HDL composition leads to suppression of the interaction with lipoproteins, which may result in an increase in

TRLs and a decrease in native-LDL with cholesterol conversion among lipoproteins. Shahrokh et al. have shown that PL uptake by LDL contributes to form larger LDL particles (Shahrokh and Nichols, 1985), suggesting that the POPC/apoA-I discs might produce a large-sized LDL particle from a small-sized LDL particle using cholesterol-poor LDL in patients with TD. Although the plasma total concentrations of cholesterol and triglycerides do not change following incubation with POPC/apoA-I discs *in vitro*, the discs may transfer the cholesterol or triglycerides, resulting in changes in the lipoprotein components. These results suggest that the formation of mature-HDL particles by adding POPC/apoA-I discs led to physiological lipoprotein patterns such as higher native-LDL and lower TRLs in circulating plasma.

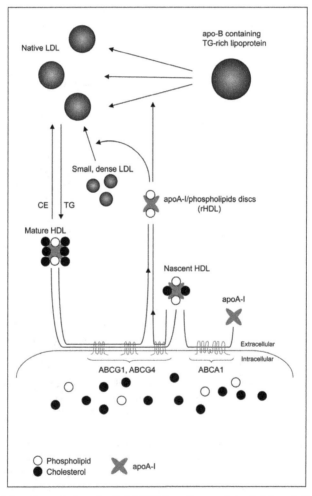

Fig. 6. Suggested function of phospholipid (PL)/apolipoprotein A-I (apoA-I) discs in HDL metabolism. apo, apolipoprotein; rHDL, reconstituted HDL; ABC, ATP-binding cassette transporter; CE, cholesteryl ester; TG, triglyceride

The suggested function of PL apoA-I discs in patients with TD is described in Fig. 6. rHDL and the apoA-I complex with PLs have beneficial effects for cholesterol efflux and lipoprotein components in patients with TD. Briefly, the PL/apoA-I discs acts to modulate lipoprotein metabolism via at least three different steps. 1) PL/apoA-I discs remove the cholesterol from peripheral cells through an ABCA1-independent pathway such as the ABCG1- and ABCG4-dependent pathway. 2) PL/ApoA-I discs form nascent HDL particles with cholesterol and PLs. 3) PL/ApoA-I discs interact with other lipoproteins such as apoB containing TRLs in circulating plasma. The discoidal apoA-I or apoA-I mimetics complex with PLs and potentially prevent or cure the symptoms of TD.

7. Conclusion

TD is a rare autosomal recessive disorder characterized by the absence or extremely low levels of HDL cholesterol and apoA-I in plasma. In addition, cholesteryl esters accumulate in many macrophage-rich tissues and organs. TD is caused by a defect in the ABCA1 gene, which is located on chromosome 9q31. ABCA1 has been identified as a pivotal gene in the regulation of plasma HDL cholesterol levels and cellular cholesterol homeostasis, which are defective in patients with TD. ABCA1 is a membrane protein that transports cholesterol and phospholipids from the membranous inner leaflet to the outer leaflet, and subsequently, lipid-free or lipid-poor apoA-I takes up the transported cholesterol and phospholipids to yield nascent HDL. Due to the ABCA1 genetic defect, patients with TD have an extremely low level of HDL cholesterol and cannot form nascent HDL particles. Namely, TD is based on a disorder of cellular cholesterol excretion as the initial step of RCT via ABCA1. If the process is able to performed in vitro, it leads to the generation of HDL particle, which can take up the excessive cholesterol from peripheral cell, and it acts as a new therapeutic target without using gene therapy in patients with TD.

8. References

Assman, G., von Eckardstein, A., Brewer, H.B.J. Eds., 1995. Familial high density lipoprotein deficiency: Tangier disease., New York: McGraw-Hill.

Baldan, A., Pei, L., Lee, R., Tarr, P., Tangirala, R.K., Weinstein, M.M., Frank, J., Li, A.C., Tontonoz, P., Edwards, P.A., 2006. Impaired development of atherosclerosis in hyperlipidemic Ldlr-/- and ApoE-/- mice transplanted with Abcg1-/- bone marrow. Arterioscler Thromb Vasc Biol. 26, 2301-7.

Bodzioch, M., Orso, E., Klucken, J., Langmann, T., Bottcher, A., Diederich, W., Drobnik, W., Barlage, S., Buchler, C., Porsch-Ozcurumez, M., Kaminski, W.E., Hahmann, H.W., Oette, K., Rothe, G., Aslanidis, C., Lackner, K.J., Schmitz, G., 1999. The gene encoding ATP-binding cassette transporter 1 is mutated in Tangier disease. Nat Genet. 22, 347-51.

Bortnick, A.E., Rothblat, G.H., Stoudt, G., Hoppe, K.L., Royer, L.J., McNeish, J., Francone, O.L., 2000. The correlation of ATP-binding cassette 1 mRNA levels with cholesterol efflux from various cell lines. J Biol Chem. 275, 28634-40.

Brooks-Wilson, A., Marcil, M., Clee, S.M., Zhang, L.H., Roomp, K., van Dam, M., Yu, L., Brewer, C., Collins, J.A., Molhuizen, H.O., Loubser, O., Ouelette, B.F., Fichter, K., Ashbourne-Excoffon, K.J., Sensen, C.W., Scherer, S., Mott, S., Denis, M., Martindale, D., Frohlich, J., Morgan, K., Koop, B., Pimstone, S., Kastelein, J.J., Hayden, M.R., et al., 1999. Mutations in ABC1 in Tangier disease and familial high-density lipoprotein deficiency. Nat Genet. 22, 336-45.

Bungert, S., Molday, L.L., Molday, R.S., 2001. Membrane topology of the ATP binding cassette transporter ABCR and its relationship to ABC1 and related ABCA transporters: identification of N- linked glycosylation sites. J Biol Chem. 276, 23539-46.

Chen, H., Rossier, C., Lalioti, M.D., Lynn, A., Chakravarti, A., Perrin, G., Antonarakis, S.E., 1996. Cloning of the cDNA for a human homologue of the Drosophila white gene and mapping to chromosome 21q22.3. Am J Hum Genet. 59, 66-75.

Costet, P., Luo, Y., Wang, N., Tall, A.R., 2000. Sterol-dependent transactivation of the ABC1 promoter by the liver X receptor/retinoid X receptor. J Biol Chem. 275, 28240-5.

Croop, J.M., Tiller, G.E., Fletcher, J.A., Lux, M.L., Raab, E., Goldenson, D., Son, D., Arciniegas, S., Wu, R.L., 1997. Isolation and characterization of a mammalian homolog of the Drosophila white gene. Gene. 185, 77-85.

Dean, M., Rzhetsky, A., Allikmets, R., 2001. The human ATP-binding cassette (ABC) transporter superfamily. Genome Res. 11, 1156-66.

Dean, M., Annilo, T., 2005. Evolution of the ATP-binding cassette (ABC) transporter superfamily in vertebrates. Annu Rev Genomics Hum Genet. 6, 123-42.

Despres, J.P., Marette, A., 1994. Relation of components of insulin resistance syndrome to coronary disease risk. Curr Opin Lipidol. 5, 274-89.

Fredrickson, D.S., Altrocchi, P.H., Avioli, L.V., Goodman, D.S., Goodman, H.C., 1961. Tangier disease combined clinical staff conference at the National Institutes of Health. Ann Intern Med. 55, 1016-1031.

Havel, R.J., Eder, H.A., Bragdon, J.H., 1955. The distribution and chemical composition of ultracentrifugally separated lipoproteins in human serum. J Clin Invest. 34, 1345-53.

Hobbs, H.H., Rader, D.J., 1999. ABC1: connecting yellow tonsils, neuropathy, and very low HDL. J Clin Invest. 104, 1015-7.

Huang, Y., von Eckardstein, A., Wu, S., Langer, C., Assmann, G., 1995. Generation of pre-beta 1-HDL and conversion into alpha-HDL. Evidence for disturbed HDL conversion in Tangier disease. Arterioscler-Thromb-Vasc-Biol. 15, 1746-54.

Ishida, B.Y., Frolich, J., Fielding, C.J., 1987. Prebeta-migrating high density lipoprotein: quantitation in normal and hyperlipidemic plasma by solid phase radioimmunoassay following electrophoretic transfer. J Lipid Res. 28, 778-86.

Kennedy, M.A., Barrera, G.C., Nakamura, K., Baldan, A., Tarr, P., Fishbein, M.C., Frank, J., Francone, O.L., Edwards, P.A., 2005. ABCG1 has a critical role in mediating cholesterol efflux to HDL and preventing cellular lipid accumulation. Cell Metab. 1, 121-31.

Klein, I., Sarkadi, B., Varadi, A., 1999. An inventory of the human ABC proteins. Biochim-Biophys-Acta. 1461, 237-62.

Klucken, J., Buchler, C., Orso, E., Kaminski, W.E., Porsch-Ozcurumez, M., Liebisch, G., Kapinsky, M., Diederich, W., Drobnik, W., Dean, M., Allikmets, R., Schmitz, G., 2000. ABCG1 (ABC8), the human homolog of the Drosophila white gene, is a regulator of macrophage cholesterol and phospholipid transport. Proc Natl Acad Sci U S A. 97, 817-22.

Kunitake, S.T., La Sala, K.J., Kane, J.P., 1985. Apolipoprotein A-I-containing lipoproteins with pre-beta electrophoretic mobility. J Lipid Res. 26, 549-55.

Langmann, T., Klucken, J., Reil, M., Liebisch, G., Luciani, M.F., Chimini, G., Kaminski, W.E., Schmitz, G., 1999. Molecular cloning of the human ATP-binding cassette transporter 1 (hABC1): evidence for sterol-dependent regulation in macrophages. Biochem Biophys-Res-Commun. 257, 29-33.

Lawn, R.M., Wade, D.P., Garvin, M.R., Wang, X., Schwartz, K., Porter, J.G., Seilhamer, J.J., Vaughan, A.M., Oram, J.F., 1999. The Tangier disease gene product ABC1 controls the cellular apolipoprotein-mediated lipid removal pathway. J Clin Invest. 104, R25-31.

Mauldin, J.P., Srinivasan, S., Mulya, A., Gebre, A., Parks, J.S., Daugherty, A., Hedrick, C.C., 2006. Reduction in ABCG1 in Type 2 diabetic mice increases macrophage foam cell formation. J Biol Chem. 281, 21216-24.

McNeish, J., Aiello, R.J., Guyot, D., Turi, T., Gabel, C., Aldinger, C., Hoppe, K.L., Roach, M.L., Royer, L.J., de Wet, J., Broccardo, C., Chimini, G., Francone, O.L., 2000. High density lipoprotein deficiency and foam cell accumulation in mice with targeted disruption of ATP-binding cassette transporter-1. Proc Natl Acad Sci U S A. 97, 4245-50.

Miller, M., Rhyne, J., Hamlette, S., Birnbaum, J., Rodriguez, A., 2003. Genetics of HDL regulation in humans. Curr Opin Lipidol. 14, 273-9.

Neufeld, E.B., Remaley, A.T., Demosky, S.J., Stonik, J.A., Cooney, A.M., Comly, M., Dwyer, N.K., Zhang, M., Blanchette-Mackie, J., Santamarina-Fojo, S., Brewer, H.B., Jr., 2001. Cellular localization and trafficking of the human ABCA1 transporter. J Biol Chem. 276, 27584-90.

Nissen, S.E., Tsunoda, T., Tuzcu, E.M., Schoenhagen, P., Cooper, C.J., Yasin, M., Eaton, G.M., Lauer, M.A., Sheldon, W.S., Grines, C.L., Halpern, S., Crowe, T., Blankenship, J.C., Kerensky, R., 2003. Effect of recombinant ApoA-I Milano on coronary atherosclerosis in patients with acute coronary syndromes: a randomized controlled trial. JAMA. 290, 2292-300.

Oram, J.F., Lawn, R.M., Garvin, M.R., Wade, D.P., 2000. ABCA1 is the cAMP-inducible apolipoprotein receptor that mediates cholesterol secretion from macrophages. J Biol Chem. 275, 34508-11.

Oram, J.F., Lawn, R.M., 2001. ABCA1. The gatekeeper for eliminating excess tissue cholesterol. J Lipid Res. 42, 1173-9.

Orso, E., Broccardo, C., Kaminski, W.E., Bottcher, A., Liebisch, G., Drobnik, W., Gotz, A., Chambenoit, O., Diederich, W., Langmann, T., Spruss, T., Luciani, M.F., Rothe, G., Lackner, K.J., Chimini, G., Schmitz, G., 2000. Transport of lipids from golgi to plasma membrane is defective in tangier disease patients and Abc1-deficient mice. Nat Genet. 24, 192-6.

Out, R., Hoekstra, M., Hildebrand, R.B., Kruit, J.K., Meurs, I., Li, Z., Kuipers, F., Van Berkel, T.J., Van Eck, M., 2006. Macrophage ABCG1 deletion disrupts lipid homeostasis in alveolar macrophages and moderately influences atherosclerotic lesion development in LDL receptor-deficient mice. Arterioscler Thromb Vasc Biol. 26, 2295-300.

Out, R., Hoekstra, M., Meurs, I., de Vos, P., Kuiper, J., Van Eck, M., Van Berkel, T.J., 2007. Total body ABCG1 expression protects against early atherosclerotic lesion development in mice. Arterioscler Thromb Vasc Biol. 27, 594-9.

Ranalletta, M., Wang, N., Han, S., Yvan-Charvet, L., Welch, C., Tall, A.R., 2006. Decreased atherosclerosis in low-density lipoprotein receptor knockout mice transplanted with Abcg1-/- bone marrow. Arterioscler Thromb Vasc Biol. 26, 2308-15.

Remaley, A.T., Rust, S., Rosier, M., Knapper, C., Naudin, L., Broccardo, C., Peterson, K.M., Koch, C., Arnould, I., Prades, C., Duverger, N., Funke, H., Assman, G., Dinger, M., Dean, M., Chimini, G., Santamarina Fojo, S., Fredrickson, D.S., Denefle, P., Brewer, H.B., Jr., 1999. Human ATP-binding cassette transporter 1 (ABC1): genomic organization and identification of the genetic defect in the original Tangier disease kindred. Proc Natl Acad Sci U S A. 96, 12685-90.

Repa, J.J., Turley, S.D., Lobaccaro, J.A., Medina, J., Li, L., Lustig, K., Shan, B., Heyman, R.A., Dietschy, J.M., Mangelsdorf, D.J., 2000. Regulation of absorption and ABC1-mediated efflux of cholesterol by RXR heterodimers. Science. 289, 1524-9.

Rust, S., Rosier, M., Funke, H., Real, J., Amoura, Z., Piette, J.C., Deleuze, J.F., Brewer, H.B., Duverger, N., Denefle, P., Assmann, G., 1999. Tangier disease is caused by mutations in the gene encoding ATP-binding cassette transporter 1. Nat Genet. 22, 352-5.

Rye, K.A., Hime, N.J., Barter, P.J., 1997. Evidence that cholesteryl ester transfer protein-mediated reductions in reconstituted high density lipoprotein size involve particle fusion. J Biol Chem. 272, 3953-60.

Santamarina-Fojo, S., Peterson, K., Knapper, C., Qiu, Y., Freeman, L., Cheng, J.F., Osorio, J., Remaley, A., Yang, X.P., Haudenschild, C., Prades, C., Chimini, G., Blackmon, E., Francois, T., Duverger, N., Rubin, E.M., Rosier, M., Denefle, P., Fredrickson, D.S., Brewer, H.B., Jr., 2000. Complete genomic sequence of the human ABCA1 gene: analysis of the human and mouse ATP-binding cassette A promoter. Proc Natl Acad Sci U S A. 97, 7987-92.

Savary, S., Denizot, F., Luciani, M., Mattei, M., Chimini, G., 1996. Molecular cloning of a mammalian ABC transporter homologous to Drosophila white gene. Mamm-Genome. 7, 673-6.

Schwartz, K., Lawn, R.M., Wade, D.P., 2000. ABC1 gene expression and ApoA-I-mediated cholesterol efflux are regulated by LXR. Biochem Biophys Res Commun. 274, 794-802.

Shahrokh, Z., Nichols, A.V., 1985. Interaction of human-plasma low-density lipoproteins with discoidal complexes of apolipoprotein A-I and phosphatidylcholine, and characterization of the interaction products. Biochim Biophys Acta. 837, 296-304.

Singaraja, R.R., Bocher, V., James, E.R., Clee, S.M., Zhang, L.H., Leavitt, B.R., Tan, B., Brooks-Wilson, A., Kwok, A., Bissada, N., Yang, Y.Z., Liu, G., Tafuri, S.R., Fievet, C., Wellington, C.L., Staels, B., Hayden, M.R., 2001. Human ABCA1 BAC transgenic mice show increased high density lipoprotein cholesterol and ApoAI-dependent efflux stimulated by an internal promoter containing liver X receptor response elements in intron 1. J Biol Chem. 276, 33969-79.

Smith, J.D., 2006. Insight into ABCG1-mediated cholesterol efflux. Arterioscler Thromb Vasc Biol. 26, 1198-200.

Uehara, Y., Engel, T., Li, Z., Goepfert, C., Rust, S., Zhou, X., Langer, C., Schachtrup, C., Wiekowski, J., Lorkowski, S., Assmann, G., von Eckardstein, A., 2002. Polyunsaturated Fatty Acids and Acetoacetate Downregulate the Expression of the ATP-Binding Cassette Transporter A1. Diabetes. 51, 2922-2928.

Uehara, Y., Miura, S., von Eckardstein, A., Abe, S., Fujii, A., Matsuo, Y., Rust, S., Lorkowski, S., Assmann, G., Yamada, T., Saku, K., 2007. Unsaturated fatty acids suppress the expression of the ATP-binding cassette transporter G1 (ABCG1) and ABCA1 genes via an LXR/RXR responsive element. Atherosclerosis. 191, 11-21.

Uehara, Y., Tsuboi, Y., Zhang, B., Miura, S., Baba, Y., Higuchi, M.A., Yamada, T., Rye, K.A., Saku, K., 2008a. POPC/apoA-I discs as a potent lipoprotein modulator in Tangier disease. Atherosclerosis. 197, 283-9.

Uehara, Y., Yamada, T., Baba, Y., Miura, S.I., Abe, S., Kitajima, K., Higuchi, M.A., Iwamoto, T., Saku, K., 2008b. ATP-binding cassette transporter G4 is highly expressed in microglia in Alzheimer's brain. Brain Res. 1217C, 239-246.

Vaisman, B.L., Lambert, G., Amar, M., Joyce, C., Ito, T., Shamburek, R.D., Cain, W.J., Fruchart-Najib, J., Neufeld, E.D., Remaley, A.T., Brewer, H.B., Jr., Santamarina-Fojo, S., 2001. ABCA1 overexpression leads to hyperalphalipoproteinemia and increased biliary cholesterol excretion in transgenic mice. J Clin Invest. 108, 303-9.

Venkateswaran, A., Laffitte, B.A., Joseph, S.B., Mak, P.A., Wilpitz, D.C., Edwards, P.A., Tontonoz, P., 2000. Control of cellular cholesterol efflux by the nuclear oxysterol receptor LXR alpha. Proc Natl Acad Sci U S A. 97, 12097-102.

von Eckardstein, A., Chirazi, A., Schuler-Luttmann, S., Walter, M., Kastelein, J.J., Geisel, J., Real, J.T., Miccoli, R., Noseda, G., Hobbel, G., Assmann, G., 1998a. Plasma and fibroblasts of Tangier disease patients are disturbed in transferring phospholipids onto apolipoprotein A-I. J Lipid Res. 39, 987-98.

von Eckardstein, A., Huang, Y., Kastelein, J.J., Geisel, J., Real, J.T., Kuivenhoven, J.A., Miccoli, R., Noseda, G., Assmann, G., 1998b. Lipid-free apolipoprotein (apo) A-I is converted into alpha-migrating high density lipoproteins by lipoprotein-depleted plasma of normolipidemic donors and apo A-I-deficient patients but not of Tangier disease patients. Atherosclerosis. 138, 25-34.

von Eckardstein, A., Nofer, J.R., Assmann, G., 2001. High density lipoproteins and arteriosclerosis. Role of cholesterol efflux and reverse cholesterol transport. Arterioscler Thromb Vasc Biol. 21, 13-27.

von Eckardstein, A., Rohrer, L., 2009. Transendothelial lipoprotein transport and regulation of endothelial permeability and integrity by lipoproteins. Curr Opin Lipidol. 20, 197-205.

Walker, J.E., Saraste, M., Runswick, M.J., Gay, N.J., 1982. Distantly related sequences in the alpha- and beta-subunits of ATP synthase, myosin, kinases and other ATP-requiring enzymes and a common nucleotide binding fold. Embo J. 1, 945-51.

Wang, N., Silver, D.L., Thiele, C., Tall, A.R., 2001. ATP-binding cassette transporter A1 (ABCA1) functions as a cholesterol efflux regulatory protein. J Biol Chem. 276, 23742-7.

Wang, N., Lan, D., Chen, W., Matsuura, F., Tall, A.R., 2004. ATP-binding cassette transporters G1 and G4 mediate cellular cholesterol efflux to high-density lipoproteins. Proc Natl Acad Sci U S A. 101, 9774-9.

Willy, P.J., Umesono, K., Ong, E.S., Evans, R.M., Heyman, R.A., Mangelsdorf, D.J., 1995. LXR, a nuclear receptor that defines a distinct retinoid response pathway. Genes Dev. 9, 1033-45.

Yang, X.P., Freeman, L.A., Knapper, C.L., Amar, M.J., Remaley, A., Brewer, H.B., Jr., Santamarina-Fojo, S., 2002. The E-box motif in the proximal ABCA1 promoter mediates transcriptional repression of the ABCA1 gene. J Lipid Res. 43, 297-306.

Zhang, B., Kaneshi, T., Ohta, T., Saku, K., 2005. Relation between insulin resistance and fast-migrating LDL subfraction as characterized by capillary isotachophoresis. J Lipid Res. 46, 2265-77.

5

Thalassemia Syndrome

Tangvarasittichai Surapon
Chronic Diseases Research Unit, Department of Medical Technology,
Naresuan University, Phitsanulok
Thailand

1. Introduction

Thalassemia is an inherited disorder of autosomal recessive gene disorder caused by impaired synthesis of one or more globin chains. The impairment alters production of hemoglobin (Hb) (Ridolfi et al., 2002). Thalassemia causes varying degrees of anemia, which can range from significant to life threatening. People of Mediterranean, Middle Eastern, African, and Southeast Asian descent are at higher risk of carrying the genes for thalassemia (Weatherall, 1997). These hereditary anemias are caused by mutations that decrease hemoglobin synthesis and red cell survival. These hereditary anemia caused by decreased or absent production of one type of globin chain either α or β globin chain. These hematologic disorders range from asymptomatic to severe anemia that can cause significant morbidity and mortality. It was first recognized clinically in 1925 by Dr. Thomas Cooley, who described a syndrome of anemia with microcytic erythrocytes. Then it was called Cooley's anemia. Later Wipple and Bradford renamed this disease as "Thalassemia". Because it was found in the region of the Mediterranean Sea (thalasa is an old Greek word for sea) (Cooley, 1946). Thalassemias can cause significant problems because these are inherited disorders, newborn screening and prenatal diagnosis are important in management of patients. This topic will review the clinical features of thalassemia while focusing on pathophysiology, clinical features, complication, management, screening and diagnosis. Formerly the distribution of thalassemia had been mainly limited to the areas from the Mediterranean basin through the Middle East and Indian subcontinent up to Southeast Asia so called "thalassemia belt" (Chernoff, 1959). However, recent migrations of people have spread thalassemia genes throughout the world.

2. Pathophysiology

Hemoglobin (Hb) is the molecule that carries and transports oxygen all through the body. Normal human hemoglobin is a tetramer formed by two pairs of globin chains attached to heme. The hemoglobin type is determined by the combination of tetra-globin chains (α, β, δ, and γ chains). Each globin chain is structurally different and thus has different oxygen affinity, electrical charge, and electrophoretic mobility. Normal adult hemoglobins are expressed as A_2, A and F (fetal). Ninety-five to ninety-eight percent of adult hemoglobin is A the major hemoglobin, which consists of two α- and two β-chains (α_2, β_2). Hemoglobin A_2 (α_2, δ_2), the remainder of hemoglobin in adults is a minor component (less than 3.3%), and 1% or less of F (α_2, γ_2) (Nathan & Oski, 1993.), the gamma hemoglobin (Hb-F) is the predominant hemoglobin found only during fetal development. The equal production of α and non-α (β, δ, γ) globin chains is necessary for normal red blood cell (RBC) function. The failure in hemoglobin synthesis is a main cause of microcytosis and anemia in many population groups around the world. Hb variants are characterized by the gene mutation of the globin chains form hemoglobin (i.e., the replacement of different amino acids at a certain position). Thalassemia occurs when there is decreased or absent production of one of the types of globin chains (most commonly either α or β), that cause insufficeient amount of normal structure globin chains. This results in an imbalance between α- and β-chains and causes the clinical features of thalassemia (Nathan & Gunn, 1966), it can be separated into two major types such as α-thalassemia and β- thalassemia.

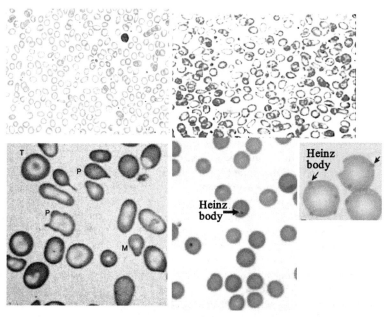

Fig. 1. Red blood cell morphology is altered in patients with all forms of thalassemia. Hypochromic microcytes and target cells are the main features in asymptomatic individuals. Patients with more severe forms of thalassemia have the anisocytosis and poikilocytosis, hypochromic microcytic, target cells, ovalocytes, occasional fragmented red blood cells

The absence or decreased of normal production of α-globin chains results in a relative excess of γ-globin chains in the fetus and newborn, and β-globin chains in children and adults. When globin chains are not produced in equal amounts, any excess chains accumulate and precipitate damaging the RBC and accelerating its destruction. The absence of normal production of α-chains results in a relative excess of γ-globin chains in the fetus and newborn, and β-globin chains in children and adults. Further, the β-globin chains are capable of forming soluble tetramers (β-4, or Hb-H); yet this form of hemoglobin is unstable and tends to precipitate within the cell forming insoluble inclusions (Heinz bodies) that damage the red cell membrane. α-Thalassemia is generally less severe because the excess unpaired β-chains that accumulate are less damaging to RBCs than the unpaired α chains. Furthermore, diminished hemoglobinization of individual red blood cells results in damage to erythrocyte precursors and ineffective erythropoiesis in the bone marrow, as well as hypochromia and microcytosis of circulating red blood cells. (Fig 1)

In β-thalassemia, reduced amount (β+) or absence (β0) of β-globin chains excess α-chains accumulate in the RBC and precipitate because they are highly insoluble. These precipitated globin chains occur in both erythroid precursors in the bone marrow and circulating RBCs. The destruction of precursor RBCs results in ineffective erythropoiesis, increased erythropoietin, and proliferation of the bone marrow. This expanded bone marrow (up 25 to 30 times normal) can result in the characteristic bony abnormalities of β-thalassemia if the process is not prevented by transfusion therapy. Prolonged and severe anemia and increased erythropoietic drive also result in hepatosplenomegaly and extramedullary erythropoiesis, leading to their premature death and hence to ineffective erythropoiesis. The degree of globin chain reduction is determined by the nature of the mutation at the β-globin gene located on chromosome 11. Peripheral hemolysis contributing to anemia is more prominent in thalassemia major than in thalassemia intermedia, and occurs when insoluble α-globin chains induce membrane damage to the peripheral erythrocytes.

Genes that regulate both synthesis and structure of different globins are organized into 2 separate clusters. The α-globin genes are encoded on chromosome 16 and the γ, δ, and β-globin genes are encoded on chromosome 11 as demonstrated in Fig 2. Each individual normally carries a linked pair of α-globin genes, 2 from the paternal chromosome, and 2 from the maternal chromosome. Therefore, each diploid human cell has four copies of the α-globin gene. The four α-thalassemia syndromes thus reflect the disease state produced by deletion or no-function of one, two, three, or all four of the α-globin genes (Higgs et al., 1989) (Table 1). The silent carrier state of α-thalassemia represents a mutation of one copy of the α-globin gene and results in no hematologic abnormalities.

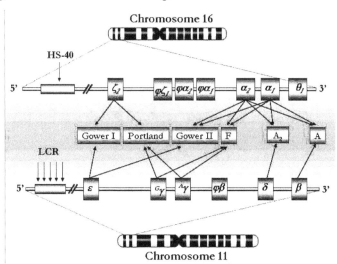

Fig. 2. Schematic represent of the globin gene loci. The upper panel shows the α-globin locus that resides on chromosome 16. Each of the four alpha globin genes contributed to the synthesis of the α-globin protein. The lower panel shows the β-globin locus that resides on chromosome 11. The two γ-globin genes are active during fetal growth and produce hemoglobin F. The "adult" gene, beta, takes over after birth

3. Geographical distribution of thalassemias and the malaria hypothesis

It is a widely accepted conclusion that the high frequency of thalassemias and sickle cell anemia observed in some tropical and subtropical areas of the world (Fig 3). This due to the resistance against malignant malaria (*Plasmodium falciparum*) conferred by these inherited defects to the heterozygous carriers (Allison, 1954). According to the malaria hypothesis, the heterozygous for HbS or a thalassemic (clinically healthy) are resistant to malaria and have a selective advantage over both homozygotes which have a higher chance of dying during the first years of life because of either malaria or anemia. The preferential survival of the heterozygote thus makes possible the persistence at polymorphic frequencies of the abnormal genes in the population, provided that the selective agent (malaria) remains present and active. Because there is a loss of both normal and abnormal genes, an equilibrium between their frequency will be reached in a period of time which depends on the extent of the selective advantage (balanced polymorphism). The malaria hypothesis is supported by the overlapping geographical distribution of these disorders and endemic malaria and by clinical and epidemiological studies showing a positive correlation between malaria endemicity and frequency of abnormal alleles (Siniscalco et al., 1966).

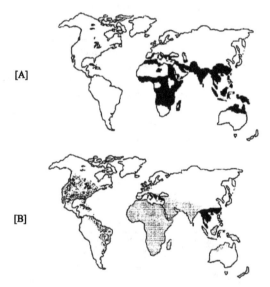

Fig. 3. The geographical distribution of [A] malaria (■) [B] thalassemia (□, α^+- thalassemia α^0- thalassemia). Because of migration, hemoglobinopathies are improved into the area where malaria has never been endemic

The α-thalassemias are most prevalent in Asian and African populations. Persons of Mediterranean and African descent have the highest incidence of β-thalassemia. Thalassemic mutations have maintained a high frequency, particularly in these areas, because the heterozygous state confers some protection against malaria (Weatherall, 1987). Other abnormalities of hemoglobin also occur with increased frequency in these populations: therefore, thalassemia may coexist with other disorders of hemoglobin such as the sickle cell syndromes, hemoglobin E (Hb-E), or hemoglobin C (Hb-C).

Syndrome	Molecular basis	Laboratory values	Clinical Feature
α- Thalassemia			
α- Thalassemia silent carrier	One α- gene deletion $(-\alpha/\alpha\alpha)$ Heterozygous α-thalassemia	No anemia or RBC morphology abnormalities; Asymptomatic may have l-2 % Hb Bart's at birth	Asymptomatic
α-Thalassemia trait (minor)	Two α-gene deletion $(--/\alpha\alpha)$ Heterozygous α-thalassemia-1 Two α-gene deletion $(-\alpha/-\alpha)$ Homozygous α-thalassemia 2	Mild anemia, microcytosis, and hypochromia; 4-6% Hb Bart's at birth	Asymptomatic
Hb H disease (Hb variants related to mutation in α-globin chain)	Three α-gene deletion $(--/-\alpha)$ α-thalassemia-1/α-thalassemia-2 Hb Constant Spring α-thalassemia-1/Hb Constant Spring	Moderate anemia, microcytosis, hypochromia, RBC fragments; Hb Bart's prominent at birth α- chain has extra 31 amino acids	Jaundice, gallstones, splenomegaly, occasionally need transfusion; antioxidant drugs can precipitate hemolysis
Hb Bart's Hydrops fetalis	Four α-gene deletion $(--/--)$ Homozygous α-thalassemia 1	Severe anemia, nucleated RRCs; only Hb H, Bart's, and Portland present	Death in utero or shortly after birth
β- Thalassemia			
β-Thalassemia trait (minor)	Point mutations Heterozygous β^0-thalassemia Heterozygous β^+-thalassemia	Mild anemia, hypochromia, and microcytosis; RBC morphologic abnormalities; Hb A_2, and F often elevated	Asymptomatic
β-Thalassemia intermedia	Point mutations - β^0-thalassemia/β^+-thalassemia -HbEβ^+-thalassemia	Moderate anemia, microcytosis, and hypochromia; RBC morphologic abnormalities; Hb A, and F increased; Hb A decreased to absent	Maintain Hb of 7 g/dL without transfusion; clinical phenotype between β-thalassemia trait and thalassemia major

Syndrome	Molecular basis	Laboratory values	Clinical Feature
β-Thalassemia major	Point mutations -Homozygous β^0 -thalassemia - HbEβ^0 -thalassemia (Thalassemia intermediate or thalassemia major)	Severe anemia, microcytosis, and hypochromia; RBC fragments and striking morphologic abnormalities; Hb A$_2$, and F ncreased; Hb A decreased to absent	Require chronic transfusion; develop iron overload resulting in endocrine abnormalities and chronic organ damage
RBC= red blood cell; Hb H = hemoglobin H			

Table 1. Characteristic of the Thalassemia Syndromes

β-thalassemia is prevalent in Mediterranean countries, the Middle East, Central Asia, India, Southern China, and the Far East as well as countries along the north coast of Africa and in South America. The highest carrier frequency is reported in Cyprus (14%), Sardinia (10.3%), and Southeast Asia (Flint et al., 1998). The high gene frequency of β-thalassemia in these regions is most likely related to the selective pressure from *Plasmodium falciparum* malaria (Flint et al., 1998). Population migration and intermarriage between different ethnic groups has introduced thalassemia in almost every country of the world, including Northern Europe where thalassemia was previously absent. It has been estimated that about 1.5% of the global population (80 to 90 million people) are carriers of β-thalassemia, with about 60,000 symptomatic individuals born annually, the great majority in the developing world. The total annual incidence of symptomatic individuals is estimated at 1 in 100,000 throughout the world and 1 in 10,000 people in the European Union. According to Thalassemia International Federation, only about 200,000 patients with thalassemia major are alive and registered as receiving regular treatment around the world (Thalassemia International Federation: Guidelines for the clinical management of thalassemia 2nd edition. 2008 (http://www.Thalassemia. org. cy)).

4. Molecular basis and classification

The thalassemia syndromes are one of the most thoroughly studied diseases at the molecular level. Consequently, some explanation for the clinical heterogeneity seen in patients can be explained at the molecular level.

4.1 α-Thalassemias

The major clinical syndromes resulting from α-thalassemia were first recognized in the mid 1950s and early 1960s through the association of the abnormal hemoglobins (Hb-H and Hb Bart's) with hypochromic microcytic anemia in the absence of iron deficiency (Minnich et al., 1954, Rigas et al., 1955), Lie-Injo & Jo, 1960). α-Thalassemia is divided into deletional and nondeletional types (Bain 2006). There are at least 40 different deletions. The size of the deletion is important and affects the clinical phenotype of hydrops fetalis. Over 95% of α thalassemia is caused by large deletions involving one or both of the α-globin genes. The α-globin gene cluster occurs on the short arm of chromosome 16, band 16 p 13.3 and includes the α-globin genes as well as the embryonic genes (as two identical α-globin genes (α_1 and α_2) that are aligned one after the other on the chromosome). Common α-thalassemia deletions that spare the embryonic gene allow for the production of functional embryonic hemoglobin early in gestation. In contrast, the large deletions (severe) lack the benefit of embryonic hemoglobin. Non-deletion mutations may have a more severe phenotype than most of the deletional mutations. The most common non-deletional α-thalassemia mutation is Hemoglobin Constant Spring; this mutation of the stop codon results in 31 amino acids being added to α chain. Depending on the production of α-globin chains, α-thalassemia determinants can be classified into two groups: $α°$ and $α^+$. In $α°$-thalassemia the production of α-chains by the affected chromosome is completely abolished; $α^+$-thalassemia is defined by the variable amounts of α polypeptide chains which can still be expressed in cis to the thalassaemic cluster. This nomenclature, which describes α-thalassemias in terms of α-globin chain expression/haplotype, has replaced the previous classification of these defects into severe (α-thalassaemia-1) and mild (α-thalassaemia-2) forms (Weatherail & Clegg, 1981).

In the passed, genetics of these syndromes were more confusing. This was because the adult carriers of α-thalassemia do not produce large amounts of either Hb-H or Hb Bart's. Although the relatives of the affected individuals do not have a readily defined phenotype, it was eventually shown that the offspring of individuals with Hb-H disease have raised levels of Hb Bart's ($γ_4$) in the neonatal period (Na-Nakorn et al., 1969), and the parents of individuals with Hb-H disease and the Hb Bart's hydrops fetalis syndrome have mildly hypochromic, microcytic red cell indices (Ali, 1969); sometimes Hb-H inclusions could be demonstrated in occasional red cells (McNiel JR, 1968). By 1969 it had been shown that Hb-H disease results from the inheritance of α-thalassemia-1 x α-thalassemia-2 and the Hb Bart's hydrops fetalis syndrome results from α-thalassemia-1 x α-thalassemia 1) (Na-Nakorn et al., 1969, Pootrakul et al., 1967).

The structural organization of the α-globin genes revealed by blot hybridization analysis (Orkin, 1978), Normal individual have two α-genes on each chromosome 16 or four copies of the α-globin gene (αα/αα) and carriers for α-thalassemia have either three (−α/αα) or two (− −/αα) α genes. Thus, the most frequently encountered genotype of Hb-H disease is −−/− α and Hb Bart's hydrops fetalis is − −/− − (Orkin, 1978, Orkin et al., 1979, Phillips 3d et al., 1980). Thus by 1980 the molecular genetics of α-thalassemia was understood. The four α-thalassemia syndromes thus reflect the disease state produced by deletion or nonfunction of one, two, three, or all four of the α-globin genes (Higgs et at., 1989). α-Thalassemia trait occurs with deletion or nonfunction of two α-globin genes. The two genes are deleted from the same chromosome (cis-deletion) or one gene is lost from each chromosome 16 (trans-deletion). The cis-deletion is most common in Asian and Mediterranean populations, whereas individuals of African descent usually have the trans-deletion (Higgs et al., 1989). Both varieties of α-thalassemia trait produce an asymptomatic, mild anemia associated with microcytosis. Hemoglobin H (Hb-H) disease, a three-gene deletion, usually results from inheritance of the cis α-thalassemia trait from one parent and the one gene deletion from the other parent. Therefore, this abnormality is rare in the black population because the cis-deletion is uncommon. Hydrops fetalis results from deletion of all four α-globin genes and generally causes death in utero because no physiologically useful hemoglobin is produced beyond the embryonic stage. Although the α-thalassemia syndromes also are of varying clinical severity, these differences cannot be explained by the number of deleted or nonfunctional genes. One of the most frequent α-thalassemia mutations is the _ _SEA deletion, which deletes both α-globin genes but spares the embryonic gene. Homozygosity for this deletion (_ _SEA) is the most common cause of hydrops fetalis (Chui & Waye 1998). The sparing of the embryonic gene allows enough functional embryonic hemoglobin (Hemoglobin Portland 1 and Hemoglobin Portland 2) to allow gestation to continue and the phenotype of hydrops fetalis to develop. In contrast, other common α-thalassemia mutations ($_{--}$FIL, $_{--}$THAI) also lack the entire embryonic α-globin cluster, and therefore do not produce the functional embryonic Hemoglobin Portland. These embryos may terminate unnoticed early in gestation (Chui & Waye 1998). Over 5% of individuals in the Philippines are carriers for the $_{-}$ $_{-}$SEA or $_{-}$ $_{-}$FIL mutation. Hydrops fetalis, while most common in Southeast Asia, is found worldwide among many ethnic groups; $_{-}$ $_{-}$MED is a common α⁰-thalassemia mutation in Mediterranean regions, particularly Greece and Cyprus. It has resulted in hydrops fetalis.

Non-deletional α-thalassemia is found throughout the world. Up to 8% of Southeast Asians are carriers of Hemoglobin Constant Spring. In the Middle East, Hemoglobin αTSaudiα is a common α-thalassemia non-deletional mutation. It is a mutation of the polyadenylation signal sequence of the α 2 gene, resulting in decreased expression of structurally normal α chains. Hemoglobin Koya Dora, another structural non-deletional mutation, is found in India. Other structural mutations, such as hemoglobin Quong Sze found in Southeast Asia, are highly unstable and result in defects in the hem pocket (Skordis, 2006, Leung et al., 2002).

4.2 α Thalassemia trait

α-Thalassaemia trait is usually caused either by the interaction of the normal haplotype with a $α^0$- or a $α^+$-thalassaemia determinant or by the homozygosity for two $α^+$ haplotypes. Much less frequently this phenotype can be the result of compound heterozygosity for a deletional $α^+$- thalassaemia and a $α^+$ determinant caused by a point mutation or even homozygosity for the latter kind of determinant. Depending on the nature and localization of the mutation, the phenotype of the trait can thus range from the silent cartier to individuals showing very pronounced haematological abnormalities.

Patients with α-thalassemia trait have microcytosis, hypochromia, and mild anemia. Small amounts of hemoglobin Bart's (a tetramer of γ chains: $γ_4$) may be noted on a newborn screen. Individuals with this disorder are asymptomatic and do not require transfusions or any other treatment. The diagnosis of α-thalassemia trait is considered when the patient has the appropriate RBC abnormalities, when iron deficiency and β-thalassemia trait have been excluded, and when family studies (CBC, hemoglobin profile, and review of the peripheral smear) are consistent with the diagnosis (Nathan & Oski 1993). To make the diagnosis with complete certainty requires characterization of gene deletions with restriction endonuclease mapping or globin chain synthesis studies showing a decreased (α:β ratio. However, this confirmation rarely is indicated clinically.

4.3 Hemoglobin H disease

Hemoglobin H (Hb-H) disease is the most severe non-fatal form of α-thalassemia syndrome, mostly caused by molecular defects of the α-globin genes in which α-globin expression is decreased, causes a moderate anemia with hypochromia, microcytosis, and red cell fragmentation. Two common genotypes lead to the phenotype of Hb-H disease are α-thalassemia-1/α-thalassemia-2 and Hb Constant Spring/α-thalassemia-1. Both genotypes are equally common but Hb Constant Spring/α-thalassemia-1 is more severe than α-thalassemia-1/α-thalassemia-2 (Fucharoen et al., 1988). Compound heterozygotes for α⁰- and α⁺- thalassemia (--/-α) with only one functional α-globin gene have a severe imbalance in globin chain synthesis with a two- to five-fold excess of β-globin chains synthesis (Nathan & Oski 1993.). Newborns have large amounts of Bart's Hb. (Higgs et al., 1989). When the switch from γ- to β-globin chain production occurs, Hb Bart's ($γ_4$) switches to Hb-H ($β_4$) and the typical picture of Hb-H disease results. The excess β-globin chains precipitate and form a characteristic abnormal hemoglobin; hemoglobin H (Hb-H) or β-globin tetramer ($β_4$). This causes a phenotype of mild to moderate chronic hemolytic anemia named Hb-H disease characterized by readily detectable Hb-H inclusion bodies in the peripheral blood cells. Hb-H is unable to transport oxygen at physiologic conditions; therefore, patients have a more severe deficit in oxygen carrying capacity than would be expected from their measured hemoglobin level (Nathan & Oski 1993). Increased red cell destruction occurs because Hb-H containing cells are sensitive to oxidative stress. Thus the complications of the disease are related to hemolysis and include jaundice, hepatosplenomegaly, gallstones, and leg ulcers. Most affected individuals have a mild disorder with an Hb concentration of 7-10 g/dL and require only symptomatic care with occasional transfusions. Therefore, iron overload is rarely a problem in these patients.

The clinical phenotypes of Hb-H disease found in nondeletional α-thalassemia (--/αTα) are often more severe than those caused by α⁺-thalassemia resulting from simple deletion (--/-α). Recent molecular analysis of more than 500 thalassemia carriers at the Department of Pediatrics, Siriraj Hospital, Thailand, revealed that the frequency of deletional α-thalassemia is significantly higher compared with non-deletional mutations (mainly Hb CS and Pakse) in Thai population (15%-20% vs 1%-2%, respectively). However, the number of symptomatic patients with Hb-H disease due to non-deletional mutations appeared to be higher than those with deletional Hb-H (60% vs 40% from 350 Hb-H disease patients), as shown in Table 1, suggesting that non-deletional Hb-H patients have more significant clinical symptoms and require more medical attention (Fucharoen & Viprakasit, 2009).

A striking clinical feature of Hb-H disease is the sudden drop in the Hb concentration with associated symptoms of acute anemia during episodes of pyrexia (Chinprasertsuk et al., 1994). It has been postulated that fever either alone or together with oxidative substances released in the process of infection, induces the unstable Hb-H to precipitate in the red cells as inclusion bodies. These red cells then either hemolyze or are rapidly destroyed by the reticuloendothelial cells. Blood transfusions should be given together with treatment for infections. Body temperature should be normalized as quickly as possible in order to reduce induction of Hb-H precipitation within the red cells. Hb Constant Spring is detected in addition to Hb-A and H in patients with Hb Constant Spring α-thalassemia-1. They are slightly more severe than classical Hb-H disease with lower Hb concentrations, larger spleens, higher levels of Hb-H and more red cells containing inclusion bodies (Fucharoen et al., 1988).

4.4 Hemoglobin Bart's Hydrops fetalis syndrome

Hydrops fetalis, the most severe form of α-thalassemia, occurs in infants whose parents both have α-thalassemia syndrome (Higgs et al., 1989). As discussed previously, these infants have deletion of all four α-globin genes and produce only Hb Bart's, Hb-H, and small amounts of embryonic hemoglobins. Therefore, they have very little physiologically useful hemoglobin and are hydropic secondary to severe anemia. These infants are usually stillborn or die shortly after delivery (Chui & Waye, 1998, Leung et al., 2008, Lorey et al., 2001, Michlitsch et al., 2009, Weatherall 2008) Advances in perinatal care and recognition of surviving homozygous thalassemia newborns have precipitated studies of long-term survivors with this disorder. Recently, the Newborn Screening Program of California reported 8 surviving α-thalassemia major newborns along with 500 Hemoglobin H babies (Michlitsch et al., 2009). In southern China, the prevalence of α⁰-thalassemia trait is 8.5% and 0.23% of births had homozygous α-thalassemia (Chui & Waye, 1998). In addition to China and Southeast Asia, Bart's hydrops fetalis is now being recognized in Greece, Turkey, Cyprus, India, Sardinia, and other parts of the world (Chui & Waye 1998, Yang & Li, 2009, Suwanrath-Kengpol et al., 2005)

Clinical and haematological examinations reveal severely anaemic infants with variable hemoglobin levels (3-10g/dl) and marked anisopoikilocytosis with large hypochromic red cells and with the presence of numerous erythroblasts. The analysis of the hemolysate shows, in the hydrops caused by the deletion of four α genes, about 80% Hb Bart's (γ_4) and 20% Hb Portland 1 ($\zeta_2 \gamma_2$) with very small amounts, if any, of Hb Portland 2 ($\zeta_2 \beta_2$) and HbH (β_4) (Kutlar et al., 1989). Lower levels of Hb Portland 1 have been observed in genetic compounds for the SEA deletion and the large Fil deletion which also eliminates the ζ gene (Kutlar et al., 1989). In the rare cases of Hb-H disease with hydrops fetalis, in addition to Hb Bart's and the embryonic Hb Portland 1 and 2, variable amounts of HbH, HbF and HbA can also be detected (Chan et al., 1997). The lack of hem-hem interaction or Bohr effect and binds oxygen irreversibly tightly and high oxygen affinity of Hb Bart's make this γ tetramer unsuitable for the delivery of oxygen to the tissues. The ensuing hypoxia is the cause of fetal hydrops and intrauterine death caused by massive organomegaly, severe albuminemia, and heart failure. This leads to gross body edema, growth failure.

4.5 β-Thalassemias

The β-thalassemias are widespread throughout the Mediterranean region, Africa, the Middle East, the Indian subcontinent and Burma, Southeast Asia including southern China, the Malay Peninsula, and Indonesia. Estimates of gene frequencies range from 3 to 10 percent in some areas. (Weatherall, 1994) Within each population at risk for β-thalassemia a small number of common mutations are found, as well as rarer ones; each mutation is in strong linkage disequilibrium with specific arrangements of restriction-fragment length polymorphisms, or haplotypes, within the β-globin cluster. A limited number of haplotypes are found in each population, so that 80 percent of the mutations are associated with only 20 different haplotypes. This observation has helped demonstrate the independent origin of β-thalassemia in several populations (Flint et al., 1993). There is evidence that the high frequency of β-thalassemia throughout the tropics reflects an advantage of heterozygotes against. *Plasmodium falciparum* malaria, (Weatherall, 1987) as has already been demonstrated in α-thalassemia (Allen et al., 1997).

The β-globin gene cluster is located on chromosome 11 and is not duplicated like the α-globin genes. Therefore, each diploid cell contains only two β-globin genes. Mutations are described that affect every step in the process of gene expression from transcription and translation to post-translational stability of the β-globin chain (Kazazian Jr., 1990) The variable clinical severity of the β-thalassemia syndromes depends on how significantly these different mutations affect β-globin synthesis. Although over ninety such mutations are known, a given mutation generally is found in one ethnic group and not another. Nearly 200 different mutations have been described in patients with β-thalassemia and related disorders. Although most are small nucleotide substitutions within the cluster, deletions may also cause β-thalassemia (Weatherall 1994). All the mutations result in either the absence of the synthesis of β-globin chains (β^0-thalassemia) or a reduction in synthesis (β^+-thalassemia) (Fig. 2). Mutations in or close to the conserved promoter sequences and in the 5' untranslated region down-regulate transcription, usually resulting in mild β^+-thalassemia. Transcription is also affected by deletions in the 5' region, which completely inactivate transcription and result in β^0-thalassemia. Both splicing of the messenger RNA (mRNA) precursor and ineffective cleavage of the mRNA transcript are result in β-thalassemia. In some mutations, no normal message is produced, whereas other mutations only slightly reduce the amount of normally spliced mRNA. Mutations within invariant dinucleotides at intron–exon junctions, critical to the removal of intervening sequences and the splicing of exons to produce functional mRNA, result in β^0 -thalassemia. Mutations in highly conserved nucleotides flanking these sequences, or in "cryptic" splice sites, which resemble a donor or acceptor splice site, result in severe as well as mild β^+-thalassemia. Substitutions or small deletions affecting the conserved AATAAA sequence in the 3' untranslated region result in ineffective cleavage of the mRNA transcript and cause mild β^+-thalassemia. Mutations that interfere with translation involve the initiation, elongation, or termination of globin-chain production and result in β^0 -thalassemia. Approximately half of all β-thalassemia mutations interfere with translation; these include frame-shift or nonsense mutations, which introduce premature termination codons and result in β^0-thalassemia. A more recently identified family of mutations, usually involving exon 3, results in the production of unstable globin chains of varying lengths that, together with a relative excess of α-globin chains, precipitate in red-cell precursors and lead to ineffective erythropoiesis, even in the heterozygous state. This is the molecular basis for dominantly inherited (β^+) thalassemia. In addition, missense mutations, resulting in the synthesis of unstable β-globin chains, cause β-thalassemia. β-thalassemia includes three main forms: Thalassemia Major, variably referred to as Cooley's Anemia and Mediterranean Anemia, Thalassemia Intermedia and Thalassemia Minor also called " β-thalassemia carrier", "β-thalassemia trait" or "heterozygous β-thalassemia". According to Thalassemia International Federation, only about 200,000 patients with thalassemia major are alive and registered as receiving regular treatment around the world (Thalassemia International Federation: Guidelines for the clinical management of thalassemia 2nd edition. 2008 [http://www.thalassemia. org.cy]). The most common combination of β-thalassemia with abnormal Hb or structural Hb variant with thalassemic properties is β-thalassemia/Hb-E which is most prevalent in Southeast Asia where the carrier frequency is around 50%.

4.6 β-Thalassemia trait

Carriers of thalassemia, individuals with this disorder are heterozygous for a mutation that affects β-globin synthesis (Kazazian Jr., 1990). They are mildly anemic with hypochromic, microcytic RBCs. Targeting and elliptocytosis are often seen. As with α-thalassemia trait, one must exclude iron deficiency to make the diagnosis. In general, patients with β-thalassemia trait have a lower mean corpuscular volume (MCV) and a higher red cell count for the degree of anemia than seen in iron deficiency. Thus, the Mentzer index (MCV/RBC) is useful as a screening test to differentiate thalassemia from iron deficiency. If the Mentzer index is < 13, thalassemia is more likely; if > 13, iron deficiency is more common. Hb electrophoresis is normal with iron deficiency, but with β-thalassemia trait the hemoglobin A_2, (Hb A_2) is often elevated. Globin chain synthesis studies show an excess of α-chains (Nathan & Oski 1993). These patients need no treatment, but should receive genetic counseling regarding the potential for having a child with β-thalassemia major or a combination of β-thalassemia trait and sickle hemoglobin (Sβ-thal). When both parents are carriers there is a 25% risk at each pregnancy of having children with homozygous thalassemia. Within the first months of life, adult hemoglobin containing 2 pairs of α and β-chain (Hb-A: $\alpha_2\beta_2$) physiologically replaces fetal hemoglobin (HbF: $\alpha_2\gamma_2$). In β-thalassemia, deficient of production structurally normal β-chain lead to anemia, largely as a consequence of ineffective hemopoiesis (Olivieri 1999, Nathan & Gunn, 1966).

4.7 Thalassemia intermedia

These β-thalassemia patients who clinically are between the extremes of thalassemia trait and thalassemia major (Nathan & Oski 1993), have milder anemia and by definition do not require or only occasionally require transfusion. The regular transfusion therapy is not required initially. These patients usually maintain a hemoglobin level of 7 g/dL without transfusions. At the severe end of the clinical spectrum, patients present between the ages of 2 and 6 years and although they are capable of surviving without regular blood transfusion, growth and development are retarded. At the other end of the spectrum are patients who are completely asymptomatic until adult life with only mild anemia. Therefore, pregnant or older patients are less able to tolerate the anemia and may need transfusion support. Hypertrophy of erythroid marrow with the possibility of extramedullary erythropoiesis, a compensatory mechanism of bone marrow to overcome chronic anemia, is common. Its consequences are characteristic deformities of the bone and face, osteoporosis with pathologic fractures of long bones and formation of erythropoietic masses that primarily affect the spleen, liver, lymph nodes, chest and spine. Enlargement of the spleen is also a consequence of its major role in clearing damaged red cells from the bloodstream.

4.8 β-Thalassemia major (Cooley's anemia)

A Detroit pediatrician, Thomas Cooley, first described this disorder in 1925 after noticing similarities in the appearance and clinical findings in several anemic children of Greek and Italian immigrants (Cooley et al., 1927). Prior to the advent of routine transfusion therapy, β-thalassemia major patients did not survive beyond the first few years of life. Survival is now improved with hypertransfusion regimens, iron chelation therapy, and bone marrow transplantation. Serious thalassemia is associated with iron overload, tissue damage, and increased risk of cardiovascular complications. β-Thalassemias are the most important among the thalassemia syndromes with an average trait prevalence of 7% in Greece, 15% among Cypriots, and 4.8% in Thailand (Weatherall, 1998, Weatherall & Clegg, 2001).

Clinical presentation of thalassemia major occurs between 6 and 24 months. Affected infants fail to thrive and become progressively pale. Feeding problems, diarrhea, irritability, recurrent bouts of fever, and progressive enlargement of the abdomen caused by spleen and liver enlargement may occur. In some developing countries, where due to the lack of resources patients are untreated or poorly transfused, the clinical picture of thalassemia major is characterized by growth retardation, pallor, jaundice, poor musculature, genu valgum, hepatosplenomegaly, leg ulcers, development of masses from extramedullary hematopoiesis, and skeletal changes resulting from expansion of the bone marrow. Skeletal changes include deformities in the long bones of the legs and typical craniofacial changes (bossing of the skull, prominent malar eminence, depression of the bridge of the nose, tendency to a mongoloid slant of the eye, and hypertrophy of the maxillae, which tends to expose the upper teeth).

In β-thalassemia major, severity of anemia requires initiation of blood tranfusions during infancy. If a regular transfusion program that maintains a minimum Hb concentration of 9.5 to 10.5 g/dL is initiated, growth and development tends to be normal up to 10 to12 years (Thalassemia International Federation: Guidelines for the clinical management of thalassemia 2nd edition. 2008 (http://www.thalassemia.org.cy)). Transfused patients may develop complications related to iron overload. Complications of iron overload in children include growth retardation and failure or delay of sexual maturation. Later iron overloadrelated complications include involvement of the heart (dilated myocardiopathy or rarely arrythmias), liver (fibrosis and cirrhosis), and endocrine glands (diabetes mellitus, hypogonadism and insufficiency of the parathyroid, thyroid, pituitary, and, less commonly, adrenal glands) (Borgna-Pignatti & Galanello, 2004).

4.9 Hemoglobin E (Hb-E)

The most common combination of β-thalassemia with abnormal Hb or structural Hb variant with thalassemic properties is Hb-E/β-thalassemia which is most prevalent in an area stretching from northern India and Bangladesh, through Laos, Carmbodia, Thailand, Vietnam, Malaysia, the Philippines, and Indonesia where the carrier frequency is around 50%. Hb-E is caused by a mutation of the 26th amino acid of a normal β-chain, glutamine, is replace by lysine. This mutation also activates a cryptic synthesis of the β-globin chain and leads to a thalassemic phenotype. Furthermore, the hemoglobin E gene, which can interact with β-thalassemic alleles and cause a broad phenotypic spectrum, reaches a frequency of up to 50% in Thailand (Weatherall 1998). These Hb-E/beta-thalassemias may be identified to three categories depending on the severity of symptoms:

4.10 Mild Hb-E/β-thalassemia

It is observed in about 15% of all cases in Southeast Asia. This group of patients maintains Hb levels between 9 and 12 g/dl and usually does not develop clinically significant problems. No treatment is required.

4.11 Moderately severe Hb-E/β-thalassemia

The majority of Hb-E/β-thalassemia cases fall into this category. The Hb levels remain at 6-7 g/dl and the clinical symptoms are similar to thalassemia intermedia. Transfusions are not required unless infections precipitate further anemia. Iron overload may occur.

4.12 Severe Hb-E/β-thalassemia

The Hb level can be as low as 4-5 g/dl. Patients in this group manifest symptoms similar to thalassemia major and are treated as thalassemia major patients.

Hb-E/β-thalassemia is more frequent than homozygous β-thalassemia in Thailand because of the high frequency of Hb-E (Fucharoen & Winichagoon, 2000) It is the most common severe thalassemia syndrome in adults. There are two types of Hb-E/β-thalassemia, classified based on the presence or absence of Hb-A, Hb-E/β+-thalassemia and Hb-E/β0-thalassemia. In patients with Hb- E/β0-thalassemia, only Hb-E and Hb-F are present without detectable Hb-A. Hb-E constitutes between 40-60% of the hemoglobin with the rest Hb-F. Hb-A is present in Hb-E/β+-thalassemia, resulting in a milder clinical picture than Hb-E/β0-thalassemia. Since Hb-E/β-thalassemia is unique to Southeast Asia in general and to Thailand in particular, details of clinical manifestations as well as variability in disease severity will be discussed. In addition, as population migrations have caused the demography of the disease to shift worldwide, this thalassemia syndrome currently has more global implications.

5. Management of β-thalassemia major

5.1 Transfusions

Goals of transfusion therapy are the primary means of treatment for patients with severe β-thalassemia (Fosburg & Nathan 1990) for correction of anemia, suppression of erythropoiesis and inhibition of gastrointestinal iron absorption, which occurs in non transfused patients as a consequence of an increased ineffective erythropoiesis. The decision to start transfusion in patients with confirmed diagnosis of thalassemia should be based on the presence of severe anemia (Hb < 7 g/dl for more than two weeks, excluding other contributory causes such as infections). However, also in patients with Hb > 7 g/dl, other factors should be considered, including facial changes, poor growth, evidence of bony expansion and increasing splenomegaly. Post-transfusion Hb level of 9 to 10 g/dl - 13 to 14 g/dl prevents growth impairment, organ damage and bone deformities, allowing normal activity and quality of life (Thalassemia International Federation: Guidelines for the clinical management of thalassemia 2nd edition. 2008 [http://www.thalassemia.org.cy], Borgna-Pignatti & Galanello, 2004). The frequency of transfusion is usually every two to four weeks. Shorter intervals might further reduce the overall blood requirement, but are incompatible with an acceptable quality of life. The amount of blood to be transfused depends on several factors including weight of the patient, target increase in Hb level and hematocrit of blood unit. Appropriate graphs and formulae to calculate the amount of blood to be transfused are available (Thalassemia International Federation: Guidelines for the clinical management of thalassemia 2nd edition. 2008 [http://www.thalassemia. org.cy]). In general, the amount of transfused RBC should not exceed 15 to 20 ml/kg/day, infused at a maximum rate of 5 ml/kg/hour, to avoid a fast increase in blood volume. To monitor the effectiveness of transfusion therapy, some indices should be recorded at each transfusion, such as pre- and posttransfusion Hb, amount and hematocrit of the blood unit, daily Hb fall and transfusional interval. These measurements enable two important parameters to be calculated: red cell requirement and iron intake. Hypertransfusion and iron chelation is the standard therapy for thalassemia major. These transfusion regimens will provide a marked improvement in survival, growth and sexual development, prevent disfiguring bony abnormalities, decrease cardiac effort, and limit the development of hepatosplenomegaly. The red blood cell transfusions are lifesavers for patients with thalassemi. They are responsible for a series of inevitable complications and expose the patients to a variety of risks of long term transfusion therapy is iron overload.

6. Complications

In developed countries, patients are now given routine transfusion therapy, which has lengthened survival and altered the clinical course of the disease. Assessment and treatment of iron overload patients maintained on a regular transfusion regimen progressively develop clinical manifestations of iron overload. Iron overload of tissue is fatal with or without transfusion if not prevented or adequately treated. It is the most important complication of β-thalassemia and is a major focus of management (Olivieri & Brittenham 1997). Iron status should be accurately assessed in order to evaluate its clinical relevance, the need for treatment, and the timing and monitoring of chelation therapy. The iron status of multitransfused patients can be assessed by several methods. Serum ferritin has in general been found to correlate with body iron stores (Brittenham et al., 1993). After approximately one year of transfusions, iron begins to be deposited in parenchymal tissues (Risdon et al., 1973), where it may cause substantial toxicity as compared with that within reticuloendothelial cells (Hershko &Weatherall 1988, Hershko et al., 1998) Morbidity and mortality are now the result of chronic transfusion induced iron overload and most patients die of heart dysfunction of iron deposition (Zurlo et al., 1989). Iron accumulation in the liver causes fibrosis and cirrhosis (Fosburg & Nathan, 1990). Endocrine abnormalities related to iron overload include diabetes mellitus and impaired glucose tolerance, adrenal insufficiency, hypothyroidism, osteoporosis, hypoparathyroidism and hypogonadism (Fosburg & Nathan, 1990).

In the presence of excess metal iron can generate reactive oxygen species (ROS) (Stohs & Bagchi, 1995) that can modify oxidant-mediated intracellular signaling and cause oxidative damage to lipids, protein, and DNA. A well-studied physiologic biochemical iron reacts with O_2 species through the Fenton and Haber-Weiss reactions to form cytotoxic hydroxyl radicals. In this reaction, ferrous (Fe^{2+}) iron reacts with hydrogen peroxide to produce ferric (Fe^{3+}) iron and highly reactive hydroxyl radicals. This reaction is of particular importance in the liver because this organ, like the heart, has high steady-state production of O_2 and H_2O_2 from abundant mitochondrial activity (Eaton & Qian 2002). In addition to reacting with H_2O_2, ferrous iron may react with O_2 to produce ferric iron and a superoxide radical. The superoxide radical may engage in a series of reactions to generate hydrogen peroxide, which may serve as a substrate in the Fenton reaction to further result in the production of hydroxyl radicals. The hydroxyl radical can non-selectively attack proteins, nucleic acids, polysaccharides and lipids. Indeed, the production of hydroxyl radicals has been demonstrated in rats exhibiting iron overload (Kadiiska et al., 1995).

As indicate iron $\qquad\qquad Fe^{3+} + O_2^{\bullet-} \rightarrow Fe^{2+} + O_2$

$$Fe^{2+} + H_2O_2 \rightarrow Fe^{3+} + OH^- + \bullet OHOO$$

Net reaction: $\qquad\qquad O_2^{\bullet-} + H_2O_2 \rightarrow \bullet OHOO + OH^- + O_2$

These free radicals cause oxidative damage via lipid peroxidation, DNA hydroxylation, and protein oxidation (Schaible & Kaufmann 2004). Oxidative stress is another prominent mechanism of vasculopathy. In hemolytic disorders, the erythrocyte may be a major determinant of the global redox environment. The thalassemias have increased concentrations of ROS compared with normal red blood cells (Aslan & Freeman, 2004, Hebbel et al., 1982, Chakraborty & Bhattacharyya, 2001). Overproduction of ROS, such as superoxide, by both enzymatic (Xanthine oxidase, NADPH oxidase, uncoupled eNOS) and nonenzymatic pathways (Fenton chemistry), promotes intravascular oxidant stress that can likewise disrupt NO homeostasis and produce the highly oxidative peroxynitrite (Wood et al., 2008). Alters cell membrane lipids and abnormal erythrocyte phosphatidylserine (PS) exposure triggered in part by oxidative stress may also contribute to the early demise of the red blood cell in circulation, making them more vulnerable to enzymatic breakdown by secretory phospholipase A2, an important lipid mediator in inflammation. PS exposure also induces binding of red cells to endothelial cells, leading to sequestration of PS-exposing cells in peripheral blood vessels. This process can contribute to vascular dysfunction, hemolysis, and a pro-thrombotic state (Neidlinger et al., 2006). In the alterations in glutathione buffering system common to these hemoglobinopathies (Chakraborty & Bhattacharyya, 2001, Chakraborty & Bhattacharyya, 2001, Reid et al., 2006) may render erythrocytes incapable of handing the increased oxidant burden, thereby predisposing them to hemolysis. Hydroxyl radical formed by iron catalyzed reactions reacts with a polyunsaturated fatty acid of a membrane lipid caused lipid peroxidation. The resulting lipid hydroperoxides can affect membrane fluidity and membrane protein function. A large number of lipid breakdown products are generated including malondialdehyde (MDA) and 4-hydroxy-2-nonenal (4-HNE). In rat models of iron overload, lipid peroxidation has been found in whole liver and also in isolated cellular fractions including mitochondria, microsomes and lysosomes (Bacon et al., 1983, Britton et al., 1987). The reactive aldehydes

(MDA and HNE) can react with proteins to form adducts. The MDA and HNE-lysine adducts have been found in hepatocytes and plasma from rats fed a diet containing carbonyl iron for 13 weeks (Houglum et al., 1990).

Iron overload causes vitamin C to be oxidized at an increased rate, leading to vitamin C deficiency in these patients. Vitamin C in children <10 years and 100 mg >10 years at the time of DFO infusion may increase the chelatable iron available in the body, thus increasing the efficacy of chelation. However there is currently no evidence supporting the use of vitamin C supplements in patients on DFP, DFX or combination treatment. Vitamin C may increase iron absorption from the gut, labile iron and hence iron toxicity and may therefore be particularly harmful to patients who are not receiving DFO, as iron mobilized by the vitamin C will remain unbound, causing tissue damage. The effectiveness and safety of vitamin E supplementation in thalassemia major has not been formally assessed and it is not possible to give recommendations about its use at this time.

7. Assessment of iron overload

Patients maintained on a regular transfusion regimen progressively develop clinical manifestations of iron overload: hypogonadism (35-55% of the patients), hypothyroidism (9-11%), hypoparathyroidism (4%), diabetes (6-10%), liver fibrosis, and heart dysfunction (33%) (Cunningham et al., 2004, Borgna-Pignatti et al., 2004). Iron status should be accurately assessed in order to evaluate its clinical relevance, the need for treatment, and the timing and monitoring of chelation therapy. The iron status of multitransfused patients can be assessed by several methods. Serum ferritin has in general been found to correlate with body iron stores (Brittenham et al 1993). However, as a single value it is not always reliable because, being an acute phase reactant, it is influenced by other factors such as inflammatory disorders, liver disease, malignant. Despite this, serial measurements of serum ferritin remain a reliable and the easiest method to evaluate iron overload and efficacy of chelation therapy. Determination of liver iron concentration in a liver biopsy specimen shows a high correlation with total body iron accumulation and is considered the gold standard for the evaluation of iron overload (Angelucci et al., 2000). However, liver biopsy is an invasive technique with the possibility (though low) of complications. Moreover, we should consider that the presence of hepatic fibrosis, which commonly occurs in individuals with iron overload and HCV infection, and heterogeneous liver iron distribution can lead to possible false negative results (Villeneuve et al., 1996). In recent years, nuclear magnetic resonance imaging (MRI) techniques for assessing iron loading in the liver and heart have been introduced (Wood et al., 2004, Tanner et al., 2006). R2 and T2* parameters have been validated for liver iron concentration. Cardiac T2* is reproducible, transferable between different scanners, correlates with cardiac function, and relates to tissue iron concentration.

As the body has no effective means for removing iron, the only way to remove excess iron is to use iron binders (chelators), which allow iron excretion through the urine and/or stool. As a general rule, patients should start iron chelation treatment once they have had 10-20 transfusions or when ferritin levels rise above 1000 ng/ml (Thalassemia International Federation: Guidelines for the clinical management of thalassemia 2nd edition. 2008 [http://www.thalassemia.org.cy]). Chelation of iron with desferoxamine is effective in reducing iron load and extending life expectancy. However, to be effective, this drug must be given by subcutaneous continuous infusion each day and is not without side effects including hearing and visual loss (Fosburg & Nathan, 1990). Several oral agents for chelation are in various stages of testing and, if effective, will improve the quality of life for chronically transfused patients (Nathan & Piomelli 1990). Other therapies such as splenectomy and vitamin and folic acid supplements are also of benefit.

The first drug available for treatment of iron overload was deferoxamine (DFO), an exadentate iron chelator that is not orally absorbed and usually as a subcutaneous 8- to 12-hour nightly infusion, 5-7 nights a week. Average dosage is 20-40 mg/kg body weight for children and 30-50 mg/kg body weight for adults (Thalassemia International Federation: Guidelines for the clinical management of thalassemia 2nd edition. 2008 [http://www.thalassemia.org.cy], Borgna-Pignatti & Galanello, 2004). In high risk cases, continuous administration of DFO via an implanted delivery system (Port-acath) or subcutaneously, at doses between 50 and 60 mg/ kg per day, were the only options to intensify the chelation treatment before the advent of the combined therapy with DFO and deferiprone (Anderson et al., 2004). Implanted delivery systems are associated with risk of thrombosis and infection. With DFO, iron is excreted both in faeces (about 40%) and in urine. The most frequent adverse effects of DFO are local reactions at the site of infusion, such as pain, swelling, induration, erythema, burning, pruritus, wheals and rash, occasionally accompanied by fever, chills and malaise.

7.1 Iron overload-related complications

Iron overload of tissue with or without transfusion is fatal, which is the most important complication of β-thalassemia if not prevented or adequately treated, which is a major focus of management (Olivieri & Brittenham, 1997). In patients who are not receiving transfusions, abnormally regulated iron absorption results in increases in body iron burden, depending on the severity of erythroid expansion (Pippard et al., 1979, Pootrakul et al., 1988). Regular transfusions may double this rate of iron accumulation. Most clinical manifestations of iron loading do not appear until the second decade of life in patients with inadequate chelation. After approximately one year of transfusions, iron begins to be deposited in parenchymal tissues, (Risdon et al., 1973) where it may cause substantial toxicity as compared with that within retic-uloendothelial cells (Hershko & Weatherall 1988, Hershko et al., 1998). As iron loading progresses, the capacity of serum transferrin, the main transport protein of iron, to bind and detoxify iron may be exceeded and a non–transferrin-bound fraction of plasma iron may promote the generation of free hydroxyl radicals, propagators of oxygen-related damage (Hershko & Weatherall 1988, Hershkoet al., 1998). The advances in free-radical chemistry have clarified the toxic properties of these and other oxygen-derived species generated by iron, which may cause widespread tissue damage (Hershkoet al., 1998). Although the body maintains a number of antioxidant mechanisms against damage induced by free radicals, including superoxide dismutases, catalase, and glutathione peroxidase, in patients with large iron burdens these may not prevent oxidative damage (Hershko & Weatherall 1988, Hershkoet al., 1998). In the absence of chelating therapy the accumulation of iron results in progressive dysfunction of the heart, liver, and endocrine glands (Olivieri & Brittenham 1997). Extensive iron deposits are associated with cardiac hypertrophy and dilatation, degeneration of myocardial fibers, and in rare cases fibrosis (Buja & Roberts 1971). In patients who are receiving transfusions but not chelating therapy, symptomatic cardiac disease has been reported within 10 years after the start of transfusion (Wolfe et al., 1985) and may be aggravated by myocarditis (Kremastinos et al., 1995) and pulmonary hypertension (Aessopos et al., 1995, Duet al., 1997). Iron-induced liver disease is a common cause of death in older patients (Zurlo et al., 1989) and is often aggravated by infection with hepatitis C virus. Within two years after the start of transfusions, collagen formation (Iancu et al., 1977) and portal fibrosis (Thakerngpol et al., 1996) have been reported; in the absence of chelating therapy, cirrhosis may develop in the first decade of life (Risdon et al., 1973, Witzleben & Wyatt 1961, Jean et al., 1984). The striking increases in survival in patients with β-thalassemia over the past decade have focused attention on abnormal endocrine function (delayed puberty, hypogonadism and assisted reproduction), now the most prevalent iron-induced complication in older patients. Iron loading within the anterior pituitary is the primary cause of disturbed sexual maturation, reported in 50 percent of both boys and girls with the condition (Italian Working Group on Endocrine Complications, 1995) and also cause growth deficiency, which therapeutic used of GH to thalassemia patients proven to have GH deficiency, who may have a satisfactory response to treatment (Karydis et al., 2004, Wu et al., 2003). Furthermore, early secondary amenorrhea occurs in approximately one quarter of female patients over the age of 15 years (Italian Working Group on Endocrine Complications, 1995).

Even in the modern era of iron-chelating therapy, diabetes mellitus is observed in about 5 percent of adults (Italian Working Group on Endocrine Complications, 1995). As the iron burden increases and iron-related liver dysfunction progresses, hyperinsulinemia occurs as a result of reduced extraction of insulin by the liver, leading to exhaustion of beta cells and reduced circulating insulin concentrations (cause diabetes and impaired glucose tolerance) (Cavallo-Perin et al., 1995). Studie reporting reduced serum concentrations of trypsin and lipase (Gullo et al., 1993) suggest that the exocrine pancreas is also damaged by iron loading. Over the long term, iron deposition also damages the thyroid (hypothyroidism), parathyroid (hypoparathyroidism), and adrenal glands (Magro et al., 1990, Sklar et al., 1987) and may provoke pulmonary hypertension, right ventricular dilatation, and restrictive lung disease (Du et al., 1997, Factor et al., 1994, Tai et al., 1996).

In most studies, bone density is markedly reduced (cause osteoporosis) in patients with β-thalassemia, particularly those with hypogonadism. Osteopenia may be related to marrow expansion, even in patients who receive transfusions, (Pootrakul et al., 1988) or to iron-induced osteoblast dysfunction, diabetes, hypoparathyroidism, or hypogonadism (Anapliotou et al., 1995).

7.2 Splenectomy

If the annual red cell requirement exceeds 180-200 ml/Kg of RBC (assuming that the Hct of the unit of red cells is about 75%), splenectomy should be considered, provided that other reasons for increased consumption, such as hemolytic reactions, have been excluded. Other indications for splenectomy are symptoms of splenic enlargement, leukopenia and/or thrombocytopenia and increasing iron overload despite good chelation (Weatherall & Clegg 2001).

8. Bone marrow and cord blood transplantation

Successful allogeneic bone marrow transplant for severe β-thalassemia was first reported in 1982 (Thomas et al., 1982). Since that time, numerous transplants have been performed with the best outcome for well chelated patients with no liver disease (Lucarelli et al., 1990). Bone marrow transplantation (BMT) from HLA-identical donors has been successfully performed worldwide. BMT remains the only definitive cure currently available for patients with thalassemia. The outcome of BMT is related to the pretransplantation clinical conditions, specifically the presence of hepatomegaly, extent of liver fibrosis, history of regular chelation and hence severity of iron accumulation. In patients without the above risk factors, stem cell transplantation from an HLA identical sibling has a disease free survival rate over 90% (Gaziev & Lucarelli, 2003). The major limitation of allogenic BMT is the lack of an HLA-identical sibling donor for the majority of affected patients. In fact, approximately 25-30% of thalassemic patients could have a matched sibling donor. BMT from unrelated donors has been carried out on a limited number of individuals with β-thalassemia. Provided that selection of the donor is based on stringent criteria of HLA compatibility and that individuals have limited iron overload, results are comparable to those obtained when the donor is a compatible sib (La Nasa et al., 2005). However, because of the limited number of individuals enrolled, further studies are needed to confirm these preliminary findings. If BMT is successful, iron overload may be reduced by repeated phlebotomy, thus eliminating the need for iron chelation. Complications include a rate of Chronic graft versus-host disease (GVHD) of variable severity may occur in 2-8% of individuals and a variable incidence of mixed chi-merism (Angelucci et al., 1997). Post-transplantation management of preexisting hepatic iron overload, iron-induced cardiac dysfunction, and viral hepatitis may prevent progression of these processes (Angelucci et al., 1997). Cord-blood transplantation, the use of unrelated phenotypically matched donors, and in utero transplantation (Westgren et al., 1996), offers a good probability of a successful cure and is associated with a low risk of GVHD (Locatelli et al., 2003, Pinto & Roberts, 2008). By this mean, for couples who have already had a child with thalassemia and who undertake prenatal diagnosis in a subsequent pregnancy, prenatal identification of HLA compatibility between the affected child and an unaffected fetus allows collection of placental blood at delivery and the option of cord blood transplantation to cure the affected child (Orofino et al., 2003). On the other hand, in cases with an affected fetus and a previous normal child, the couple may decide to continue the pregnancy and pursue BMT later, using the normal child as the donor. At present this therapy is of limited applicability because only a small number of patients have a related, human leukocyte antigen matched donor. Improvements in transplantation from unrelated donors may expand the use of this treatment in the future.

9. Genetic counseling and prenatal diagnosis

Prevention of β-thalassemia is based on carrier identification, genetic counseling and prenatal diagnosis (Cao et al., 1998). Carrier detection has been previously described. Genetic counseling provides information for individuals and at risk couples (i.e. both carriers) regarding the mode of inheritance, the genetic risk of having affected children and the natural history of the disease including the available treatment and therapies under investigation. Prenatal diagnosis for pregnancies at increased risk is possible by analysis of DNA extracted from fetal cells obtained by amniocentesis, usually performed at approximately 15-18 weeks gestation or chorionic villi sampling (CVS) at 10-11 weeks gestation. Both disease-causing alleles must be identified before prenatal testing can be performed. Analysis of fetal cells in maternal blood and analysis of fetal DNA in maternal plasma for the presence of the father's mutation are currently under investigation (Mavrou et al., 2007, Lo 2005). Pre-implantation genetic diagnosis may be available for families in which the disease-causing mutations have been identified.

10. Screening and diagnosis for hemoglobin variants and thalassemia

There are many techniques that have been used to screen and diagnose for hemoglobin variants and thalassemia, mostly done in combinations. These techniques were ranging from screening to extensive analysis, including a few indirect studies. Screening techniques can indicate a defect in hemoglobin synthesis. Positive results from these tests need confirmation by a more extensive analysis technique. Negative results normally help in cutting down the number of subjects that need to be further diagnosed by a more advanced and complicated testing. Extensive analysis techniques can give more precise information in types of thalassemia or types of Hb variants. They normally perform with higher instruments and technologies, and therefore are more expensive than screening techniques. The flow chart shown in Fig 4 summarizes the techniques for diagnosis of thalassemia and hemoglobinopathies that are commonly used in most laboratories.

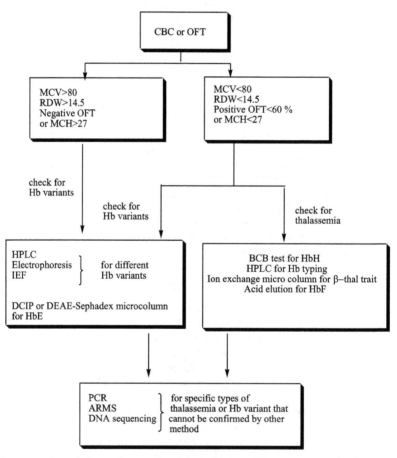

Fig. 4. The summerised chart of normal process of hemoglobin variants and thalassemia

10.1 Screening techniques for thalassemia

Screening techniques are defined as simple techniques and low cost which can indicate the possibility of having thalassemia. These techniques should involve the least sample pretreatment and be rapid, and may not need special instrumentation. These techniques could be used in any primary health care setting. This would lead to low cost and high sample throughput analysis. Positive samples need further confirmatory test while negative samples can be eliminated from further complicated and expensive testing. These screening techniques cannot provide the information on the exact type of hemoglobinopathies, but can help in cutting down the number of samples from unnecessary complicated and expensive testing.

10.1.1 Complete blood count (CBC)

Complete blood count, a primary screening for thalassemia used an electronic blood-cell counter to provide accurate erythrocyte indices as the characteristics of the blood (Hillman & Ault, 1980). The main features of the blood tested in the CBC are the total white blood cell count (WBC), red blood cell count (RBC), hematocrit (Hct), hemoglobin (Hb), red cell distribution width (RDW), peripheral blood smear and other important erythrocyte indices (EI), included mean corpuscular volume (MCV), mean corpuscular hemoglobin (MCH), and mean corpuscular hemoglobin concentration (MCHC) (Klee et al., 2000). Among these parameters, MCV and MCH are the most important indicies that can indicate the existence of thalassemia trait, i.e., when individuals who have hypochromic microcytosis with MCV< 80 fL and MCH< 27 pg should be investigated further.

Parameter	Normal range
RBCs (x10^{12}/L)	3.8 – 5.8
Hb (g/dL)	11.5 – 16.5
Hct (%)	37.0 – 47.0
MCV (fL)	76 – 96
MCH (pg)	27 – 32
MCHC (g/dL)	30.0 – 35.0
RDW (%)	11.5 – 14.5

Table 2. The normal ranges of each parameter

In table 2 summarizes the tests performed in the CBC, the calculation needed for each parameters and the approximate normal cutoff level. However, due to the similar lowed blood cell count between the patients with thalassemia and the ones with iron deficiency, it has been suggested that in the geographic regions where iron deficiency rate is high, the cutoffs for thalassemia interpretation should be adjusted to more suitable values by using a receiver operator char acteristic (ROC) curve (Kotwal et al., 1999), which in this case should better differentiate thalassemic microcytosis from non-thalassemic ones (i.e., iron deficiency patients). As the study in Thailand, they used the combination of MCH (25) pg, RDW (14.5%) and OFT (<55%) with the lower cutoff to increase the screening specificity in those area (Tangvarasittichai et al., 2004). Many laboratories use a CBC autoanalyzer which can provide many blood parameters (such as MCH, MCV, RDW) also be added along with osmotic fragility test an alternative screening test for specific thalassemia testing.

Combined red blood cells indices for α-Thalassemia-1 Screening

1. Red blood cells (RBC) indices included hemoglobin (Hb), hematocrit (Hct), mean corpuscular volume (MCV), mean corpuscular hemoglobin (MCH), MCHC, and RDW from the automated blood cell analyzer

2. In the study of Tangvarasittichai et al. (2004) used the ROC curve and the AUC of each parameters showed the % specificity of each parameter and their combination for screening the α-thalassemia-1 elute as in the table below.

Parameters (Cut-off point)	% Specificity
MCH/OFT/RDW (25 pg/55%/14.5%)	92.4
MCH/OFT/MCV (25 pg/55%/75 fL)	91.9
MCH/OFT (25 pg/55%)	91.7
MCH/RDW/MCV (25 pg/14.5%/75 fL)	90.0
MCH/RDW (25 pg/14.5%)	89.6
MCH/MCV (25 pg/75 fL)	88.5

Table 3. The combined red blood cells indices to increase the specificity for screening α-thalassemia 1

10.1.2 Osmotic fragility test (OFT)

The main purpose of this technique is used as a diagnostic test for the hereditary spherocytosis and it is also useful for screening of thalassemia. This simple technique utilizes osmosis, the movement of water from lower to higher salt concentration region, to test for the osmotic resistance of the red blood cell (Fernandez-Alberti et al., 2000). A single hypotonic saline solution can be prepared from dilution of a Tyrode's solution, which is composed of NaCl, KCl, $CaCl_2$ $6H_2O$, $MgCl_2$ $6H_2O$, $NaHCO_3$, NaH_2PO_4, glucose and distilled water (Electron Microscope Sciences Catalog, Available: http://www.emsdiasum. com/ems/chemicals/ salt. html (October 16, 2003). Different laboratories may be using slightly different recipes for preparation of hypotonic salt solution, but all are normally based on the same concept of kinetic osmotic fragility. The most simple of a single hypotonic saline solution can be prepared which is composed of 0.45% glycerine and 0.36% sodium chlorine in phosphate buffer (pH7.4) (Sirichotiyakul et al., 2004). Whole blood is thoroughly mixed with this solution. In a hypotonic condition, the concentration of salt on the outside of a cell is lower than that on the inside, resulting in net water movement into cells. Normal red blood cells are broken within 1–2 min and the mixture then turns clear and reddish. Abnormal red blood cells have deviated osmotic resistances as compared to normal red cells. Spherocytes and erythrocytes with various membrane defects may show decreased osmotic resistance. However, red blood cells of thalassemia have higher osmotic resistance and thus have slower rupture rate, therefore the mixture remains turbid even after 1–2 h (Silvestroni & Bianco 1983). The OFT is a quick preliminary and very economic test before performing further studies of the blood cells. The percent hemolysis of more than 60% was considered normal (no α-thalassmia-1 or β-thalassemia trait). The screening test (OFT) was considered abnormal or positive test when the percent hemolysis is of 60% or less [β-thalassemia trait= 30.5±1.4%; α-thalassmia 1 = 30.8±1.2%] and the positive test of gold standard or final diagnosis was considered either when HbA2 levels of 4.1–9% or positive PCR (SEA type).

10.2 Conventional confirmatory tests for thalassemia and Hb variants

These are useful tests to confirm the existence of certain Hb variants or abnormal level of some Hb types. Confirmatory tests for Hb variants include deoxyhemoglobin solubility test (DST) for detection of HbS and dichlorophenol indophenol precipitation test (DCIP) for detection of HbE. HbH disease which relates to α-thalassemia can be detected by DCIP and brilliant cresyl blue test (BCB). Alkaline resistant hemoglobin test (ART) and acid elution stain (AES) are used for detection of abnormal levels of HbF, which can help identify some types of thalassemia. The ion exchange microcolumn technique is used to quantify the amount of HbA2 and HbF to identify β-thal trait, E-trait and EE homozygotes. These conventional techniques are relatively low cost and do not require complicated instrumentation. However, some of these techniques may need a highly experienced operator to translate the results. Therefore, availability of more modern instrumentation that can provide more precise information with little requirement of an experienced operator and less usage of toxic chemicals diminishes the use of some of these conventional techniques such as DST and ART.

10.2.1 Deoxyhemoglobin solubility test

Deoxyhemoglobin solubility test for HbS based on its insolubility in a potassium phosphate saponin buffer solution (composed of K_2HPO_4, KH_2PO_4, saponin and distilled water). Turbidity would be observed within 5 min if the whole blood containing HbS were mixed with sodium hyposulfite and saponin buffer. This test can discriminate samples with HbS from samples with almost all other hemoglobins except Hb Bart's and some rare sickle Hb, if a positive test result is shown (i.e., high enough turbidity that newsprint cannot be seen through the test mixture when placed behind the tube), then a follow-up test by electrophoresis is recommended. A false-negative result may be from a high anemic condition (Fairbanks, 1980, Nalbandian et al., 1971, Greenberg et al., 1972).

10.2.2 Hemoglobin precipitation test

Some hemoglobin variants such as HbH ($\beta 4$ with α- thalassemia) and Hb Koln (β $^{98Val \rightarrow Met}$) are classified as unstable hemoglobins which can be precipitated by heating or adding a chemical such as isopropanol or dichlorophenol indophenol (Dispenzieri, 2001, Winichagoon et al., 2002).

10.2.2.1 The heat instability test

Test can be carried out at either medium temperature (50°C) for 1–2 h or at high temperature (68°C) with chemical reaction aids for 1 min. Although taking longer time, the medium temperature stability test is very simple. The clear supernatant of erythrocyte hemolysate in Tris buffer medium, obtained after removing plasma, hemolyzing with distilled water and removing stroma, is placed in the 50 °C water bath for 1 h. Normal hemolysates remain completely clear, while unstable hemoglobins cause flocculation of various turbidities. The test can be done much faster by using chemicals, i.e., KCN and K_3Fe $(CN)_6$, to form hemolysate cyanmethemoglobin. In a phosphate buffer medium, this hemolysate cyanmethemoglobin is agitated rapidly in the 68 °C hot water bath. After 1 min, normal hemolysate may show slight cloudiness and therefore this high temperature method, even though very fast, may need high experience in interpretation in order to avoid a false-positive interpretation (Klee, 1980, Dacie et al., 1964).

Hemolysate preparation (For heat, isopropanol precipitation)

Reagent: (i) 0.9% NaCl, (ii) Transformation solution (TS): consist with 0.2 g $K_3Fe(CN)_6$ and 0.2 g KCN in 1000 ml distill water (DW) (iii) Carbon tetrachloride (CCl_4) solution
Sample: EDTA whole blood. **Reagent:** 0.15 M Tris-HCl buffer.

Type	%Hb instability
Normal	2.3±1.2
HbH	9.7±2.4
α-Thalassemia trait	4.3±1.7
Homozygous β-thalassemia	5.4±1.6
β-Thalassemia trait	4.3±2.3
β-Thalassemia/HbE	6.4±2.2

Table 4. % Hb instability value by Heat Precipitation

10.2.2.2 Isopropanol precipitation test

Another way to demonstrate the Hb instability is with isopropanol precipitation. Packed erythrocytes, cold deionized water and CCl_4 (1:1:1.5 ratio) are placed in a closed tube and vortexed for a few minutes, followed by centrifugation. The clear supernatant is then mixed with isopropanol–Tris buffer at a control temperature of about 37 ∘C. Unstable hemoglobins cause more turbidity over time, while normal hemoglobins remain clear for at least 30 min. The isopropanol test is reported to have some limitations on the subjects that contain ≥5% HbF, and those that are inappropriately preserved (i.e., unrefrigerated or too old samples) may give false positive results. Adding anticoagulating reagent can help reduce the false reading but it is suggested that the samples with high HbF should be tested by heat stability, as it is not interfered by HbF (Klee, 1980, Brosious et al., 1976, Carrell & Kay, 1972).

Reagent: 0.1 M Tris-HCl buffer pH 7.4; Isopropanol buffer: as a mixture of 17 ml isopropanol with 83 ml of Tris-HCl buffer

Type	%Hb instability
Normal	1.2±1.1
HbH	16.1±5.2
α-Thalassemia trait	3.5±1.9
Homozygous β-thalassemia	4.2±3.0
β-Thalassemia trait	3.2±2.1
β-Thalassemia/HbE trait	2.9±1.7

Table 5. % Hb instability value by Isopropanol Precipitation

10.2.2.3 Dichlorophenol indophenol (DCIP) precipitation test

The dichlorophenol indophenol (DCIP) precipitation test is also used widely to screen for HbE and HbH. DCIP can oxidize HbE and HbH faster than any other type of hemoglobin, and therefore it can be used to screen for HbE and HbH. Interpretation of results can be difficult since it involves observing the cloudiness in a deep blue color of DPIC solution. However, a reducing agent may be added to overcome this problem. For example, in the AOAC standard titration method for ascorbic acid, the color of an oxidant DCIP is changed from dark blue to light blue on the way to the end point pink (Helrich, 1995). Therefore, if a small amount of ascorbic acid were added to the DCIP thalassemia test, then the observation could be made more accurately under the light blue condition.

Reagents: DCIP reagent: Tris base 4.36 g, EDTA $Na_2.2H_2O$ 2.68 g, DCIP (Sigma) 0.0276 g, Saponin 0.05 g dissolve in DW adjusted pH 7.5 by 6M HCl , then DW to 500 ml store at 4°C.

Interpretation results: Negative = Clear; Positive = cloudiness in a deep blue color of DCIP solution. Hemoglobin precipitation tests can be used to screen for some hemoglobin variants but they may not be able to speciate the types of hemoglobins (i.e., HbE and HbH show similar results). Further tests are needed to pinpoint the exact type.

10.2.3 Brilliant cresyl blue test or new methylene blue test

Both simple colorimetric tests are based on the same procedures with different reagents, specifically performed for HbH diagnosis. HbH is unstable and it precipitates in the red cells, giving the appearance of many small golf balls inside the cells that can be observed when staining the blood film with brilliant cresyl blue ($C_{17}H_2OClN_3O$) or new methylene blue ($C_{18}H_{22}ClN_3S:SClZnCl_2$) (Brilliant cresyl blue MSDS sheet, Available: http://www.proscitech. com/ catalogue/ msds/ c085.pdf (April 14, 2003), New Methylene,

Blue MSDS Sheet. Available: http://www.jtbaker.com/ msds/ englishhtml/n2700.htm (April 20, 2003)). The incubation time of blood and the reagents (brilliant cresyl blue in sodium citrate media) takes about 1 h in a controlled temperature setting of about 37 ∘C (Rigas et al., 1961). This test is very useful to confirm for α-thalassemia involving HbH inclusion body. However, the technique yields low sensitivity for α-thal trait and therefore it should only be used as a confirmatory test, but not for screening of α-thalassemia.

10.2.4 Alkaline resistant hemoglobin test

This is a test for abnormal level of fetal hemoglobin (HbF). Normally hemoglobins are denatured at alkaline pH such as in NaOH solution and they can be precipitated readily with saturated ammonium sulfate ($(NH_4)_2SO_4$) solution. However, HbF is not denatured as easily and remains soluble. Differences in alkaline resistance of the normal Hb and fetal Hb allow for rapid testing for the amount of HbF in blood. The procedure consists of a few experimental and calculation steps (Klee, 1980, Singer et al., 1951, Betke et al., 1959). A suspended mixture of Hb-cyanide–ferricyanide (or cyanmethemoglobin) is prepared by adding packed red cells, obtained from centrifugation of whole blood in isotonic saline solution, into a cyanide–ferricyanide solution (KCN and $K_3Fe(CN)_6$ in distilled water). Then NaOH is added and the solution is mixed for a few minutes before adding the saturated $(NH_4)_2SO_4$ solution. Coagulated protein can be removed by filtering the mixture until a clear filtrate is obtained. The percent of alkaline resistant hemoglobin is calculated based on the absorbance of the filtrate (Df) and the absorbance of the 1:10 dilution of the original cyanmethemoglobin without NaOH and $(NH_4)_2SO_4$ added (Db) at 540 nm, using the following equation: (100 Df)/(10 Db).

In a normal person more than 1 year old, the percentage of HbF should be expressed as being less than 1-2% by using this method. Higher levels of HbF will be suspected of having a hemoglobin disorder of some kind. Although the method was found to mistakenly yield lower results for a subject with HbF higher than 30% of total hemoglobin, such as in umbilical cord blood of newborns, this method was sufficiently sensitive and reproducible for measuring 1-10% HbF, providing that final cyanmethemoglobin concentration is higher than 480 mg/100 ml (Pembrey et al., 1972). In the cases where high amount of HbF is present, an alternative method such as immunological determination of HbF, e.g., by the gel precipitation or immuno-diffusion, involving the use of monoclonal antibody against HbF, may be used (Weatherall & Clegg, 2001, Yuregir 1976, Dover et al., 1979).

Reagent: (i) TS as 0.2 g $K_3(FeCN)_6$ and 0.2 g KCN in 100 ml DW (ii) 1.2 N NaOH (iii) saturated (sat) $(NH_4)2SO_4$

Type	%HbF
Normal	<1
β-Thalassemia trait	1- 10 %
β-Thalassemia major	>50%

Table 6.

10.2.5 Acid elution stain (modified Kleihauer–Betke test)

This is a simple test for HbF and Hb Bart's. After smearing a blood sample on the slide and letting it dry, the slide is immersed in an 80% alcohol solution (ethyl, methyl or propyl alcohol) for 2–3 min. After that, the slide is immersed in a staining solution of Amido Black 10B ($C_{22}H_{14}N_6O_9S_2Na_2$) prepared in alcohol with pH adjusted to 2.0. After 3 min, the slide is washed under running water for 1 min. In the acidic condition, HbA, HbA$_2$, HbE, and HbH will be eluted out of the blood cells, leaving the cells empty (ghost cells) and showing no color. HbF and Hb Bart's can tolerate acid and are stained by the Amido Black 10B, showing dark blue color of the cells which can be observed under the microscope. There are a few precautions that need to be taken when working with this technique. If the slide is left dry for too long, HbA will not be eluted out. The concentration of alcohol is also important because alcohol higher than 85% will cause HbA to stay in the cell, while lower than 65% will cause vacuolization of HbF. In addition, if the pH of the solution is higher than 2.5, HbA will not be eluted. All these cases will show false results (Research Organics. Available: http://www.resorg.com/(October 17, 2003), Betke & Sanguansermsri, 1972). The drawbacks of this technique are time consuming and subjected to human error. Another possible way of detection of HbF is flow cytometry which is more precise as described later.

10.2.6 Ion exchange micro-column

In the regions where economic restriction does not allow for the use of a relatively higher cost instrument such as HPLC, a cheaper method such as this ion exchange microcolumn along with other inexpensive tests can be used in combination to diagnose the type of thalassemia. This technique is based on ion exchange chromatography as a simplified version of high performance liquid chromatography. The use of diethylaminoethyl DEAE anion exchanger, packed in a relatively cheap and small syringe, and Tris–HCl mobile phase can be adapted to separate HbA2 and HbF effectively. The relative amounts of these Hbs can be estimated by calculating the peak areas of the absorbance, measured at 415 nm, of fractions eluted from the column. It has been shown that the results obtained from the batchwise micro-column are in agreement with those from HPLC, though the method lacks automation and yields lower precision (Dozy et al., 1968, Brosious et al., 1978, Srisawang et al., 2003). However, the result from ion exchange micro-column technique is acceptably accurate and precise and can be used to confirm some types of thalassemias such as β-thalassemia trait. In addition, with its simplicity and low cost, some laboratories perform this technique together with the OF tests as regular screening techniques, especially where thalassemia cases related to abnormal ratio of HbA2 and HbF is commonly found such as in Thailand. It has been estimated that the cost for chemicals and materials per test of the micro-column technique is approximately five times less than that of HPLC. Even though the total analysis time per run is longer than automated HPLC (4 h versus 20 min), many ion exchange micro-columns can be set up and run at the same time. Therefore, the total analysis time of, e.g., 50 tests using multiple micro-columns at one time is less than performing 50 continuous HPLC runs (16 h using HPLC and 4 h using ion exchange micro-columns). In addition, an attempt to reduce the analysis time per run and to make the micro-column technique more automated has been carried out. A flow injection analysis system was joined together with a much smaller ion exchange column to improve the analysis time for hemoglobin typing as compared to the batch process (Srisawang et al., 2003). More work needs to be done, but the preliminary results have suggested that the flow based and reduced volume ion exchange column system has the potential to improve the analysis time per run and to greatly reduce the amount of blood sample needed for the analysis.

Hemoglobin E detection: DEAE Sepharose Microcolumn (GE Healthcare BioSciences, Uppsala, Sweden)

Sufficient DEAE Sepharose was added to columns of 10x1.5 cm to produce a 2 cm Sepharose layer (Figure 5), was saturated with buffer A (0.05 M Tris, pH 8.5). Hemolysate was loaded in the column (40μl of EDTA blood sample to 10 ml 0.05 M, pH 8.0 Tris buffer B. Hb E, which is a weak anion, eluted first from the microcolumn by using buffer B as the elution buffer. The Hb E positive blood samples produced an orange eluted. Hb E negative sample produced a colorless. This Hb E microcolumn testing was approximately 10-15 minutes.

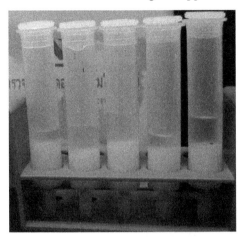

Fig. 5. DEAE Sepharose Microcolumn after preparation for hemoglobin E detection

10.3 Instrumental techniques for determination of thalassemia and Hb variants

These techniques involve modern technologies of complicated instrumentation. They can be automated and are usually faster and more reliable but more expensive than the conventional techniques. Even though these techniques can provide detailed information and can help in diagnosis of many types of Hb variants, there are a few exceptional Hb variant cases that cannot be identified with these techniques, and more extensive confirmatory tests are needed. Most instrumental techniques can perform qualitative and quantitative analysis, but with limited ways to accurately quantitate the signals, such as in gel electrophoresis, these techniques have be used mainly for diagnosis of Hb variants rather than for detection of abnormal level of Hbs in thalassemia diagnosis, as shown in the flow chart in Fig. 4.

10.3.1 High performance liquid chromatography

High-performance liquid chromatographic (HPLC) methods with high sensitivity and specificity have been developed for both screening and confirmation of hemoglobinopathies and thalassemia in newborns. The HPLC technique requires a very small amount of blood samples (μl), therefore, it is very suitable for prenatal diagnosis of thalassemia (Maiavacca et al., 1992, Sanguansermsri et al., 2001, Rao et al., 1997), where sample may be limited and difficult to obtain. In HPLC, particle size of the stationary phase packed in the column is quite small (about 2–5μm). The degree of interactions determines the degree of migration and separation of the components (Skoog & Leary, 1992, Christian, 2004). However, in most laboratories, HPLC has been used for diagnosis of Hb variants rather than for quantification of normal Hb or thalassemia diagnosis. There are many reports showing the agreement of results obtained from HPLC and those obtained from other techniques such as the globin synthesis technique, isoelectrofocusing, carboxymethylcellulose chromatography and DNA sequencing (Sanguansermsri et al., 2001, Rao et al, 1997, Fucharoen et al., 1998).

Cation exchangers, such as CM-cellulose (CMC) and silica supported with carboxylic acid residues with bis-Tris–KCN developer, can also be used for the same purpose (Rouyer-Fessard et al, 1989, Papadea & Cate, 1996, Wilson et al., 1983). The ratio of different globin chains (e.g., $\beta:\gamma$ for β- thalassemia diagnosis) can also be determined with HPLC using a reverse phase C18 column and shows similar results to those obtained from CMC which is normally employed for this purpose (Congote, 1981). HPLC was become the preferred method for thalassemia screening because of its speed and reliability. An automated HPLC system has been developed primarily detection of β-thalassemia carriers, HbS, and HbC. In the study of Fucharoen et al. (1998), they used automatic HPLC system (VARIANT ™, Bio-Rad) set up with the α-thalassemia short (ATS) program and β-thalassemia shot (BTS) program to detect various types of thalassemias in both prenatal and postnatal specimens. HPLC has an overall performance better than electrophoresis.

Analyses were performed with a HPLC machine interfaced with a computer program, with an autoinjector or manual injector, and a UV detector at 415 nm. A 3.5 x 0.46 cm cation exchanger column packed with porous (100-nm pore size) 5-gm microparticulate polyaspartic acid-silica (Poly CAT Atm) or Poly LC (Columbia, MD).

Sample preparation by using 100 µl of EDTA whole blood was washed with isotonic saline (NaC1 9 g/L). The cells were then lysed by adding two to three volumes of water, vortex-mixed, and centrifuged at 3000 x g for 5 min. Added 50 µl of hemolysate to 1 mL of mobile phase A, of which 20 µl was injected onto the column. The column effluent was monitored at 415 nm and the peak areas were used for the individual quantitative hemoglobin peaks.

The gradient programwas made up of a mobile phase A (10 mmol/L Bis-Tris, 1 mmol/L KCN, pH 6.87) and mobile phase B (10 mmolIL Bis-Tris, 1 mmolJL KCN, 200 mmol/L NaCl, pH 6.57). With a flow rate of 1.5 ml/min (a new column should be rinsed with water for 10 mm and with mobile phase B for at least 20 min, and should then be equilibrated with 12% B for another 20 min before sample application). Elution of hemoglobins was performed by increasing the mobile phase B to 40% and to 100% at 8 and 12 min, respectively, and then decreasing to 12% at 13 min. The column was re-equilibrated with 12% mobile phase B for at least 7 min before application of next sample.

Anion exchange resin DEAE and gradient Tris–HCl buffer solution, pH 8.5–6.0, is a widely used stationary–mobile phase system for HbA_2 and HbF quantification to effectively diagnose β-thalassemia and Hb Bart's hydrop fatalis that occur frequently in Southeast Asia (Sanguansermsri et al., 2001, Sanguansermsri et al., 2001). The system can also separate other Hb variants such as HbS, HbC and HbJ (Huisman & Dozy, 1962, Huisman & Dozy, 1965). In the study of Tangvarasittichai et al. (2009), they modified the fast protein liquid chromatography (FPLC) method from microcolumn chromatographic techniques for HbA_2 determination. The FPLC, a general system was used for protein purification and separation. However, they used the method for FPLC application for separation HbA_2, as the diagnosis of β-thalassemia (Tangvarasittichai et al., 2009).

10.3.2 Fast protein liquid chromatography (FPLC) technique for the diagnosis of β-Thalassemia (as demonstrated by Tangvarasittichai et al. (2009)

Hemolysate was prepared by mixing 50 µl of EDTA blood sample with 10.0 ml of Tris buffer A. 0.5 ml of hemolysate was passsed through a 5 x 0.5 cm (1ml) column of diethylaminoethyl (DEAE) sepharose, Hi Trap ™ (GE Healthcare, Sweden) connected to the FPLC (AKTA prime, Amersham Biosciences, USA) with flow rate 2 ml/min. Elluent from column was monitored by a single path ultraviolet monitor at 280 nm in a 10 min path-length high resolution flow cell, and the histogram was saved in the computer. The reagents for FPLC were as linear gradient of buffer A [50 ml of stock Tris buffer (as Tris 60.57 g mixed with 500 ml distilled water, adjusted pH 9.0 with 4 M HCl) was diluted in distilled water 1,000 ml, added 0.1 g KCN (adjusted pH 8.1 with 4 M HCl)], and buffer B (diluted 500 ml of buffer A with 500 ml 1M NaCl). The gradient profile to achieve the separation as in the table

Linear gradient profile of buffer A and B	
Buffer A, volume (ml)	Buffer b, %
10.0	0
11.0	10
12.0	30
13.0	50
14.0	70
15.0	90
15.5	100
20.0	0

Table 7. The gradient profile of FPLC technique
The fractions were then separated to HbA_2 or HbE (in the same fraction, HaA_2/E), HbA and HbF

The cut-off values of FPLC for HbA2/E diagnosiswere as follows: Normal (<6%), β-thalassemia (7-10%), He-trait (>10-40%), homozygous HbE (>60%), and β-thalassemia/He (40-60%)

10.3.3 Electrophoresis

Electrophoresis is one of the widely used techniques for analyzing hemoglobin variants based on the movement of different Hb or different globin chains, containing different charges, in the electric field. At an alkaline pH, Hb is negatively charged and will move toward the anode (positively charged) terminal. Electrophoresis of total Hb is different from electrophoresis of separated globin chains. Electrophoresis of hemolysates on cellulose acetate membrane is mainly used in alkaline pH electrophoresis, is a simple, reliable method for detecting abnormal hemoglobin, and capable of separating common hemoglobin variants such as S, f, a, and C. Normal operating voltage is about 250mV and the approximate run time is about 90 min. After that, the membrane needs to be stained, de-stained and air dried before separation of globin chains can be observed. The main limitation of electrophoresis at alkaline pH is a inability to differentiate HbA_2, HbC, HbO and HbE from one another, nor can HbD, HbG and Hb Lepore be differentiated from HbS (Fairbanks, 1980, Rich et al., 1979, Salmon et al., 1978). Therefore, it is normally used to screen for some types of Hb variants. The confirmatory test can be done using electrophoresis in acidic media. At a lower pH of about 6.0, a better separation of different hemoglobins is obtained. Those Hbs that co-migrate in alkaline pH electrophoresis can be separated in acidic media. Nevertheless, the main technique for Hb quantification by densitometric scanning of the gel is still somewhat difficult and unreliable (Fairbanks, 1980) and therefore electrophoresis technique has been used mainly for detection of Hb variants rather than measuring level of Hb in thalassemia diagnosis. It is highly specific in the detection of certain Hb disorders such as sickle cell disease. Even though the electrophoresis in acidic media is quite a powerful technique in separation of many types of Hbs, please keep in mind that not all Hb variants can be separated by electrophoresis in acidic media. For example, Hb Okayama cannot be separated using electrophoresis, but can be done so in HPLC (Frers et al., 2000). Capillary electrophoresis is the new format of electrophoresis where separation takes place in a small fused silica capillary. It is rapid, easily automated and consumes low amounts of reagents, as compared to conventional gel electrophoresis. It also offers much higher throughput as compared to HPLC (Doelman et al., 1997). However, some researchers found that CE has higher instrumentation cost and is less accurate as compared to automated HPLC (Jenkins & Ratnaike, 2003). To perform electrophoresis of globin chains, a few steps need to be done in order to obtain free globin chains. First, heme is removed from hemoglobin by treating with mercaptoethanol. Then the four globin chains are split apart without denaturing them using 8 M urea.

10.3.4 Electrophoresis of hemolysates on cellulose acetate (alkaline buffers)
In this method, erythrocyte hemolysate is electrophoresed on cellulose acetate in urea-2-mercaptoethanol buffers in the presence of additional 2-mercaptoethanol. The latter severs heme from globin, while the urea severs the a- and non-a-globin chains, which migrate on the cellulose acetate according to their electrical charge. The method requires very small amounts of hemolysate, yet it provides excellent resolution of globin chains in alkaline (Ueda & Schneider, 1969).

The electrophoresis apparatus and sample plate, aligning base, applicator, dispenser, and cellulose acetate. Some prepared reagents-such as the pH 8.5 buffer (Supreheme),

Solutions: De-ionized water is used throughout. Concentrated citric acid: 300 g/liter.

Hemolyzing reagent was 1.0 g of tetrasodium ethylenediaminetetraacetate per liter of water containing 0.2 g of KCN per liter. Staining solution was 5 g of Ponceau S per liter of tri-chloroacetic acid solution (50 g/liter). Dilute acetic acid was 3 ml of glacial acetic acid plus 97 ml of water. Buffer solutions, All pH measurements are made at room temperature.

Alkaline-urea-mercaptoethanol-buffer solutions:

(i) Barbital buffer, pH 8.6, (ii) Tris-EDTA-boric acid buffer, pH 8.5, containing 10.2 g of Tris (about 80 mmol/liter), 0.6 g of EDTA, and 3.2 g of boric acid/liter, (iii) Tris-EDTA-boric acid buffer, pH 8.6, containing 18 g of Tris (about 150 mmol/liter), 2.3 g of EDTA, and 3 g of boric acid/liter.

To about 70 ml of each of these buffers, add 36 g of urea and stir on a mechanical stirrer until the urea dissolves. Adjust the volume (now about 98 ml) to 100 ml with additional buffer. In each case the final pH is about 8.9. These urea-containing buffers are used to dilute the hemolysate and soak the Titan III cellulose acetate. Just before placing buffers into the electrophoresis chambers, add 5 ml of 2-mercaptoethanol per liter.

Collect blood samples by venipuncture into a syringe with anticoagulant, or by finger stick into heparinized hematocrit tubes. Prepare hemolysates by adding one volume of water and 0.4 volume of toluene to one volume of saline-washed, packed erythrocytes. A more rapid alternative is to add three volumes of hemolyzing reagent to one volume of unwashed and sedimented or centrifuged cells (Titan III cellulose acetate plates). In most cases, however, erythrocyte hemolysates (5-10 g of hemoglobin per 100 ml) were electrophoresed directly. Add one volume of the appropriate urea buffer and one-half to one volume of undiluted 2-mercaptoethanol to one volume of hemolysate. (The additional mercaptoethanol is needed for removal of heme from globin.) Convenient volumes are 20 µl each of hemolysate and urea-buffer, and 10 to 20 µl of 2 mercaptoethanol. About 2 µl of this mixture, after it has stood at room temperature for about 0.5 h but not longer than 4 h, are placed into the sample wells.

Electrophoresis

Preparation of cellulose acetate: Mercaptoethanol may soften the Mylar backing of cellulose acetate gels, so soak the Titan III plates for several hours (or longer) in the appropriate urea-buffer without mercaptoethanol. Drain and soak for about 1 h in the corresponding urea-mercaptoethanol buffer, and finally drain and blot before applying samples. Soak Titan II sheets overnight (or longer) in the desired urea-mercaptoethanol buffer. Drain and blot. Application of samples and electrophoresis: Depress the tips of the sample applicators into the wells containing the hemolysate-urea-buffer-mercaptoethanol mixtures and wipe them off, then depress again. Make several trial applications on paper towels, until the lines formed are sufficiently thin. Then hold the applicator down for about 20 s on the Titan III plate positioned in the aligning base. When acid buffers are being used, apply samples about 1 cm from the anodal end of the plate; apply those in alkaline buffers centrally. Always include at least one control sample, usually Hb AS. In the electrophoresis chamber, rest the plates on wicks of filter paper; two or three plates may be analyzed simultaneously (200 to 350 V for 1 to 1.5 h), with a glass plate on each to weight it down.

10.3.5 Isoelectric focusing (IEF)

This technique is based on the electrophoresis technique but with a higher degree of separation. Different Hbs migrate in a pH gradient to the point where their net charges are zero. The order of migration is the same as in alkaline electrophoresis but the narrower bands obtained from this method (IEF) allow for the resolution of HbC, HbE, HbO, HbS, HbD and HbG (Laosombat et al., 2001, Gwendolyn et al., 2000). Two different formats of IEF, thin layer gel and capillary, have been reported (Hempe & Craver, 1994, Hempe et al., 1997). Cossu et al. (1982) applied the immobilized pH gradient method (IPG) with a thin layer gel that has a pH range of 6.7–7.6 to differentiate heterozygous from homozygous β-thalassemia in newborns. The group suggested the use of umbilical cord blood because it contains only HbF, HbA and acetylated HbF (HbFac) and the ratio of HbA:HbFac or HbF:HbA is used instead of the conventional β:α ratio in the IEF of globin chains.

Isoelectric focusing ((IEF) Hicks & Hughes, 1975)

Preparation of hemolysates for isoelectro focusing

The blood used for isoelectrofocusing was collected in vacutainers (Becton-Dickinson, Rutherford, N.J. 07070) with disodium ethylenediaminetetraacetate as anticoagulant. The erythrocytes were washed three times with NaCl solution (154 mmol/liter) and lysed with an equal volume of distilled water and 0.4 ml of toluene per milliliter of erythrocytes. The mixture was shaken for 5 mm and the hemoglobin solution was cleared of cellular debris by centrifugation (20 mm, 4586 x g). Isoelectric focusing was used to obtain purified hemoglobin biopolymers for our sensitivity studies, the procedure being essentially that recommended by Svensson (1962) and Ui (1971), performed at 4°C with use of carrier ampholytes (Ampholine, 10 g/liter; LKB-Produkter AB, Stockholm, Sweden) and an electrofocusing column (Model 8101, LKB-Produkter AB) of 440-ml capacity. Solutions and linear density gradients in the column were prepared manually. The dense solution used was a sucrose solution (670 g/liter) containing carrier ampholytes (20 g/liter); less-dense solution contained 4 g of carrier ampholytes per liter, with no sucrose. (i)The protein load applied varied from 60 to 80 mg, and the sample was introduced onto the column between the dense solution and the less-dense solution. (ii) The initial voltage was 200 V, the final voltage 750 V. The voltage was increased at 2-h intervals by 200-V increments to the final voltage. (iii) Equilibrium was usually reached in 48 h. (iv) pH range from 6 to 8 was used, this range was used for isoelectrofocusing hemoglobins S, C, F, A, and D or G. (v) Fractions of 2 to 2.5 ml were collected and the absorbance of each fraction was read at 280 nm to identify the various isolated hemoglobin peaks. (vi) The pH of each fraction was determined at 25 °C with a pH meter. (vii) The separated hemoglobins were quantitated by measuring the absorbance at 415 nm with a spectrophotometer.

10.3.6 Capillaries Isoelectric focusing (cIEF)

Capillary IEF showed very promising performance both in qualitative and quantitative aspects. A single IEF run can replace the main tests that normally have to be carried out in combination for qualitative and quantitative analysis of Hbs, for instance, alkaline and acid electrophoresis for major Hb variants, ion exchange chromatography for HbA2 quantification and alkaline resistant test for HbF (Hempe et al., 1997). It has been proven to have a comparable performance to chromatography or radioactive globin chain methods (Dubart et al., 1980) and can be used for analysis of hemoglobin variants in adult and newborn (Mario et al., 1998).

10.3.7 Flow cytometry

Even though acid elution stain test seems to be simple, it is rather time consuming and subject to human error. The more precise and sensitive quantification of HbF can be done using the instrumental based flowcytometric technique (Mundee et al., 2000). The interested component of the cell is bound to a fluorescence label. Light scattering can identify the cell population of interest. Fluorescence intensity is measured to quantify the component of interest. The discovery of monoclonal antibody production has extended the use of flow cytometry. Antibody against HbF tagged with fluorescent dye can be used to specifically determine the amount of HbF. It has been demonstrated that detection of both a fetal cell surface antigen and HbF using two different monoclonal antibodies and two colored dyes is a precise way to identify the fetal cells (van Weeghel et al., 2000, Presented by Purdue University Cytometry Laboratories, Available: http://www. wiley. com/legacy/products/subject/life/cytometry/isac2000/6730.htm). The technique called gradient centrifugation has been proved to enrich the fetal cells from the adult blood and can extend the sensitivity of the flow cytometric analysis of HbF (Chen & Davis, 1997).

10.4 Advanced techniques for thalassemia and Hb variants

These are advanced techniques used to detect thalassemia and Hb variants. They are complicated and expensive techniques which are used in the cases for which there are no other ways to accurately identify or confirm the types of thalassemia or Hb variants. They involve DNA technology that can provide in-depth detailed information of gene mutation.

10.4.1 Polymerase chain reaction (PCR)

PCR selectively amplifies mutant or normal alleles using specific oligonucleotide primers. PCR is a technique that allows a small amount of DNA to be amplified in vitro. The process is composed of cycles of the three following steps: (i) perform heat denaturing to separate the DNA sequence target into two strands, (ii) anneal each strand to the specific primers and (iii) then extend the polymerase chain from the primer termini (Mathews & Holde, 1996). Once there are enough of the DNA target sequences produced for further analysis. DNA fragments can be separated by gel electrophoresis. That is commonly done following the

PCR to different DNA fragments. Many additional methods can be coupled with gel electrophoresis and PCR to obtain better information. Direct DNA sequencing of PCR products is quite a straight forward method to indicate the mutation site (Chern & Chen, 2000). Methods for the detection of point mutations were based on restriction fragment length polymorphism (RFLP) analysis (Saiki et al., 1985), and the effects of base-pair changes on DNA fragment melting temperature (denaturing gradient gel electrophoresis) (Fischer & Lerman, 1983). The RFLP technique can differentiate between different DNA sequences based on the length of fragments yielded by a particular enzyme restriction and can indicate the mutation point of a gene in thalassemia patients (Lee et al., 2002). The detection techniques have utilized allele-specific oligonucleotide (ASO) (Saiki et al., 1986, Conner et al., 1983) hybridization, the single-stranded conformational polymorphism (SSCP) (Orita et al 1989), amplification refractory mutation system (ARMS) (Newton et al., 1989), Primer-guided nucleotide incorporation assays (Hargrove et al., 1990, Takatsu et al., 2004), oligonucleotide ligation assaya (Li et al., 2005), real time PCR (Cheng et al., 2004, Johnson et al., 2004), and DNA microarray technology (Wong et al., 2004, Meaburn et al., 2006). The ARMS-PCR, also known as allele specific PCR, is another technique that has been introduced to be used for thalassemia diagnosis. This technique utilizes two PCR reactions: one contains a primer specific for the normal allele and the other contains one for the mutant allele. Gel electrophoresis is then employed to separate specific DNA bands. The PCR products were separated in 2% agarose gel. The samples were mixed with gel loading buffer and then were slowly loaded into the slots of the agarose gel, which pre-stained with ethidium bromide. The gel then electrophoresed at 150 volts, 15 min for α-thalassemia-1 (SEA type, THAI type), HbCS and HbPS and 150 volts, 25 min for α-thalassemia-2 (3.7 and 4.2 kb deletion) to check the size of PCR product. The size of DNA fragment was checked by comparing the 100 bp or 1 Kb DNA size standard (New England BioLabs) at the same gel. The images were captured using gel documentation (Bio-Rad) under ultraviolet light. Diagnosis of genotyping is based on whether there is amplification in one or both reactions (i.e., the band in normal reaction only indicates normal allele, the band in mutant reaction only indicates mutant allele, and bands in both reactions indicate a heterozygote) (Kanavakis et al., 1997, Old et al., 2000, Simsek et al., 1999). ARMS-PCR is more accurate as compared to RFLP. Single stranded conformation polymorphism (SSCP) is the technique that was developed based on the fact that the mobility in gel electrophoresis of single strands of DNA drastically depends on nucleotide sequence. Single strandedDNA is produced by adding one primer at a concentration higher than another primer in the PCR step. After the primer with lower amount is used up, the reaction will continue producing only the product of the excess primer. The mobilities of single strands are then compared (Takahashi-Fujii et al., 1994). Single stranded DNA may also be produced by denaturing double stranded DNA, as in the technique called denaturing gradient gel electrophoresis (DGGE) (Kanavakis et al., 1997, Vrettou et al., 1999, Losekoot et al., 1990). Table 8 showed some examples of PCR primers for used in thalassemia diagnosis and table 9 summarized of common genotype in thalassemia syndrome in Thailand.

10.4.2 DNA sequencing analysis for β-thalassemia mutation

DNA polymerase amplifies single-stranded DNA templates, by adding nucleotides to a growing chain (extension product). Chain elongation occurs at the 3' end of a primer, an oligonucleotide that anneals to the template. The deoxynucleotide added to the extension product is selected by base-pair matching to the template. When a dideoxynucleotide is incorporated at the 3′ end of the growing chain, chain elongation is terminated selectively at A, C, G or T because the chain lacks a 3′-hydroxyl group. With 3′-dye labeled dideoxynucleotide (dye terminators), DNA sequencers detect fluorescence from four different dyes that are used to identify the A,C,G and T extension reactions. All four colors and therefore all four bases can be detected and distinguished in a single gel lane and displaed vary in color peak of bases.

Primers	Diagnosis	Reference
P1 (sense): 5′-GCGATCTGGGCTCTGTGTTCT-3′ **P2 (antisense):** 5′-GTTCCCTGAGCCCCGACATG-3′ **P3 (antisense):** 5′-GCCTTGAACTCCTGGACTTAA-3′	α^0-thalassemia (SEA type), (--SEA)	2008; 54:281
P1 (sense): 5′-CCTCCTGGGATTACATCTGG-3′ **P2 (antisense):** 5′-GCACCTCTGGGTAGGTTCTG-3′ **P3 (sense):** 5′-CCCCTGACAATCTCATCATCT-3′	α^0-thalassemia (THAI type), (--THAI)	2005; 8(3): 241
P1 (sense): 5′-AAGTCCACCCCTTCCTTCCTCACC-3′ **P2 (antisense):** 5′-ATGAGAGAAATGTTCTGGCACCTGCACTTG-3′ **P3 (antisense):** 5′-TCCATCCCCTCCTCCCGCCCCTGCCTTTTC-3′	α^+-thalassemia (3.7 kb deletion), (-α3.7)	2005; 8(3): 241
P1 (sense): 5′-TCCTGATCTTTGAATGAAGTCCGAGTAGGC-3′ **P2 (antisense):** 5′-TGGGGGTGGGTGTGAGGAGACAGGAAAGAGAGA-3′ **P3 (antisense):** 5′-ATCACTGATAAGTCATTTCCTGGGGGTCTG-3′	α^+-thalassemia (4.2 kb deletion), (-α4.2)	2005; 8(3): 241
P1 (sense): 5′-GCTGACCTCCAAATACCGTC-3′ **P2 (antisense):** 5′-GTAAACACCTCCATTGTTGG-3′	ARMS for HbCS	2005; 8(3): 241
P1 (sense): 5′-GCTGACCTCCAAATACCGTTAT-3′ **P2 (antisense):** 5′-GTAAACACCTCCATTGTTGG-3′	ARMS for HbPS	2005; 8(3): 241

Table 8. Some examples of PCR primers for used in thalassemia diagnosis

10.4.3 DNA technology: DNA probe/DNA microchip

Analysis of nucleic acids has led to the understanding of the gene expression that controls Hbs formation. This information is more detailed as compared to information obtained from protein analysis that normally only suggests type and amount of different Hbs production. The advance of DNA studies and fabrication technology together has led to the development of methods for diagnosis using a DNA microchip. Normally the segment of a gene of interest first has to be amplified by PCR to obtain a sufficient amount prior to hybridization with allele specific oligonucleotide probes that are immobilized on the solid phase or chip (Bianchi et al., 1997, Saiki et al., 1988, Fotin et al., 1998). The bound target gene can be detected using either labels such as fluorescent substances (Kurg et al., 2000, Kobayashi et al., 1995) or electronic transducers such as piezoelectronic and ion sensitive field effect transistors (ISFETs) (Cailloux, Novel DNA Chips. Patent No. WO/ 2001/064945 (2001)). One example of devices that has been used commonly is a cytometer. Cytometry is a laser based technique that allows for analysis of physical properties and fluorescence intensity of an individual cell in a heterogeneous environment. The image can differentiate different types of cells or DNA sequences that are labeled with different colors by comparing the ratios of fluorescence of different targets. With the aid of a computer, detection and visualization of many different probes can be done simultaneously (Osterhout et al., 1996, Janssen & Hoffmann, 2002).

Phenotype	Common genotype	
α-Thalassemia		
Thalassemia minor	$--/\,\alpha\alpha$	Heterozygous α-thalassemia-1
Silent Carrier	$-\alpha\,/\alpha\,\alpha$	Heterozygous α-thalassemia-2
Hb Bart's hydrops fetalis	$--/--$	Homozygous α-thalassemia-1
Thalassemia minor	$-\alpha/-\alpha$	Homozygous α-thalassemia-2
Hb H disease	$--/-\alpha$	α-thalassemia 1/ α-thalassemia-2
Hb H disease	$--/\,\alpha^{CS}\,\alpha$	α-thalassemia 1/Hb Constant spring
β-Thalassemia		
Thalassemia minor	Heterozygous β^0-thalassemia	
Thalassemia minor	Heterozygous β^+-thalassemia	
Thalassemia major	Homozygous β^0-thalassemia	
Thalassemia intermedia	β^0-thalassemia/ β^+-thalassemia	
Thalassemia intermedia or Thalassemia major	Hb E-β^0-thalassemia	
Thalassemia intermedia	Hb E-β^+-thalassemia	

Table 9. Summarized of common genotype in thalassemia syndromes in Thailand

10.5 Indirect thalassemia indication and treatment follow-up

These studies are not to be used for thalassemia diagnosis. However, the relevance of the variable of interest and the existence of thalassemia may help treatment follow-up or a new way to economically test for thalassemia.

10.5.1 Ferritin

Ferritin is the iron storage protein serves to store iron in a non-toxic form, to deposit it in a safe form, and to transport it to areas where it is required. Ferritin level in serum directly relates to the amount of iron stored in the body, which is important for red blood cell production. If ferritin is high, there is iron in excess. Ferritin is also used as a marker for iron overload disorders. Normal ranges of ferritin are 12–300 and 12–150 ng ml−1 for male and female, respectively (Medlineplus, Medical Encyclopedia, The US National Library of Medicine and the National Institutes of Health. Available: http://www.nlm.nih.gov/medlineplus/ency/article/003490.htm (October 16, 2003). The technique commonly used to quantify ferritin is immunoassay (Konjin et al., 1981). A significantly high level of ferritin is found in patients with iron overload and this may help differentiate thalassemia patients from those with iron deficiency, both of which will have a low red blood cell count (Arosio et al., 1981). In addition, any inflammatory disorder can cause a high level of ferritin, act as an acute phase protein. Therefore, long term monitoring of ferritin would be necessary, to gain any additional information for thalassemia diagnosis or treatment follow-up (Telfer et al., 2000).

10.5.2 Nuclear magnetic resonance spectroscopy

The nuclear magnetic resonance technique is the determination of the transverse relaxation time of hepatic water. That is based on the magnetic properties of some nuclei that when placed in the magnetic field, would take up radio frequency energy that matches the magnetic field strength and later re-emit that energy (Gunzler & Williams, 2001). The phenomenon is known as nuclear magnetic resonance (NMR) because it involves the nucleus in a magnetic field that has its strength in resonance with the applied radio frequency. NMR spectroscopy was used for the study of composition of chemical compounds. Later, the technique was developed into the imaging technology, magnetic resonance imaging (MRI), that became a major breakthrough in medical fields because it can reveal the image of the parts of the body and seems to be the most sensitive means at present.. NMR has been widely applied to study body iron overload (Jensen et al., 1994, Mazza et al., 1995, Dixon et al., 1994). NMR spectroscopy has been employed mainly for study of iron level in the fraction of tissue in vitro such as liver, spleen, heart, while NMR imaging has been used mainly for determination of iron in vivo, it is an accurate method of measuring liver iron content, especially when the iron content is below 3% (Dixon et al., 1994). So far, there has been no report on health hazards directly related or side effects to NMR and therefore the NMR technique is considered a safe and non-invasive way to study body iron content with an excellent means of assessing the effectiveness of the various therapeutic strategies used in the management of patients with iron overload.

10.5.3 Whatman 3 MM dried blood spots for identifying α-Thalassemia-1 (as demonstrated by Tangvarasittichai et al., (2008)

This method using small samples spotted onto Whatman 3 MM paper (Whatman chromatography paper, Whatman International Ltd, UK) for measurement of α-Thalassemia-1 by polymerase chain reaction (PCR) method. Forty-microliters of whole blood were multiple spotted onto Whatman 3 MM paper, and let dry at room temperature for a minimum of 3 hours, stored in sealed plastic bag at room temperature until the day of assay everymonth for 6 months. DNA extraction was extraced by Chelex method. The dried blood spot was cut into 3 pieces while for the whole blood test 40 μl of whole EDTA blood was used. Added 1 ml of lysis buffer (1% triton X-100) in a 1.5 ml tube, vortexed and centrifuged at 10,000 g for 1 min, discharged the supernatant and washed the pellets by using 1 ml distilled water and the resuspended in 100 μl of distilled water with the addition of 1 drop of Chelex ® solution. Mixtures were incubated at 56°C for at least 2 hr befor being boiled for 5-10 minutes, Samples were spun down by brief centrifugation. Extracted DNA was stored at 4°C until used. PCR reaction had a volume of 10 μl and contained 1 μl of 10x Tris buffer, 1 μl of 25 mmol/l KCl, 1 μl of glycerol, 1 μl of 2 mmol/l of each dATP, dCTP, dGTP, dTTP, 1 μl of 5 μmol/l of 3 primers, 5 μl of DNA solution and 0.1 μl of 5 U/μl *Taq* polymerase. The composition of the 3 primers is

P1: 5'-GCGATCTGGGCTCTGTGTTCT-3',

P2: 5'-GTTCCCTGAGCCCCGACACG-3',

P3: 5'-GCCTTGAACTCCTGGATTAA-3'

The cycling conditions 94 °C for 5 min followed by 40 cycles of amplification, denaturing at 94°C for 40 sec, annealing at 56°C for 40 sec and extension at 72°C for 40 sec. The last cycle extension time was 5 min. The PCR was analyzed by electrophoresis on 2% agarose gel and DNA bands were detected with ethirium bromide by UV transluminator. α-Thalassemia-1 trait (SEA-type) showed a specific 188 bp fragment in addition to a 314 bp fragment obtained from the normal DNA sequence.

11. Conclusion

The rapid increase in understanding of the pathophysiology of thalassemia, diseases of the globin gene have served as a model for the understanding of gene expression and regulation at the molecular level and this knowledge forms the basis for therapeutic interventions, such as gene therapy and augmentation of abnormal hemoglobin levels. Clinical interventions for the treatment of thalassemia patients have also progressed. We have a better knowledge of the optimal amount and method of treatment to provide (such as transfusions and desferrioxamine), as well as of the side-effects of these treatments. Then, the early or prenatal diagnosis of thalassemia is very important, it may base on hematologic and molecular genetic testing. There are many different techniques available for thalassemia diagnosis, but used alone they may not be able to ensure the diagnostic result. Therefore, it is quite common to utilize more than one technique for thalassemia diagnosis. In Fig. 4 summarizes techniques commonly used for diagnosis of Hb variants and thalassemia in most laboratories. If MCV, MCH or OFT screening test reveals a normal result, the possibility of having thalassemia can be eliminated, but analysis of Hb variants should be done. If an abnormal result is obtained from the screening test, there is a possibility of having either Hb variants or thalassemia case. If Hb variants tests do not show any abnormal results, thalassemia tests should still be performed. Choices of techniques depend mainly on budget and equipment available. It should be pointed out that even in laboratories equipped with high technology and many years of experience, quite a few false diagnoses were reported, which resulted in the births of thalassemia children or to have genetic counseling for abortions the unaffected fetuses. It is very important to take precaution in every step of the diagnostic procedures to ensure the most accurate diagnosis. Developments in chemical analysis methodologies are still very useful to this field.

12. References

Aessopos, A, Stamatelos, G, Skoumas, V, Vassilopoulos G, Mantzourani M, et al. (1995). Pulmonary hypertension and right heart failure in patients with β-thalassemia intermedia. *Chest*, 107, p.p.50-53.

Ali, SA. (1969). Hemoglobin H disease in Arabs in Kuwait. *J Clin Pathol*, 22, p.p. 226 - 228.

Allen, S. J., O'Donnell, A., Alexander, N. D. E., Alpers, M. P., Peto, T. E. A., et al. (1997). α+-Thalassemia protects children against disease caused by other infections as well as malaria. *PNAS*, 94, p.p.14736 – 14741.

Allison, A.C. (1954). Protection Afforded by Sickle-cell Trait Against Subtertian Malarial Infection. *Br Med J*, 1, p.p. 290 - 294.

Anapliotou, M.L.G., Kastanias, I.T., Psara, P., Evangelou, E.A., Liparaki, M., et al. (1995). The contribution of hypogonadism to the development of osteoporosis in thalassaemia major: new therapeutic approaches. *Clin Endocrinol (Oxf)*, 42, p.p. 279-287.

Anderson, L.J., Westwood, M.A., Holden, S., Davis, B., Prescott, E.,et al. (2004). Myocardial iron clearance during reversal of siderotic cardiomyopathy with intravenous desferrioxamine: a prospective study using T2* cardiovascular magnetic resonance. *Br J Haematol*, 127(3), p.p. 348-355.

Angelucci, E., Giovagnoni, A., Valeri, G., Paci, E., Ripalti, M., et al. (1997). Limitations of Magnetic Resonance Imaging in Measurement of Hepatic Iron. *Blood*, 90, p.p. 4736-4742.

Angelucci, E., Brittenham, G.M., McLaren, C.E., Ripalti, M., Baronciani, D., et al. (2000). Hepatic iron concentration and total body iron stores in thalassemia major. *N Engl J Med*, 343(5), p.p. 327-331.

Arosio, P., Iacobello, C., Montesoro, E., & Albertini, A. (1981). Serum ferritin evaluation with radioimmunoassays specific for HeLa and liver ferritin types. *Immunol Lett*, 3(5), p.p. 309-313.

Aslan, M. & Freeman, B.A. (2004). Oxidant-mediated impairment of nitric oxide signaling in sickle cell disease-mechanisms and consequences. *Cell Mol Biol*, 50(1), p.p. 95-105.

Bacon, B.R., Tavill, A.S., Brittenham, G.M., Park, C.H., & Recknagel, R.O. (1983). Hepatic lipid peroxidation in vivo in rats with chronic iron overload. *J Clin Invest*, 71(3), p.p. 429-439.

Bain, B.J. (2006). *Hemoglobinopathy Diagnosis*. 2nd ed. Malden, Mass.: Blackwell Publishing, p. 66.

Betke, K. & Sanguansermsri, T. (1972). Cytological differentiation of blood pigments. Possibilities, results and practical application. *Munch Med Wochenschr*, 114(23), p.p. 1099-1104.

Betke, K., Marti, H.R., & Schlicht, I. (1959). Estimation of small percentages of foetal hemoglobin. *Nature*, 184(Suppl 24), p.p. 1877-1878.

Bianchi, D.W., Williams, J.M., Sullivan, L.M., Hanson, F.W., Klinger, K.W., et al. (1997). PCR quantitation of fetal cells in maternal blood in normal and aneuploid pregnancies. *Am J Hum Genet*, 61(4), p.p.822-829.

Borgna-Pignatti, C. & Galanello, R. (2004). *Thalassemias and related disorders: quantitative disorders of hemoglobin synthesis*. In Wintrobe's Clinical Hematology Volume 42. 11th edition. Lippincott Williams & Wilkins. Philadelphia, p.p. 1319-1365.

Borgna-Pignatti, C., Rugolotto, S., De Stefano, P., Zhao, H., Cappellini, M.D., et al. (2004). Survival and complications in patients with thalassemia major treated with transfusion and deferoxamine. *Haematologica*, 89, p.p. 1187 - 1193.

Brilliant cresyl blue MSDS sheet, Available: http://www.proscitech.com/ catalogue/ msds/c085.pdf (April 14, 2003).

Brittenham, G.M., Cohen, A.R., McLaren, C.E., Martin, M.B., Griffith, P.M., et al. (1993). Hepatic iron stores and plasma ferritin concentration in patients with sickle cell anemia and thalassemia major. *Am J Hematol*, 42(1), p.p. 81-85.

Britton, R.S.; Bacon, B.R. & Recknagel, R.O. (1987). Lipid peroxidation and associated hepatic organelle dysfunction in iron overload. *Chem Phys Lipids*, 45(2-4), p.p. 207-239.

Brosious, E.M., Wright, J.M., Baine, R.M., & Schmidt, R.M. (1978). Micro-chromatographic methods for hemoglobin A2 quantitation compared. *Clin. Chem*, 24, p.p. 2196 - 2199.

Brosious, E.M., Morrison, B.Y., & Schmidt, R.M. (1976). Effects of hemoglobin F levels, KCN, and storage on the isopropanol precipitation test for unstable hemoglobins. *Am J Clin Pathol*, 66(5), p.p. 878-882.

Buja, L.M. & Roberts, W. (1971). Iron in the heart: etiology and clinical significance. *Am J Med*, 51, p.p.209-221.

Cailloux, F. *Novel DNA Chips*. Patent No. WO/ 2001/064945 (2001).

Cao, A.; Galanello, R. & Rosatelli, M.C. (1998). Prenatal diagnosis and screening of the hemoglobinopathies. *Baillieres Clin Haematol*, 11(1), p.p. 215-238.

Carrell, R.W. & Kay, R. (1972). A simple method for the detection of unstable hemoglobins. *Br J Haematol*, 23(5), p.p. 615-619.

Cavallo-Perin, P., Pacini, G., Cerutti, F., et al. (1995). Insulin resistance and hyperinsulinemia in homozygous β-thalassemia. *Metabolism*, 44, p.p. 281-286.

Chakraborty, D. & Bhattacharyya, M. (2001). Antioxidant defense status of red blood cells of patients with beta-thalassemia and Ebeta-thalassemia. *Clin Chim Acta*, 305(1-2), p.p. 123-129.

Chan, V., Chan, V.W., Tang, M., Lau, K., Todd, D.,et al. (1997). Molecular defects in Hb H hydrops fetalis. *Br J Haematol*, 96(2), p.p. 224-228.

Chen, J.C. & Davis, B.H. (1997). Characterization of fetal hemoglobin containing cells by density gradient centrifugation and flow cytometric analysis. *Clinical Immunology Newsletter*, 17(6), p. 88.

Cheng, J.; Zhang, Y. & Li, Q. (2004). Real-time PCR genotyping using displacing probes. *Nucleic Acids Res*, 32, p. e61.

Chern, S.R. & Chen, C.P. (2000). Molecular prenatal diagnosis of thalassemia in Taiwan. *Int J Gynaecol Obstet*, 69(2), p.p. 103-106.

Chernoff, AI. (1959). The Distribution of the Thalassemia Gene: A Historical Review. *Blood*, 14, p.p. 899 - 912.

Chinprasertsuk, S., Wanachiwanawin, W. & Piankijagum, A. (1994). Effect of pyrexia in the formation of intraerythrocytic inclusion bodies and vacuoles in haemolytic crisis of hemoglobin H disease. *Eur J Haematol*, 52, p.p.87-91.

Christian, G.D. (2004). *Analytical Chemistry*, 6th ed., Wiley, New York.

Chui, D.H.K. & Waye, J.S. (1998). Hydrops Fetalis Caused by α-Thalassemia: An Emerging Health Care Problem. *Blood*, 91, p.p. 2213 - 2222.

Congote, L.F. (1981). Rapid procedure for globin chain analysis in blood samples of normal and beta-thalassemic fetuses. *Blood*, 57, p.p. 353 – 360.

Conner, B.J., Reyes, A.A., Morin, C., Itakura, K., Teplitz, R.L., et al. (1983). Detection of Sickle Cell ß S-globin Allele by Hybridization with Synthetic Oligonucleotides. *PNAS*, 80, p.p. 278 - 282.

Cooley, T.B.; Witwer, E. R. & Lee, P. (1927). Anemia in children: With splenomegaly and peculiar changes in the bones report of cases. *Am J Dis Child*, 34, p.p. 347 - 363.

Cooley, TB. (1946), M.D. 1871-1945. *Am J Dis Child*, 71, p.p. 77 - 79.

Cossu, G., Manca, M., Pirastru, M.G., Bullitta, R., Bosisio, A.B., et al. (1982). Neonatal screening of beta-thalassemias by thin layer isoelectric focusing. *Am J Hematol*, 13(2), p.p. 149-157.

Cunningham, M.J., Macklin, EA., Neufeld, E.J., Cohen, A.R., & the Thalassemia Clinical Research Network. (2004). Complications of β-thalassemia major in North America. *Blood*, 104, p.p. 34 - 39.

Dacie, J.V, Grimes, A.J., Meisler, A., Stiengold, L., Hemsted, E.H., et al. (1964). Hereditary heinz-body znaemia. A report of studies on five patients with mild anaemia. *Br J Haematol*, 10, p.p. 388-402.

Dispenzieri, A. (2001). *Primary Hematology*, Humana Press, NJ.

Dixon, R.M., Styles, P., al-Refaie, F.N., Kemp, G.J., Donohue, S.M., et al. (1994). Assessment of hepatic iron overload in thalassemic patients by magnetic resonance spectroscopy. *Hepatology*, 19(4), p.p. 904-910.

Doelman, C.J.A, Siebelder, C.W.M., Nijhof, W.A., Weykamp, C.W., Janssens, J., et al. (1997). Capillary electrophoresis system for hemoglobin A1c determinations evaluated. *Clin Chem*, 43, p.p. 644 – 648.

Dover, G.J., Boyer, S.H., & Zinkham, W.H. (1979). Production of erythrocytes that contain fetal hemoglobin in anemia. Transient in vivo changes. *J Clin Invest*, 63(2), p.p. 173-176.

Dozy, A.M., Kleihauer, E.F., & Huisman, T.H. (1968). Studies on the heterogeneity of hemoglobin. 13. Chromatography of various human and animal hemoglobin types on DEAE-Sephadex. J Chromatogr, 32(4), p.p. 723-727.

Du, Z.D., Roguin, N., Milgram, E., Saab, K., & Koren, A. (1997). Pulmonary hypertension in patients with thalassemia major. *Am Heart J*, 134, p.p.532-537.

Dubart, A., Goossens, M., Beuzard, Y., Monplaisir, N., Testa, U., et al. (1980). Prenatal diagnosis of hemoglobinopathies: comparison of the results obtained by isoelectric focusing of hemoglobins and by chromatography of radioactive globin chains. *Blood*, 56: p.p. 1092 - 1099.

Eaton, J.W. & Qian, M. (2002). Molecular bases of cellular iron toxicity. *Free Radic Biol Med*, 32(9), p.p. 833-840.

Electron Microscope Sciences Catalog, Available: http://www.emsdiasum. com/ems/ chemicals/salt.html (October 16, 2003).

Factor, J.M., Pottipati, S.R., Rappaport, I., Rosner, I.K., Lesser M.L., et al. (1994). Pulmonary function abnormalities in thalassemia major and the role of iron overload. *Am J Respir Crit Care Med*, 149, p.p.1570-1574.

Fairbanks, V.J. (1980). *Hemoglobinopathies and Thalassemia Laboratory Methods and Clinical Cases*, Brian C. Decker, New York.

Fernandez-Alberti A. & Fink, N.E. (2000). Red blood cell osmotic fragility confidence intervals: a definition by application of a mathematical model. *Clin Chem Lab Med*, 38(5), p.p. 433-436.

Fischer, S.G. & Lerman, L.S. (1983). DNA Fragments Differing by Single Base-Pair Substitutions are Separated in Denaturing Gradient Gels: Correspondence with Melting Theory. *PNAS*, 80, p.p. 1579 - 1583.

Flint, J, Harding, R.M, Boyce, A.J. & Clegg, J.B. (1998). The population genetics of the hemoglobinopathies. *Baillieres Clin Haematol*, 11(1), p.p. 1-51.

Fosburg, M.T. & Nathan, D.G. (1990). Treatment of Cooley's anemia. *Blood*, 76, p.p. 435 - 444.

Fotin, A.V, Drobyshev, A.L., Proudnikov, D.Y., Perov, A.N., & Mirzabekov, A.D. (1998). Parallel thermodynamic analysis of duplexes on oligodeoxyribo- nucleotide microchips. *Nucleic Acids Res*, 26, p.p. 1515 - 1521.

Frers, C.R., Dorn, S., Schmidt, W., Kochhan, L., Simon-Schultz, J., et al. (2000). Falsely increased HbA1c values by HPLC and falsely decreased values by immunoassay lead to identification of Hb Okayama and help in the management of a diabetic patient. *Clin Lab*, 46(11-12), p.p. 569-573.

Fucharoen, S. & Winichagoon, P. (2000). Clinical and hematologic aspects of hemoglobin E beta-thalassemia. *Curr Opin Hematol*, 7(2), p.p. 106-112.

Fucharoen, S., Winichagoon, P., Wisedpanichkij, R., Sae-Ngow, B., Sriphanich, R.,et al. (19980. Prenatal and postnatal diagnoses of thalassemias and hemoglo-binopathies by HPLC. *Clin Chem*, 44: p.p.740 - 748.

Fucharoen, S., Winichagoon, P., Pootrakul, P., Piankijagum, A., & Wasi, P. (1988). Difference between two types of Hb H disease, α-thalassemia 1/α-thalassemia 2 and α-thalassemia 1/Hb Constant Spring. *Birth Defect.* ;23 (5A), p.p. 309-315.

Fucharoen, S. & Viprakasit, V. (2009) Hb H disease: clinical course and disease modifiers *Hematology*, 2009, p.p. 26 - 34.

Gaziev, J. & Lucarelli G. (2003). Stem cell transplantation for hemoglobino-pathies. *Curr Opin Pediatr*, 15(1), p.p. 24-31.

Greenberg, M.S., Harvey, H.A. & Morgan, C. (19720. A simple and inexpensive screening test for sickle hemoglobin. *N Engl J Med*, 286(21), p.p. 1143-1144.

GU¨nzler, H. & Williams A. (2001). *Handbook of Analytical Techniques*, vol.1, Wiley VCH, Germany, p. 509.

Gullo, L., Corcioni, E., Brancati, C., Bria, M., Pezzilli, R., et al. (1993). Morphologic and functional evaluation of the exocrine pancreas in β-thalassemia major. *Pancreas*, 8, p.p.176-80.

Gwendolyn, M.C, Clarke, G.M. & Higgins, T.N. (2000). Laboratory Investigation of Hemoglobinopathies and Thalassemias: Review and Update. *Clin Chem*, 46, p.p. 1284 - 1290.

Hargrove, J.L., Hulsey, M.G., Schmidt, F.H., and Beale, E.G. (1990). A computer program for modeling the kinetics of gene expression. *Biotechniques*, 8(6), p.p. 654-659.

Hebbel, R.P., Eaton, J.W., Balasingam, M., & Steinberg, M.H. (1982). Spontaneous oxygen radical generation by sickle erythrocytes. *J Clin Invest*, 70(6), p.p. 1253-1259.

Helrich, K. (1995). Association of Official Analytical Chemists, AOAC Inc., Virginia.

Hempe, J.M. & Craver R.D. (1994). Quantification of hemoglobin variants by capillary isoelectric focusing. *Clin Chem*, 40, p.p. 2288 - 2295.

Hempe, J.M., Granger, J.N., & Craver, R.D. (1997). Capillary isoelectric focusing of hemoglobin variants in the pediatric clinical laboratory. *Electrophoresis*, 18(10), p.p. 1785-95.

Hershko, C, Konijn, A.M. & Link, G. (1998). Iron chelators for thalassaemia. *Br J Haematol*, 101, p.p.399-406.

Hershko C, Weatherall DJ. (1988). Iron-chelating therapy. *Crit Rev Clin Lab Sci*, 26, p.p.303-345.

Hicks, E.J. & Hughes, B.J. (1975). Comparison of electrophoresis on citrate Agar, cellulose acetate, or starch for hemoglobin identification. *Clin Chem*, 21(8), p.p. 1072-1076

Higgs, D.R., Vickers, M.A., Wilkie, A.O., Pretorius, I.M., Jarman, A.P., et al. (1989). A review of the molecular genetics of the human alpha-globin gene cluster. *Blood*, 73, p.p. 1081 - 1104.

Hillman, R.S. & Ault, K.A. 1995). Hematology in Practical Practice, a Guide to Diagnosis and Management, McGraw-Hill, New York,

Houglum, K, Filip, M., Witztum, J.L., & Chojkier, M. (1990). Malondialdehyde and 4-hydroxynonenal protein adducts in plasma and liver of rats with iron overload. J Clin Invest, 86(6), p.p. 1991-1998.

Huisman, T.H.J. & Dozy, A.M. (1965). Studies on the heterogeneity of hemoglobin: IX. The use of tris(hydroxymethyl)aminomethane−HCl buffers in the anion-exchange chromatography of hemoglobins. *J Chromatography A*, 19, p.p. 160-169

Iancu, T.C, Neustein, H.B. & Landing, B.H. (1977). *The liver in thalassaemia major: ultrastructural observations.* In: Iron metabolism: Ciba Symposium 51. Amsterdam: Elsevier, p.p. 293-309.

Italian Working Group on Endocrine Complications in Non-endocrine Diseases. (1995). Multicentre study on prevalence of endocrine complications in thalassaemia major. *Clin Endocrinol (Oxf)*, 42, p.p.581-586.

Janssen, W.C. & Hoffmann, J.J. (2002). Evaluation of flow cytometric enumeration of foetal erythrocytes in maternal blood. *Clin Lab Haematol*, 24(2), 89-92.

Jean, G., Terzoli, S., Mauri, R., et al. (1984). Cirrhosis associated with multiple transfusions in thalassaemia. *Arch Dis Child*, 59, p.p. 67-70.

Jenkins, M. & Ratnaike, S. (2003). Capillary electrophoresis of hemoglobin. *Clin Chem Lab Med*, 41(6), p.p. 747-54.

Jensen, P.D., Jensen, F.T., Christensen, T., & Ellegaard, J. (1994). Non-invasive assessment of tissue iron overload in the liver by magnetic resonance imaging. *Br J Haematol*, 87(1), p.p. 171-184.

Johnson, M.P., Haupt, LM. & Griffiths, L.R. (2004). Locked nucleic acid (LNA) single nucleotide polymorphism (SNP) genotype analysis and validation using real-time PCR. Nucleic Acids Res, 32, p. e55.

Kadiiska, M.B., Burkitt, M.J., Xiang, Q.H., & Mason, R.P. (1995). Iron supplementation generates hydroxyl radical in vivo. An ESR spin-trapping investigation. *J Clin Invest*, 96(3), p.p. 1653-1657.

Kanavakis, E., Traeger-Synodinos, J., Vrettou, C., Maragoudaki, E., Tzetis, M., et al. (1997). Prenatal diagnosis of the thalassaemia syndromes by rapid DNA analytical methods. *Mol Hum Reprod*, 3: p.p. 523 - 528.,

Karydis, I., Karagiorga-Lagana, M., Nounopoulos, C., & Tolis, G. (2004). Basal and stimulated levels of growth hormone, insulin-like growth factor-I (IGF-I), IGF-I binding and IGF-binding proteins in beta-thalassemia major. *J Pediatr Endocrinol Metab*, 17(1), p.p. 17-25.

Kazazian, Jr. H.H. (1990). The thalassemia syndromes: molecular basis and prenatal diagnosis in 1990. *Semin Hematol*, 27(3), p.p. 209-228.

Klee, G.G., Behrman, R.E.,. Kliegman, R. & Jenson, H.B. (2000). *Nelson Textbook of Pediatrics*, W.B. Saunders.

Klee, G.G. (1980). *Role of Morphology and Erythrocyte Indices in Screening and Diagnosis*, Brian C. Decker, a Division of Thieme-Stratton Inc, New York.

Kobayashi, M., Rappaport, E., Blasband, A., Semeraro, A., Sartore, M., et al. (1995). Fluorescence-based DNA minisequence analysis for detection of known single-base changes in genomic DNA. *Mol Cell Probes*, 9(3), p.p. 175-182.

Konjin, A.M., Levy, R., Link, G. & Hershko C. (1982). A rapid and sensitive ELISA for serum ferritin employing a fluorogenic substrate. *J Immunol Methods*, 54(3), p.p. 297-307.

Kremastinos, D.T., Tiniakos, G., Theodorakis, G.N., Katritsis, D.G. & Toutouzas, P.K. (1995). Myocarditis in β-thalassemia major: a cause of heart failure. *Circulation*, 91, p.p. 66-71.

Kurg, A., Tonisson, N., Georgiou, I., Shumaker, J., Tollett, J., et al. (2000). Arrayed primer extension: solid-phase four-color DNA resequencing and mutation detection technology. Genet Test, 4(1), p.p. 1-7.

Kutlar, F, Reese, A.L., Hsia, Y.E., Kleman, K.M.& Huisman, T.H. (1989). The types of hemoglobins and globin chains in hydrops fetalis. Hemoglobin, 13(7-8), p.p. 671-183.

La-Nasa, G., Argiolu, F., Giardini, C., Pession, A., Fagioli, F., et al. (2005). Unrelated bone marrow transplantation for beta-thalassemia patients: The experience of the Italian Bone Marrow Transplant Group. *Ann NY Acad Sci*, 1054, p.p. 186-195.

Laosombat, V, Wongchanchailert, M., Sattayasevana, B., Wiriyasateinkul, A. & Fucharoen, S. (2001). Clinical and hematologic features of beta⁰-thalassemia (frameshift 41/42 mutation) in Thai patients. *Haematologica*, 86, p.p. 138 - 141.

Lee, Y.J., Park, S.S., Kim, J.Y. & Cho, H.I. (2002). RFLP haplotypes of beta-globin gene complex of beta-thalassemic chromosomes in Koreans. *J Korean Med Sci*, 17(4), p.p. 475-478.

Leung, W.C., Leung, K.Y., Lau, E.T., Tang M.H. & Chan, V. (2008). Alpha-thalassaemia. *Semin Fetal Neonatal Med*, 13(4), p.p. 215-222.,

Leung, W.C., Oepkes, D., Seaward, G. & Ryan, G. (2002) Serial sonographic findings of four fetuses with homozygous alpha-thalassemia-1 from 21 weeks onwards. *Ultrasound Obstet Gynecol*, 19(1), p.p. 56-59.

Li, J., Chu, X., Liu, Y., Jiang, J.H., He, Z., et al. (2005). A colorimetric method for point mutation detection using high-fidelity DNA ligase. *Nucleic Acids Res*, 33, p. e168.

Lie-Injo, L & Jo, B.H. (1960) A fast-moving hemoglobin in hydrops foetalis. *Nature*, 185, p. 698.

Lo, Y.M.D. (2005). Recent Advances in Fetal Nucleic Acids in Maternal Plasma. *Journal of Histochemistry & Cytochemistry*, 53, p.p. 293 - 296.

Locatelli, F., Rocha, V., Reed, W., Bernaudin, F., Ertem, M., et al. (2003). Related umbilical cord blood transplantation in patients with thalassemia and sickle cell disease. *Blood*, 101, p.p. 2137 - 2143.

Lorey, F., Cunningham, G., Vichinsky, E.P., Lubin, B.H.,Witkowska H.E. et al. (2001). Universal newborn screening for Hb H disease in California. *Genet Test*, 5(2), p.p. 93-100.

Losekoot, M., Fodde, R., Harteveld, C.L., van Heeren, H., Giordano, P.C., et al. (1990). Denaturing gradient gel electrophoresis and direct sequencing of PCR amplified genomic DNA: a rapid and reliable diagnostic approach to beta thalassaemia. *Br J Haematol*, 76(2), p.p. 269-274.

Lucarelli, G., Galimberti, M., Polchi, P., Angelucci, E., Baronciani, D., et al. (1990). Bone marrow transplantation in patients with thalassemia. *N Engl J Med*, 322(7), p.p. 417-21.

Magro, S., Puzzonia, P., Consarino C., et al. (1990). Hypothyroidism in patients with thalassemia syndromes. *Acta Haematol*, 84, p.p.72-76.

Maiavacca, R., Tedeschi, S., Mosca, A., Calmi, S., De Leonardis, P., et al. (1992). Nonradioactive quantification of low concentrations of hemoglobin A by HPLC for midtrimester prenatal diagnosis of beta-thalassemia. *Clin Chem*, 8, p.p. 1906 - 1908.

Mario, N, Baudin, B. & Giboudeau, J. (1998). Qualitative and quantitative analysis of hemoglobin variants by capillary isoelectric focusing. *J Chromatogr B Biomed Sci Appl*, 706(1), p.p. 123-129.

Mathews, C.K. & Holde, K.E.V. (1996). *Biochemistry, The Benjamin/Cummings*. Publishing Company, New York.

Mavrou, A., Kouvidi, E., Antsaklis, A., Souka, A., Kitsiou Tzeli, S., et al. (2007). Identification of nucleated red blood cells in maternal circulation: a second step in screening for fetal aneuploidies and pregnancy complications. Prenat Diagn, 27(2), p.p. 150-153.

Mazza, P., Giua, R., De Marco, S., Bonetti, M.G., Amurri, B., al et. (1995). Iron overload in thalassemia: comparative analysis of magnetic resonance imaging, serum ferritin and iron content of the liver. *Haematologica*, 80, p.p. 398 - 404.,

McNiel, J.R. (1968). *The inheritance of hemoglobin H disease* (abstr). XII Congress of the International Society of Hematology, p. 52.

Meaburn, E, Butcher, L.M., Schalkwyk, L.C. & Plomin, R. (2006). Genotyping pooled DNA using 100K SNP microarrays: a step towards genomewide association scans. *Nucleic Acids Res*, 34, p. e28.

Medlineplus, Medical Encyclopedia, The US National Library of Medicine and the National Institutes of Health. Available: *http://www.nlm.nih.gov/medlineplus/ency/article/003490.htm* (October 16, 2003).

Michlitsch, J., Azimi, M., Hoppe, C., Walters, M.C., Lubin, B., et al. (2009). Newborn screening for hemoglobinopathies in California. *Pediatr Blood Cancer*, 52(4), p.p. 486-490.

Minnich, V., Na-nakorn, S., Chongchareonsuk, S., & Kochaseni, S. (1954). Mediterranean Anemia: A Study of Thirty-two Cases in Thailand. *Blood*, 9, p.p.1 - 23.

Mundee, Y, Bigelow, N.C., Davis, B.H.& Porter, J.B. (2000). Simplified flow cytometric method for fetal hemoglobin containing red blood cells. *Cytometry*, 42(6), p.p. 389-393.

Nalbandian, R.M., Nichols, B.M., Camp, Jr. F.R., Lusher, J.M., Conte, N.F., et al. (1971). Dithionite Tube Test-A Rapid, Inexpensive Technique for the Detection of Hemoglobin S and Non-S Sickling Hemoglobin. *Clin Chem*, 17, p.p.1028 - 1032.

Na-Nakorn, S., Wasi, P., Pornpatkul, M. & Pootrakul, S.N. (1969). Further evidence for a genetic basis of hemoglobin H disease from newborn offspring of patients. *Nature*, 223(5201), p.p. 59-60.

Nathan, D.G. & Gunn, R.B. (1966). Thalassemia: the consequences of unbalanced hemoglobin synthesis. *Am J Med*, 41(5), p.p. 815-830.

Nathan, D.G. & Piomelli, S. (1990). Oral iron chelators. *Semin Hematol*, 27(2), p.p. 83-5.

Nathan, D.G. & Oski, F.A. (1993). *Hematology of infancy and childhood*, 4th ed. Philadelphia: W B Saunders Co.

Neidlinger, N.A., Larkin, S.K., Bhagat, A., Victorino, G.P. & Kuypers, FA. (2006). Hydrolysis of Phosphatidylserine-exposing Red Blood Cells by Secretory Phospholipase A2 Generates Lysophosphatidic Acid and Results in Vascular Dysfunction. *J. Biol. Chem.*, 281, p.p. 775 - 781.

New Methylene, Blue MSDS Sheet. Available: *http://www.jtbaker.com/ msds/englishhtml/n2700.htm* (April 20, 2003)

Newton, C.R., Graham, A., Heptinstall, L.E., Powell S.J., Summers, C.,et al. (1989). Analysis of any point mutation in DNA. The amplification refractory mutation system (ARMS). *Nucleic Acids Res*, 17, p.p. 2503 - 2516.)

Old, J., Petrou, M., Varnavides, L., Layton, M., & Modell, B. (2000). Accuracy of prenatal diagnosis for hemoglobin disorders in the UK: 25 years' experience. *Prenat Diagn*, 20(12), p.p. 986-991.

Olivieri, N.F. & Brittenham, G.M. (1997). Iron-chelating therapy and the treatment of thalassemia. *Blood*, 89, p.p. 739-761.

Olivieri, N.F. (1999). Correction: The (beta)-Thalassemias. N Engl J Med 1999; 341: 99-109 July 8, 1999. *N Engl J Med*, 341(18), p. 1407.

Orita, M., Iwahana, H., Kanazawa, H., Hayashi, K. & Sekiya, T. (1989). Detection of Polymorphisms of Human DNA by Gel Electrophoresis as Single-Strand Conformation Polymorphisms. *PNAS*, 86, p.p. 2766 - 2770.

Orkin, S.H. (1978). The duplicated human globin genes lie close together in cellular DNA. *PNAS*, 75, p.p. 5950 - 5954.

Orkin, S.H., Old, J., Lazarus, H., Altay, C., Gurgey, A., et al. (1979). The molecular basis of alpha-thalassemias: frequent occurrence of dysfunctional alpha loci among non-Asians with Hb H disease. *Cell*, 17(1), p.p. 33-42.

Orofino, M.G., Argiolu, F., Sanna, M.A., Rosatelli, M.C., Tuveri, T., et al. (2003). Fetal HLA typing in beta thalassaemia: implications for haemopoietic stem-cell transplantation. *Lancet*, 362(9377), p.p. 41-42.

Osterhout, M.L., Ohene-Frempong, K. & Horiuchi, K. (1996). Identification of F-reticulocytes by two-stage fluorescence image cytometry. *J Histochem Cytochem*, 44, p.p. 393 - 397.

Papadea, C. & Cate, J.C. (1996). Identification and quantification of hemoglobins A, F, S, and C by automated chromatography. *Clin Chem*, 42, p.p. 57 - 63.

Pembrey, M.E., McWade, P. & Weatherall, D.J. (1972). Reliable routine estimation of small amounts of foetal hemoglobin by alkali denaturation. *J Clin Pathol*, 25, p.p. 738 - 740

Phillips, 3d J.A., Vik, T.A., Scott, A.F.,Young, K.E., Kazazian, Jr H.H., et al. (1980). Unequal crossing-over: a common basis of single alpha-globin genes in Asians and American blacks with hemoglobin-H disease. *Blood*, 55, p.p. 1066 - 1069.

Pinto, F.O. & Roberts, I. (2008). Cord blood stem cell transplantation for hemoglobinopathies. *Br J Haematol*, 141(3), p.p. 309-324.

Pippard, M.J., Callender, S.T., Warner, G.T. & Weatherall, D.J. (1979). Iron absorption and loading in beta-thalassaemia intermedia. *Lancet*, 2, p.p. 819-821.

Pootrakul, P., Kitcharoen, K., Yansukon, P., et al. (1988). The effect of erythroid hyperplasia on iron balance. *Blood*,71, p.p.1124-1129.

Pootrakul, S, Wasi, P, & Na-Nakorn, S. (1967). Hemoglobin Bart's hydrops foetalis in Thailand. *Ann Hum Genet*, 30(4), p.p. 293-311.

Rao, V.B., Natrajan, P.G., Lulla, C.P. & Bandodkar, S.B. (1997). Rapid mid-trimester prenatal diagnosis of beta-thalassaemia and other hemoglobinopathies using a non-radioactive anion exchange HPLC technique-an Indian experience. *Prenat Diagn*, 17(8), p.p. 725-731.

Reid, M., Badaloo, A., Forrester, T. & Jahoor, F. (2006). In vivo rates of erythrocyte glutathione synthesis in adults with sickle cell disease. *Am J Physiol Endocrinol Metab*, 291, p.p. E73 - E79.

Research Organics. Available: *http://www.resorg.com/* (October 17, 2003).

Rich, S.A., Ziegler, F.D., & Grimley, P.M. (2002). Prevention of homozygous beta thalassemia by carrier screening in pregnancy. *Haema*, 5 (3), p.p. 242-245.

Rigas, D.A., Koler, R.D., Cummings, G., Duerst, M.L., Malm, D.R., et al. (1961). Decreased Erythrocyte Survival in Hemoglobin H Disease As a Result of the Abnormal Properties of Hemoglobin H: The Benefit of Splenectomy. *Blood*, 18, p.p. 1 – 17.

Rigas, D.A., Koler, R.D. & Osgood, E.E. (1955). New Hemoglobin Possessing a Higher Electrophoretic Mobility than Normal Adult Hemoglobin. *Science*, 121, p. 372

Risdon, R.A., Flynn, D.M. & Barry, M. (1973). The relation between liver iron concentration and liver damage in transfusional iron overload in thalassaemia and the effect of chelation therapy. *Gut*, 14, p. 421.

Rouyer-Fessard, P., Plassa, F., Blouquit, Y., Vidaud, M., Varnavides, L., et al. (1989). Prenatal diagnosis of hemoglobinopathies by ion exchange HPLC of hemoglobins. *Prenat Diagn*, 9(1), p.p. 19-26.

Saiki, R.K., Chang, C.A., Levenson, C.H., Warren, T.C., Boehm, C.D., et al. (1988). Diagnosis of sickle cell anemia and beta-thalassemia with enzymatically amplified DNA and nonradioactive allele-specific oligonucleotide probes. *N Engl J Med*, 319(9), p.p. 537-541.

Saiki, R.K., Scharf, S., Faloona, F., Mullis, K.B., Horn, G.T., et al.(1985). Enzymatic amplification of beta-globin genomic sequences and restriction site analysis for diagnosis of sickle cell anemia. *Science*, 230, p.p. 1350 - 1354.

Saiki, R.K., Bugawan, T.L., Horn, G.T., Mullis, K.B. & Erlich, H.A. (1986). Analysis of enzymatically amplified beta-globin and HLA-DQ alpha DNA with allele-specific oligonucleotide probes. *Nature*, 324(6093), p.p. 163-166.

Salmon, J.E., Nudel, U., Schiliro, G., Natta, C.L., & Bank, A. (1978). Quantitation of human globin chain synthesis by cellulose acetate electrophoresis. *Anal Biochem*, 91(1), p.p. 146-157.

Sanguansermsri, T., Thanaratanakorn, P., Steger, H.F., Tongsong, T., Sirivatanapa, P.,et al. (2001). Prenatal diagnosis of hemoglobin Bart's hydrops fetalis by HPLC analysis of hemoglobin in fetal blood samples. *Southeast Asian J Trop Med Public Health*, 32(1), p.p. 180-185.

Sanguansermsri, T., Thanarattanakorn, P., Steger, H.F., Tongsong T, Chanprapaph, P., et al. (2001). Prenatal diagnosis of beta-thalassemia major by high-performance liquid chromatography analysis of hemoglobins in fetal blood samples. *Hemoglobin*, 25(1), p.p. 19-27.

Schaible, U.E. & Kaufmann, S.H. (2004). Iron and microbial infection. *Nat Rev Microbiol*, 2(12), p.p. 946-53.

Silvestroni, E. & Bianco, I. (1983). A highly cost effective method of mass screening for thalassaemia. *Br Med J (Clin Res Ed)*, 286, p.p. 1007 - 1009.

Simsek, M., Daar, S., Ojeli, H. & Bayoumi, R. (1999). Improved diagnosis of sickle cell mutation by a robust amplification refractory polymerase chain reaction. *Clin Biochem*, 32(8), p.p. 677-680.

Singer, K., Chernoff, A.I. & Singer, L. (1951). Studies on Abnormal Hemoglobins: I. Their Demonstration in Sickle Cell Anemia and Other Hematologic Disorders by Means of Alkali Denaturation. *Blood*, 6, p.p. 413 - 428.,

Siniscalco, M., Bernini, L., Filippi, G., Latte, B., Khan, M., et al. (1966). Population genetics of hemoglobin variants, thalassaemia and glucose-6-phosphate dehydrogenase deficiency, with particular reference to the malaria hypothesis. *Bull World Health Organ*, 34(3), p.p. 379-393.

Sirichotiyakul, S., Tantipalakorn, C., Sanguansermsri, T., Wanapirak, C. & Tongsong, T. (2004). Erythrocyte osmotic fragility test for screening of alpha-thalassemia-1 and beta-thalassemia trait in pregnancy. *Int J Gynaecol Obstet*, 86(3), p.p. 347-350.

Sklar, C.A., Lew, L.Q., Yoon, D.J., David, R. (1987). Adrenal function in thalassemia major following long-term treatment with multiple transfusions and chelation therapy: evidence for dissociation of cortisol and adrenal androgen secretion. *Am J Dis Child*, 141, p.p. 327-330.

Skoog, D.A. & Leary, J.J. (1992). *Principles of Instrumental Analysis*, Saunders College Publication, New York.

Skordis, N. (2006). The growing child with thalassaemia. *J Pediatr Endocrinol Metab*, 19(4), p.p. 467-469.

Srisawang, B., Kongtawelert, P., Hartwell, S.K., Jakmunee, J. & Grudpan, K. (2003). A simple flow injection-reduced volume column system for hemoglobin typing. *Talanta*, 60(6), p.p. 1163-1170.

Stohs, S.J. & Bagchi, D. (1995). Oxidative mechanisms in the toxicity of metal ions. *Free Radic Biol Med*, 18(2), p.p. 321-336.

Suwanrath-Kengpol, C., Kor-anantakul, O., Suntharasaj, T. & Leetanaporn, R. (2005). Etiology and outcome of non-immune hydrops fetalis in southern Thailand. *Gynecol Obstet Invest*, 59(3), p.p. 134-137.

Svensson, H. (1962). Isoelectric fractionation, analysis and characterization of ampholytes in natural pH gradients. III, Description of apparatus for electrophoresis in columns stabilized by density gradients and direct determination of isoelectric points. *Arch Biochem*, Suppl.I, p. 132.

Tai, D.Y.H., Wang, Y.T., Lou, J., Wang, W.Y., Mak KH., et al. (1996). Lungs in thalassaemia major patients receiving regular transfusion. *Eur Respir J*, 9, p.p. 1389-1394.

Takahashi-Fujii, A., Ishino, Y., Kato, I. & Fukumaki, Y. (1994). Rapid and practical detection of beta-globin mutations causing beta-thalassemia by fluorescence-based PCR-single-stranded conformation polymorphism analysis. *Mol Cell Probes*, 8(5), p.p. 385-393.

Takatsu, K., Yokomaku, T., Kurata, S. & Kanagawa, T. (2004). A new approach to SNP genotyping with fluorescently labeled mononucleotides. *Nucleic Acids Res*, 32, p. e60.

Tangvarasittichai, O., Jongjitwimol, J. & Tangvarasittichai, S. (2008). Whatman 3 MM dried blood spots for identifying alpha-thalassemia-1. *Clin Lab*, 54(7-8), p.p. 281-283.

Tangvarasittichai, O., Jeenapongsa, R., Sitthiworanan, C.& Sanguansermsri, T. (2004). Diagnostic value of combined parameters for α-thalassemia 1 screening in pregnant women. *Naresuan University Journal*, 12, p.p. 19-24.

Tangvarasittichai, S., Tangvarasittichai, O. & Jermnim, N. (2009). Comparison of fast protein liquid chromatography (FPLC) with HPLC, electrophoresis & microcolumn chromatography techniques for the diagnosis of α-thalassemia. *Indian J Med Res*, 129, p.p. 242-248

Tanner, M.A., He, T., Westwood, M.A., Firmin, D.N., Pennell, D.J. & Thalassemia International Federation Heart T2* Investigators. (2006). Multi-center validation of the transferability of the magnetic resonance T2* technique for the quantification of tissue iron. *Haematologica*, 91, p.p. 1388 - 1391.

Telfer, P.T., Prestcott, E., Holden, S., Walker, M., Hoffbrand A.V., et al. (2000). Hepatic iron concentration combined with long-term monitoring of serum ferritin to predict complications of iron overload in thalassaemia major. *Br J Haematol*, 110(4), 971-977.

Thakerngpol, K., Fucharoen, S., Boonyaphipat, P., et al. (1996). Liver injury due to iron overload in thalassemia: histopathologic and ultrastructural studies. *Biometals*, 9, p.p. 177-183.

Thalassemia International Federation. (2008). Guidelines for the clinical management of thalassemia 2nd edition. [*http://www .thalassemia.org.cy*]

Thomas, E.D., Buckner, C.D., Sanders, J.E., Papayannopoulou, T., Borgna-Pignatti, C., et al. (1982). Marrow transplantation for thalassaemia. *Lancet*, 2(8292), p.p. 227-229.

Ueda, S. & Schneider, R.G. (1969). Rapid identification of polypeptide chains of hemoglobin by cellulose acetate electrophoresis of hemolysates. *Blood*, 34, p. 230.

Ui, N. (1971). Isoelectric points and conformation of proteins. I. Effect of urea on the behavior of some proteins in isoelectric focusing. *Biochim Biophys Acta*, 229, p.567.

van Weeghel, R., Steunebrink, G. & Suk, R., (2000). Proceedings of the International Society for Analytical Cytology ISAC2000 International Congress, Poster abstract No. 6730, May 19–35, Presented by Purdue University Cytometry Laboratories,Available: *http://www.wiley.com/legacy/products/ subject/life/cytometry/isac2000/6730.htm*.

Villeneuve, J.P., Bilodeau, M., Lepage, R., Cote, J. & Lefebvre, M. (1996).Variability in hepatic iron concentration measurement from needle-biopsy specimens. *J Hepatol*, 25(2): 172-177.

Vrettou, C., Palmer, G., Kanavakis, E., Tzetis, M., Antoniadi, T., et al. (1999). A widely applicable strategy for single cell genotyping of beta-thalassaemia mutations using DGGE analysis: application to preimplantation genetic diagnosis. *Prenat Diagn*, 19(13): 1209-1216.

Weatherall, D.J. (1987). Common genetic disorders of the red cell and the malaria hypothesis. *Ann Trop Med Parasitol*, 81(5), p.p. 539-548.

Weatherall, D.J. (1994). *The thalassemias*. In: Stamatoyannopoulos, G., Nienhuis, A.W., Majerus, P.H., Varmus, H. eds. The molecular basis of blood diseases. 2nd ed. Philadelphia: W.B. Saunders, p.p. 157-205.

Weatherall, D.J. (1997). Fortnightly review: The thalassaemias *BMJ*, 314, p. 1675.

Weatherall, D.J. (1998). Thalassemia in the next millennium. *Ann N Y Acad Sci*, 850, p.p. 1-9.

Weatherall, D.J. (2008). Hemoglobinopathies worldwide: present and future. *Curr Mol Med*, 8(7), p.p. 592-599.

Weatherail, D.J. & Clegg, J.B. (1981). *The Thalassaemia Syndromes*, 3rd edn. Oxford: Blackwell

Weatherall, D.J. & Clegg, J.B., (2001). *The Thalassemia Syndromes*, 4th ed., Blackwell Science, USA, ,

Weatherall, D.J. & Clegg, J.B. (2001). *The β and δβ thalassemia association with structural hemoglobin variants*. In: Weatherall DJ, Clegg JB. Eds. The Thalassemia syndromes. 4th ed. Oxford, UK: Blackwell scientific Publications, p.p.393-449.

Westgren, M., Ringden, O., Eik-Nes, S., Ek, S., Anvret, M., et al. (1996). Lack of evidence of permanent engraftment after in utero fetal stem cell transplantation in congenital hemoglobinopathies. *Transplantation*, 61(8), p.p. 1176-1179.

Wilson, J.B., Headlee, M.E., & Huisman, T.H. (1983). A new high-performance liquid chromatographic procedure for the separation and quantitation of various hemoglobin variants in adults and newborn babies. *J Lab Clin Med*, 102(2), p.p. 174-86.

Winichagoon, P., Thitivichianlert, A., Lebnak, T., Piankijagum, A. & Fucharoen, S. (2002). Screening for the carriers of thalassemias and abnormal hemoglobins at the community level. *Southeast Asian J Trop Med Public Health*, 33 Suppl 2,p.p. 145-150.

Witzleben, C.L. & Wyatt, J.P. (1961). The effect of long survival on the pathology of thalassaemia major. *J Pathol Bacteriol*, 82, p.p.1-12.

Wolfe, L., Olivieri, N., Sallan, D, et al. (1985). Prevention of cardiac disease by subcutaneous deferoxamine in patients with thalassemia major. *N Engl J Med*, 312, p.p. 1600-1603.

Wong, K.K., Tsang, Y.T.M., Shen, J., Cheng, R.S., Chang, Y.M., et al. (2004).Allelic imbalance analysis by high-density single-nucleotide polymorphic allele (SNP) array with whole genome amplified DNA. *Nucleic Acids Res*, 32, p. e69.

Wood, K.C., Hsu, L.L. & Gladwin, M.T. (2008). Sickle cell disease vasculopathy: a state of nitric oxide resistance. *Free Radic Biol Med*, 44(8), p.p. 1506-1528.

Wood, J.C., Tyszka, J.M., Carson, S., Nelson, M.D. & Coates, T.D. (2004). Myocardial iron loading in transfusion-dependent thalassemia and sickle cell disease. *Blood*, 103, p.p. 1934 - 1936.

Wu, K.H., Tsai, F.J. & Peng, C.T. (2003). Growth hormone (GH) deficiency in patients with beta-thalassemia major and the efficacy of recombinant GH treatment. *Ann Hematol*, 82(10), p.p. 637-640.

Yang, Y. & Li, D.Z. (2009). A survey of pregnancies with Hb Bart's disease in Mainland China. *Hemoglobin*, 33(2), p.p. 132-136.

Yuregir G.T. (1976). Determination of fetal hemoglobin in various age groups by the immunological method of Kohn and Payne. *Clin Chim Acta*, 72(2), p.p. 181-185.

Zurlo, M.G., De Stefano, P., Borgna-Pignatti, C., Di Palma, A., Piga, A., et al. (1989). Survival and causes of death in thalassaemia major. *Lancet*, 2(8653), p.p. 27-30.

6

Alström Syndrome

Cristina Maria Mihai[1], Jan D. Marshall[2] and Ramona Mihaela Stoicescu[3]
[1]"Ovidius" University, Faculty of Medicine, Constanta,
[2]The Jackson Laboratory, Bar Harbor, ME,
[3]"Ovidius" University, Faculty of Pharmacy, Constanta
[1,3]Romania
[2]USA

1. Introduction

Recent advancements in genetic research that have elucidated the function of some of the rare disease-causing genes have suggested that a large number of genetic disorders with widely divergent phenotypes, that were not previously identified as related, may be, in fact, highly related in cellular function or common pathways. A classic example of this is the recent category of disorders called ciliopathies. Cilia and flagella are ancient, evolutionarily conserved organelles that project from cell surfaces to perform diverse biological roles, including whole-cell locomotion; movement of fluid; chemo-, mechano-, and photosensation; and sexual reproduction. Over the past ten years, several studies demonstrated the connections between cilia, basal bodies and human diseases with a wide phenotypic spectrum, including randomization of body symmetry, obesity, cystic kidney diseases and retinal degeneration. Defects in ciliary structure or function can lead to a broader set of developmental and adult phenotypes, with mutations in ciliary proteins now associated with nephronophthisis, Joubert Syndrome, Meckel-Gruber Syndrome, Bardet-Biedl Syndrome, and Alström Syndrome (ALMS), [Badano et al., 2006]. Further study of these diverse ciliopathies could lead to an understanding of the phenotypic patterns that could potentially have predictive and therapeutic value. Alström Syndrome (ALMS; MIM #203800), first described by Carl-Henry Alström, in 1959 [Alström et al., 1959], is a rare condition that affects many body systems. ALMS is characterized by a constelation of serious or life-threatening medical problems including sensory deficits, obesity, type 2 diabetes mellitus, and multiple organ failure. The signs and symptoms of ALMS vary in severity, and not all affected individuals have all of the characteristic features of the disorder, making the diagnosis more difficult. Additionally, many of the signs and symptoms of this condition begin in infancy or early childhood, although some appear later in life. The major phenotypes usually observed in children with ALMS include cone–rod retinal dystrophy beginning in infancy and leading to juvenile blindness, sensorineural hearing impairment, insulin resistance, and obesity, and congestive heart failure (CHF) due to dilated cardiomyopathy (DCM). As patients reach adolescence, more of the major phenotypes develop, including type 2 diabetes mellitus, hypertriglyceridemia, hypothyroidism, and short adult stature. Males and females have hypogonadism and are infertile. Pulmonary, hepatic, and renal phenotypes are progressive [Marshall et al. 1997,

2005]. The primary cause of mortality among young affected patients is cardiac involvement from dilated cardiomyopathy whereas renal failure is the major cause of death among the older subgroup [Marshall et al., 1997]. Systemic fibrosis is commonly observed [Marshall et al., 2005]. About 700 affected individuals have been identified worldwide. The estimated prevalence is of <1: 5,000,000 [JD.Marshall, Personal communication]. Ethnically or geographically isolated populations have a higher-than-average frequency of Alström syndrome [Deeble et al., 2000 & Ozgül et al., 2007].

2. Diagnosis

2.1 Clinical diagnosis

The diagnosis of ALMS is usually established by clinical findings. Diagnosis may be delayed because some features begin at birth and others emerge as the child develops. Diagnosis can also be difficult due to variable expression of the severity of the clinical features both within and among families. It is important to note that, although some of the features are seen frequently, affected individuals may not have all of the symptoms discussed below.

2.1.1 Major features

Cone-rod dystrophy. The first symptoms are pendular or searching nystagmus and extreme photodysphoria or light sensitivity. The retinal dystrophy in ALMS often develops within a few weeks after birth and virtually all children exhibit low vision within the first year of life [Malm et al., 2008; Russell-Eggitt et al., 1998]. Fundus examination in the first decade may be normal or may show a pale optic disc and narrowing of the retinal vessels. Electroretinography (ERG), required to establish the diagnosis of cone-rod dystrophy, is abnormal from birth, eventually with impairment of both cone and rod function. Rod function is preserved initially but deteriorates as the individual ages. By 9 – 10 years of age, visual acuity is severely impaired. There is increasing constriction of visual fields, leading to total blindness with no light perception by age 16- 20 years [Marshall et al., 2007a, Michaud et al., 1996]. The severity and age of onset of the retinal degeneration vary among ALMS patients [Malm et al., 2008]. Retinal changes include attenuated vessels, pale optic discs, and partial atrophy of the retinal pigment epithelium. Pathological studies show a reduction of cell layers in the posterior retina and depletion of peripheral cells, the outer nuclear layer, and photoreceptors [Sebag et al., 1984, Vingolo et al., 2010]. Exudative retinopathy was described in Alström Syndrome [Gogi et al., 2007]. Vision may be aided in the first few years if the child is given prescription dark, red-tinted glasses. Cataract is a common finding and some patients might transiently benefit from its treatment/removal [Marshall et al., 2005, 2007, Satman et al., 2002].

Progressive bilateral sensorineural hearing impairment

Most patients develop mild-to-moderate bilateral sensorineural hearing loss in early childhood (<10 years) that is slowly progressive, particularly in the high-frequency range [Van den Abeele et al., 2001; Welsh 2007]. There is a high incidence of otitis media and fluid retention along with a high susceptibility to glue ear, which compounds the existing sensorineural impairment [Marshall et al. 2005, Michaud et al., 1997]. Hearing loss may be detected as early as age one year in some patients, although wide differences in acuity exist. Although bilateral hearing aids generally benefit most children, about 10% progress to profound deafness and must rely on tactile signing for communication [Marshall et al.,

2007a]. There is evidence that vestibular function is abnormal in some patients. [Möller, 2005]. Because hearing loss develops gradually and the onset is post-lingual, children typically do not experience the speech problems often associated with deafness. These early changes in neurosensory capabilities can have tremendous impact not only on the social development of the child but also on his/her adaptation to the external environment [Joyet al., 2007, Van den Abeele et al., 2001].

Obesity

Obesity in Alström Syndrome is an early and consistent feature observed in nearly all affected children [Marshall et al., 2005, 2007a]. Body Mass Index (kg/m²) is typically greater than 25 or >95th centile, with the distribution of adipose tissue predominantly viscerally and subcutaneously [Paisey et al., 2008]. Birth weight is normal, but rapid weight gain usually begins at approximately 6 months to 1 year of age. In some individuals body weight tends to normalize, decreasing into the high-normal to normal range after adolescence. The moderation of weight does not seem to be correlated with the onset of other serious complications such as CHF, T2DM, or renal failure [Minton et al., 2006]. Wide shoulders, a barrel chest, a 'stocky' build, and truncal obesity are typical [Marshall et al., 2007a]. However, both waist circumference and body fat percentage (as measured using dual-energy X-ray absorptiometry) negatively correlated with age, and was independent of Body Mass Index, indicating the possible recruitment of more metabolically active fat stores [Minton et al., 2006]. The presence of hyperphagia has been controversial, although both hyperphagia and food obsession are common anecdotal complaints [Marshall et al., 1997, 2005].

Growth and development

Children grow rapidly and are initially tall for their age with a height >50th centile, with 2–3 years advanced bone age prior to puberty. However, early closure of the growth plates results in height below the 50th centile by age 14–16 years [Michaud et al., 1996]. Thoracic and lumbar scoliosis and kyphosis commonly develop in the early teenage years and can progress rapidly. Many patients have a 'buffalo hump' of increased fatty tissue above the shoulders [Marshall et al., 2005, 2007a]. Abnormalities of the insulin-like growth factor system (IGFs) of affected patients have been demonstrated [Maffei et al., 2007, Mihai et al., 2008, 2009]. Yet, the exact reasons for short stature remain to be determined.

Dilated cardiomyopathy

DCM can occur at any age, but is seen most typically during infancy. Onset, progression, and clinical outcome of the DCM vary, even within families [Hoffman et al., 2005, Makaryus et al., 2003]. Approximately 40% of affected infants have a transient but severe DCM with onset between age three weeks and four months [Marshall et al., 2005, Worthley & Zeitz, 2001]. Most of these children survive and make an apparently full recovery in infancy. The proportion of those with ALMS who develop infantile-onset DCM may be underestimated because some infants who succumb early may have undiagnosed Alström syndrome.

A subset of 10-15% of patients does not experience infantile DCM, but develop cardiomyopathy for the first time as adolescents or adults. These patients present with a progressive restrictive cardiomyopathy [Worthley & Zeitz, 2001], identified between the teens to late 30s. Although DCM is the most common underlying cause of death in the infantile period, survival for children with infantile-onset tends to be better than that for

adult-onset. Marshall et al showed that while one-third of adult-onset DCM patients died, ~74% of infantile-onset DCM patients survived [Marshall et al., 2005]. As these children grow older, their cardiac function tends to be low-normal, and they remain at risk for a recurrence of CHF as adolescents or adults, with a poor prognosis. Postmortem myocardial fibrosis has been described [Minton et al., 2006]. Cardiac magnetic resonance imaging suggests myocardial fibrosis may be present both in clinically affected and asymptomatic individuals [Loudon et al., 2009].
Augmented aortic systolic pressure may also contribute to heart failure [Smith et al., 2007].
 DCM in infants in the presence of nystagmus and photophobia should be a strong indicator of a diagnosis of ALMS.

Pulmonary disease

Chronic respiratory illness is one of the most frequent complaints and ranges in severity from frequent bronchial infections to chronic asthma, sinusitis/bronchitis, alveolar hypoventilation, and frequent episodes of pneumonia. The chronically inflamed airways are hyper-reactive and highly sensitive to triggering or irritating factors. In some patients, as inflammation continues, the lungs are infiltrated by fibrotic lesions and moderate to severe interstitial fibrosis has been reported [Marshall et al., 2005]. Pulmonary disease can be quite severe and include chronic obstructive pulmonary disease and pulmonary hypertension, secondary to pulmonary fibrosis. Respiratory infections with sudden reduced blood oxygen saturation have triggered sudden death. Acute hypoxia and acute respiratory distress syndrome in some older patients probably results from a combination of pulmonary fibrosis and severe scoliosis [Khoo et al., 2009; Florentzson et al., 2010].

Insulin resistance/type 2 diabetes mellitus

Two of the earliest metabolic changes in ALMS, insulin resistance and hyperinsulinemia, have been observed in patients as young as 1 year of age, sometimes before the onset of obesity [Marshall et al., 2005, 2007a]. Most children will eventually develop T2DM, some as early as age 4, but there is wide variability in the age of onset. The median age of onset is 16 years. T2DM in Alström syndrome is the result of tissue resistance to the actions of insulin, as demonstrated by an elevated plasma insulin concentration and glucose intolerance that usually present in childhood [Marshall et al., 2005, 2007a]. *Acanthosis nigricans,* a common feature in ALMS, consistent with severe insulin resistance, obesity, hyperinsulinemia, is described in about one-third of patients, whether or not they have diabetes [Marshall et al., 2005, 2007a]. However, in a small study of 12 unrelated individuals with ALMS, severe childhood obesity, BMI and waist circumference decreased with age, whereas insulin resistance increased [Minton et al., 2006]. Interestingly, ALMS patients with T2DM do not appear to develop typical peripheral sensory neuropathy symptoms and maintain good protective sensation despite comparable hyperglycemia and dyslipidemia seen in other types of diabetes. This suggests the *ALMS1* mutations might in some way protect against hyperglycemia-induced sensory neuropathy [Paisey et al., 2009]. However, studies of nerve conduction in these patients are needed to confirm these findings.

Hepatic disease

 Nearly all patients with ALMS may have some degree of liver involvement that first presents with fatty liver. Initially, overt clinical manifestations are absent, but transaminases and gamma-glutamyl transpeptidase could be elevated. Ultrasound may show evidence of steatosis, steatohepatitis, and enlarged liver and spleen, which can progress in ALMS patients as they grow older. In some individuals, hepatic inflammation and fibrosis develops, with a highly variable age of onset, clinical course, and prognosis. As the disease progresses, liver function tests are further disturbed with altered prothrombin values or elevated International normalized ratio (INR) and ammonia. Progression to hepatic failure can occur in childhood [Quiros-Tejeira et al., 2001], but usually worsens in the second to third decades. Portal hypertension, hepatosplenomegaly, cirrhosis, esophageal varices, ascites, and liver failure are among the late clinical signs and the upper gastro-intestinal hemorrhage due to portal hypertension is a cause of death in some patients [Marshall et al., 2005, 2007a]. It is not yet known why the hepatic function becomes serious in some children, while others remain stable [Awazu et al., 1995, 1997, Connolly et al., 1991 & Marshall et al., 2005].

Liver biopsies and postmortem examination have revealed varying degrees of steatohepatitis, hepatic fibrosis, cirrhosis, chronic nonspecific active hepatitis with lymphocytic infiltration, patchy necrosis, [Marshall et al., 2005, Quiros-Tejeira et al., 2001]. Macrovesicular steatosis can be present or absent [Marshall et al., 2005]. Other gastrointestinal manifestations include upper gastrointestinal pain, chronic diarrhea, constipation, cecal volvulus, and gastroesophageal reflux [Marshall et al., 2005; Khoo et al., 2009].

Renal disease

The age of onset, progression rate, and severity of renal involvement are variable in ALMS, but most often becomes serious in adolescents or adults. Slowly progressive nephropathy, progressive glomerulofibrosis, and a gradual destruction of the kidneys are a major feature in adult patients with ALMS. Whether hypertension is a consequence of or contributes to renal dysfunction is uncertain, but it is present in ~30% of individuals [Marshall et al., 2005]. Patients may have symptoms ranging from chronic, mild kidney dysfunction to end-stage renal failure. Histopathologic changes include hyalinization of tubules and interstitial fibrosis [Goldstein and Fialkow, 1973, Marshall et al., 2005, 2007a]. There is evidence suggesting that the position of the alteration in *ALMS1* may play a role in the severity of the renal disease [Marshall et al., 2007b].

Hypogonadotropic hypogonadism

Male hypogonadotropic hypogonadism results in low plasma testosterone secondary to low plasma gonadotropin concentration. Males often have a small penis and testes, usually with gynecomastia in adolescence. Atrophic fibrotic seminiferous tubules are described [Marshall et al., 2007a]. Secondary sexual characteristics such as axillary and pubic hair are normal in both males and females. In female adolescents, sexual development usually progresses normally and menarche is not delayed (average age 12 years). In a few patients, precocious puberty has occurred (age 6–10) and breast development has been delayed. The external genitalia, uterus, and fallopian tubes are normal, but menstruation is often scant, sporadic, or irregular, sometimes accompanied by endometriosis. There can be reduced plasma gonadotropin concentrations. Baseline FSH and LH in female adolescents are usually in the normal range; however, some evidence of primary hypogonadism has been reported [Quiros-Tejeira et al., 2001]. Increased androgen production and hirsuitism are common [Kocova et al., 2010]. A relatively high frequency (>20% of female patients) of ovarian cysts is reported, which may be associated with obesity and hyperinsulinemia. No ALMS patients have been known to reproduce – the few cases where this is „reported" are in patients without a confirmed molecular diagnosis [Boor et al., 1993].

Hypertriglyceridemia

Hyperlipidemia, particularly hypertriglyceridemia, can be present from early childhood. In some patients, a sudden, rapid rise in triglycerides places them at risk for pancreatitis [Paisey et al., 2009, Wu et al., 2002]. Other features in Alström Syndrome, such as hyperinsulinemia, may also contribute to the elevated triglycerides [Maffei et al., 2002, 2007].

2.1.2 Minor features

Hypothyroidism

A hypothyroid condition, mostly primary (low free thyroxine (FT4), high thyroid-stimulating hormone (TSH)), is observed in approximately 20% of patients [Michaud et al., 1996]. Subclinical hypothyroidisms in about 30% of patients and isolated incidents of hyperthyroidism have been observed [Ozgül et al., 2007]. The mechanism of the hypothyroidism remains unknown, although it could be hypothesized that fibrotic infiltrations in the thyroid gland play a role.

Dental abnormalities

Dental anomalies include discolored teeth, gingivitis, a large space between the front teeth, and extra or missing teeth [Koray et al., 2001].

Hands and feet

Most children have characteristic wide, thick, flat feet, and short stubby fingers and toes with no polydactyly or syndactyly. Rare cases of digit anomalies have been reported [Marshall et al., 2007a].

Urological dysfunction

Males and females with ALMS can experience varying degrees of urinary problems. Minor symptoms include urinary urgency, difficulty initiating or poor flow, long intervals between voiding, incomplete voiding (urinary retention) or abdominal pain before or during urination [Marshall et al., 2005]. There can be an unusual changing presentation, switching from retention to increased frequency, and incontinence. Recurrent urinary tract infections or cystitis are common in both males and females. Urethral strictures have also been described and fibrotic infiltrations have been noted histopathologically. A subset of patients have developed more severe complications such as marked frequency and urgency, incontinence, and significant perineal or abdominal pain requiring surgical intervention [Charles et al., 1990, Marshall et al., 2005, 2007a]. Anatomical abnormalities can also occur in ALMS, including calyceal deformities, narrowed ureteropelvic angles, dilated ureters, and misalignment of the kidneys [Ozgül et al., 2007].

Developmental delay

Although delay of cognitive impairment is not a common feature of ALMS, delay in early developmental milestones is seen in ~45% of affected children. Motor milestones, in particular sitting, standing, and walking, are typically delayed by 1–2 years and there may be deficits in coordination, balance, and fine motor skills. Hearing and vision deficits probably contribute to the early developmental, expressive and receptive language, and learning delays seen in many young children with ALMS. Children with a receptive language deficit also tend to have an expressive language delay. Intellectual delays and behavioral issues in rare cases have resulted in a diagnosis of mental retardation. A range of autism-spectrum behavior has been observed in a subset of patients [Marshall et al., 2005, 2007a].

Other neurologic manifestations may include absence seizures and general sleep disturbances [Marshall et al., 2005, 2007a]. The frequency of mood and psychiatric disorders in ALMS-affected individuals has not been determined [Joy et al., 2007].

The combined effect of hearing loss and an accompanying multiple disabilities present a unique and complex problem to professionals and parents, different from the problems usually associated with any disability alone. A review of the literature yields surprisingly little specific information on educational programs for such children. The fact that there are many differences among children with multiple disabilities adds to the difficulties of providing appropriate programs.

2.2 Diagnostic criteria in Alström Syndrome

A major problem in arriving at a diagnosis of ALMS is the high phenotypic heterogeneity that can occur even within the same affected family [Ozgül et al., 2007, Hoffman et al., 2005 & Titomanilo et al., 2004]. Marshall and co-workers [Marshall et al., 2007a] provided a comprehensive guidance for diagnostic criteria in their 2007 publication, as summarized below:

Birth – 2 years: Diagnosis requires 2 major or 1 major and 2 minor criteria

Major criteria:	1) *ALMS1* mutation in 1 allele and/or family history of Alström Syndrome
	2) Vision pathology (nystagmus, photophobia).
Minor criteria:	1) Obesity
	2) DCM with CHF.
Other variable supportive evidence	Recurrent pulmonary infections, normal digits, delayed developmental milestones.

3-14 years of age: diagnosis requires 2 major criteria or 1 major and 3 minor criteria

Major criteria:	1) *ALMS1* mutation in 1 allele and/or family history of Alström Syndrome
	2) Vision pathology (nystagmus, photophobia, diminished acuity). If old enough for testing: cone dystrophy by ERG.
Minor criteria:	1) Obesity and/or insulin resistance and/or T2DM
	2) History of DCM with CHF
	3) Hearing loss
	4) Hepatic dysfunction
	5) Renal failure
	6) Advanced bone age

| Other variable supportive evidence | Recurrent pulmonary infections, normal digits, delayed developmental milestones, hyperlipidemia, scoliosis, flat wide feet, hypothyroidism, hypertension, recurrent urinary tract infections, growth hormone deficiency |

15 years – adulthood: 2 major and 2 minor criteria or 1 major and 4 minor criteria	
Major criteria:	1) ALMS1 mutation in 1 allele and/or family history of Alström Syndrome
	2) Vision pathology (history of nystagmus in infancy/childhood, legal blindness, cone and rod dystrophy by ERG).
Minor criteria:	1) Obesity and/or insulin resistance and/or T2DM
	2) History of DCM with CHF.
	3) Hearing loss
	4) Hepatic dysfunction
	5) Renal failure
	6) Short stature
	7) Males: hypogonadism. Females: irregular menses and/or hyperandrogenism
Other variable supportive evidence	Recurrent pulmonary infections, normal digits, history of developmental delay, hyperlipidemia, scoliosis, flat wide feet, hypothyroidism, hypertension, recurrent urinary tract infections/urinary dysfunction, growth hormone deficiency, alopecia.

Table 1.

In conclusion, ALMS is a very complex disorder, being characterized by a constellation of progressive and highly variable disease symptoms. Diagnosis is made on the basis of clinical features observed, usually without genetic confirmation. Delay of onset of some of the characteristic features (type 2 diabetes mellitus, DCM/chronic heart failure, hepatic dysfunction, pulmonary, and renal disease) makes early differential diagnosis very difficult in young children, as many of the cardinal features do not become apparent until the teenage years. As the child grows, the characteristic pattern of ALMS evolves and the clinical picture becomes clearer.

2.3 Age of onset and incidence of common features of Alström Syndrome

Marshall and co-workers [Marshall et al., 2005] described the age of onset and the incidence of common features of Alstrom syndrome. Cone-rod dystrophy was diagnosed in 100% of ALMS patients between birth and 15 months. Obesity usually begins to develop during the first year, birth weight being normal. Hearing loss is progressive and presents in 88% of cases during the first 9 years. Dilated cardiomyopathy could be diagnosed in 42% of infants under 4 months of age. In adolescents and adults the pattern is often restrictive cardiomyopathy, with an overall incidence of 18%. Insulin resistance/type 2 diabetes can be diagnosed in children as young as 4 years of age. While urologic dysfunction can be seen at any age, chronic renal failure begins in adolescents and adults. About 25-30 % of ALMS patients are diagnosed with developmental delay, based on the assessment of early development milestones. Liver involvement develops variabily, between 8 and 30 years of age, in 23-98% of patients. Over 98% are diagnosed with short stature after puberty or in adulthood. Among the endocrine abnormalities, hypogonadotropic hypogonadism was diagnosed in 78% of males.

2.4 Genetic diagnosis

Alström Syndrome is the consequence of recessively inherited mutations in a single gene, *ALMS1*, located on the short arm of chromosome 2 [Collin et al., 2002, Hearn et al., 2002]. Parents are obligate carriers of a single copy of the altered gene and have no reported heterozygous phenotypic characteristics. Males and females are affected with equal probability (1:1 ratio). Although the incidence is greater in isolated or consanguineous communities, there is no one ethnic group more likely to carry *ALMS1* mutations [Marshall et al, 2007a].

ALMS1 is comprised of 23 exons. The longest *ALMS1* transcript potentially encodes a 461 kDa protein of 4169 amino acids. Exon 1 contains a tract of glutamic acid residues (aa 13–29), followed by a stretch of seven alanine residues (aa 30–36) [Collin et al., 2002, Hearn et al., 2002]. Exon 8, a large 6-kb exon, contains a large tandem repeat domain encoding 34 imperfect repeats of 45–50 amino acids. This domain constitutes 40% of the protein, a short polyglutamine segment, a leucine zipper domain and a conserved motif near the C-terminus.

The *ALMS1* protein is ubiquitously expressed and at least one isoform localizes to centrosomes and basal bodies of ciliated cells, perhaps playing an important role in cilia function and intraflagellar transport [Collin et al., 2005, Hearn et al., 2005; Knorz et al., 2010]. RNA interference knockdown experiments indicate that a total lack of *ALMS1* impairs cilia formation [Li G et al., 2007].

To date, the mutations reported in *ALMS1* have been nonsense and frameshift variations (insertions or deletions) and one reciprocal translocation that are predicted to cause premature protein truncation [Collin et al., 2002, Hearn et al., 2002]. Since 2002, more than 100 different mutations in *ALMS1* have been identified. The variants are primarily clustered in exons 16, 10, and 8, but less common mutations also occur in exons 12 and 18 [Marshall et al., 2007a; Joy et al., 2007; Pereiro, et al., 2010]. Founder effects are reported in families of English and Turkish descent. In addition, numerous single-nucleotide polymorphisms have been identified, the functional significance of which is unclear [Marshall et al., 2007a]. The mechanisms by which disease alleles of *ALMS1* cause the various pathologies observed in Alström Syndrome remain unknown and identification of pathogenic mutations in *ALMS1* has not led to any genotype-specific treatments [Hearn et al., 2005, Kinoshita et al., 2003, Li G et al., 2007, Minton et al., 2006 & Patel et al., 2006].

ALMS1 RNA is widely expressed by many tissues. Splice variants have been identified from human brain and testis which may suggest differing functions of theALMS1 protein between organs [Hearn et al., 2002].

The ubiquitous expression of *ALMS1* correlates with the wide range of organ dysfunction in ALMS and suggests that the C-terminal portion of the Alms1 protein that is missing in ALMS patients plays a critical role in disease causation [Girard & Petrovsky, 2010]. Because *ALMS1* is a very large gene, complete sequencing is time consuming and expensive. Therefore, we recommend a screening strategy that targets the regions of *ALMS1* where most of the mutations are seen (exons 16, 10, part of 8). If no mutation is identified in these

132   Handbook of Genetic Disorders

areas, the remaining genomic regions can be sequenced on a research basis. The sensitivity of this approach is approximately 65%, that is, in about 42% of all patients both mutations will be detected, in about half of the patients, only one of the two mutations will be found, and in about 10% of the patients, none of the mutations will be found. The recent development of an-ALMS mutation array to detect known mutations in *ALMS1* (Asper Biotech (www.asperbio.com) can be used as an efficient and cost-effective first pass screening for known mutations *ALMS1* and 10 known Bardet-Biedl Syndrome (BBS) genes [Pereiro et al.,2010]. New technological developments including target capture and next generation sequencing will offer the possibility of efficient and cost-effective identification of novel *ALMS1* mutations and for carrier testing [Bell et al., 2011]

The possible results of genetic testing must be interpreted within the context of the clinical picture [Marshall et al., 2007a]:

- 2 mutations identified in ALMS1. Diagnosis: ALMS.
- 1 mutation in *ALMS1* together with clinical signs of Alström Syndrome. Diagnosis: very strong evidence for the confirmation of ALMS (although about 0.25% of all healthy individuals could also show this result).
- No ALMS1 mutation identified. This does not exclude the diagnosis, in the presence of clinical manifestations suggestive for ALMS.

3. Differential diagnosis of Alström Syndrome [Marshall et al., 2007a]

	Alström Syndrome	Bardet–Biedl Syndrome (BBS #1-14)	Congenital achromatopsia	Leber congenital amaurosis (LCA)	Wolfram (DIDMOAD)	Cohen Syndrome	Biemond II Syndrome
OMIM	203800	209900	216900 262300 139340	204000	222300	216550	210350
Vision	Cone dystrophy, photophobia	Night blindness, rod–cone dystrophy (age 10-16)	Cone dystrophy	Cone dystrophy (infancy)	Optic atrophy	Rod–cone dystrophy >5 years myopia, bulls-eye maculopathy, peripheral vision loss	Coloboma, microphthalmia, aniridia, cataract
Cardiac	Yes	Congenital heart defects (5–10%)	No	No	No	No	No

	Respiratory	Neurosensory hearing loss	Renal	Obesity	Diabetes	Hypogonadism	Mental development
Alström Syndrome	Pulmonary failure, recurrent cough	Yes (90%)	Glomerulo-sclerosis	Yes	T2DM (90%)	Yes	Normal/delayed
Bardet–Biedl Syndrome (BBS #1-14)	No	Yes (5–20%)	Structural renal abnormalities	Yes	T2DM (5–15%)	Yes	Mental retardation (50%)
Congenital achromatopsia	No	No	No	No	No	No	Normal/delayed
Leber congenital amaurosis (LCA)	No	No	No	No	No	No	Normal/delayed
Wolfram (DIDMOAD)	No	Yes	Diabetic nephropathy	No	Diabetes insipidus, insulin-dependent diabetes mellitus	No	Normal, behavior problems
Cohen Syndrome	No	No	No	Yes, abdominal obesity, thin arms and legs	No	No	Moderate-to-severe delay
Biemond II Syndrome	No	No	No	Yes	No	Yes	Mental retardation

Genetic	Head	Orthopedic	Urologic	Hepatic	
ALMS1 (2p13)	No	Short fingers, wide flat feet, scoliosis	Varying degrees of urinary problems (25%)	Steatosis cirrhosis	*Alström Syndrome*
BBS1, BBS2, ARL6/BBS3, BBS4, BBS5, MKKS/BBS6, BBS7, TTC8/BBS8, B1/BBS9, BBS10, TRIM32/BBS11, BBS12, MKS1/BBS13, CEP290/BBS14.	High-arched palate, hypodontia	Poly-, brachy-, and syndactyly		Steatosis	*Bardet–Biedl Syndrome (BBS #1-14)*
CNGA3 CNGB3GNAT2	No	Normal		No	*Congenital achromatopsia*
GUCY2D (LCA1), RPE65 (LCA2), SPATA7 (LCA3), AIPL1 (LCA4), LCA5 (LCA5), RPGRIP1 (LCA6), CRX (LCA7), CRB1 (LCA8), CEP290 (LCA10), IMPDH1 (LCA11), RD3 (LCA12), and RDH12 (LCA13).	No	Normal		No	*Leber congenital amaurosis (LCA)*
WFS1 (4p16)	No	Normal	Urinary atony	No	*Wolfram (DIDMOAD)*
COH1 (8q22)	Characteristic facial features	Narrow hands and feet, tapered fingers		No	*Cohen Syndrome*
	Absent incisors, microcephaly, characteristic facial features	Postaxial polydactyly, scoliosis		No	*Biemond II Syndrome*

Table 2.

4. Management

There is no treatment at this time that can cure ALMS or prevent or reverse the medical complications.
Early diagnosis is important to allow counseling of parents and institution of appropriate supportive medical treatment. In the absence of specific therapy to correct the underlying genetic defect, ALMS remains a progressive disease and regular intensive medical management is essential to track progression and to anticipate the emergence of new symptoms and disease manifestations.
Cardiac, renal and liver review should be routinely performed in all ALMS patients, even if asymptomatic.
The main causes of death in ALMS are from cardiomyopathy, pulmonary, kidney or liver failure [Marshall et al., 2005, Benso et al., 2002]. In the end stage, multiple organs are compromised, and sudden multiple organ failure is common.

4.1 Management of sensory deficits

Vision and hearing loss can impact the social and educational success of the child, so, management of the multiple sensory deficits in young children diagnosed with ALMS and social support at school are crucial [Marshall et al., 2007a].

4.1.1 Rod-cone dystrophy

Photophobia and nystagmus are serious problems, particularly in younger children. Regular ophthalmologic evaluations should be sought as soon as possible [Gogi et al., 2007]. Red-tinted prescription glasses are helpful in alleviating the distress children experience in bright lighting. No therapy for the progressive vision loss exists, but early evaluation of visual acuity facilitates the provision of visual aids and helps prepare the child for a future with little or no sight. Educational planning should anticipate future blindness, therefore, early mobility training and Braille or other non-visual language skills is critically important for the learning environment of the child. Computing skills (including voice recognition and transcription software), and the use of large print reading materials early on while vision is still present are crucial [Marshall et al 2010].

4.1.2 Progressive sensorineural hearing loss

Hearing evaluation should begin early in childhood, as otoacoustic emissions and audiometry may reveal subclinical hearing loss. Conductive loss is common in children as a result of chronic otitis media. Hearing can usually be effectively managed with bilateral digital hearing aids, but should be monitored regularly. Myringotomy has been helpful in individuals with recurrent "glue ear". Cochlear implantation has benefitted some patients, but surgeons should be aware of the risk of sudden hypoxia for these patients undergoing procedures requiring anesthesiology [Florentzson et al., 2010].

4.2 Obesity. Insulin resistance/Type 2 diabetes

The major clinical treatment focus is on control of obesity and T2DM.
Candidate therapeutic intervention to treat severe insulin resistance and possibly prevent the transition from insulin resistance to overt diabetes include insulin-sensitizing drugs (metformin and thiazolidinediones) [Sinha et al., 2007 as cited in Atabek, 2007, Nag S et al.,

2003] and beta cell-preserving drugs (incretins, thiazolidinediones) [Pagano et al., 2008, Paisey et al., 2009]. However, this requires close monitoring of liver, cardiac, and renal function. Glitazones are added to further reduce insulin resistance but must be avoided in the presence of active or treated heart failure and when the serum creatinine concentration exceeds 200 µmol/L. Exenatide, an incretin mimetic, an injectable analogue of glucagon-like peptide 1(GLP- 1) could be promising in adults with ALMS.

Weight loss exercises should play a pivotal role in weight reduction plan for ALMS patients, as in other patients diagnosed with dibetes and obesity, although could be challenging. Walking, hiking, biking, and swimming with partners and adaptations for the blind have been helpful. Peripheral sensor-motor neuropathy is a common complication of T2DM, but in a small clinical testing study in ALMS, a full preservation of protective foot sensation was demonstrated [Paisey et al., 2009]. The responsiveness to treatment of hyperglycemia is variable. Younger patients rarely require insulin, but some patients require insulin in very-high doses long term [Marshall et al., 2007a].

Caloric restriction helps control obesity, glucose tolerance and hyperinsulinemia [Holder et al., Lee et al., 2009 & Paisey et al. 2008], although as with children with other genetically acquired obesity syndromes, dietary compliance may be a major problem. Reducing dietary carbohydrates may prove more effective than fat restriction in control of hyperglycemia and hyperinsulinemia [Paisey et al., 2008]. No clinical experience has been reported in ALMS of use of specific appetite suppressant medication, such as duramine or sibutramine.

4.3 Hypertriglyceridemia

Insulin resistance, T2DM, dyslipidaemia and associated cardiac, renal and hepatic consequences coexist from a young age with considerable morbidity and reduction in life expectancy. ALMS patients can have potentially harmfully increased lipid levels. Hypertriglyceridemia can often be normalized by diet, exercise and Metformin. Some patients with severe hypertriglyceridemia responded to a combination of low-fat diet, statins and nicotinic acid [Paisey et al., 2004], very little data existing, however, about the safety and efficacy of such treatments before puberty.

Early introduction of preventative nutrition with low-carbohydrates, exercise and drug therapies (niacin extended-release and incretins) in ALMS could be beneficial [Paisey, 2009].

Pancreatitis should be treated as in the general population, but it is a challenge to treat a patient with multiple system involvement such as ALMS patients [Marshall et al., 2010, Paisey, 2009, Wu WC et al., 2003].

4.4 Impaired growth hormone (GH)-IGF1 axis function

There is an impaired growth hormone (GH)-IGF1 axis function in ALMS (Maffei et al., 2000, 2002), therefore, therapy with recombinant human Growth Hormone (rhGH) has been attempted in a small series of patients and isolated cases and has been reported to be beneficial for some metabolic parameters. Demonstrating growth hormone deficiency in a patient with ALMS, Tai and co-workers assessed the metabolic effects of growth hormone therapy concluding that rhGH therapy might have beneficial effects on body composition, liver fat content, lipid profiles, and insulin resistance in Alström Syndrome patients, with improvement of the glucose homeostasis [Tai et al., 2003]. Also, Maffei et al. found a reduction of ALS (acid labile subunit) and the increase of IGFBP-2 as expression of growth hormone deficiency condition in 15 young adults with ALMS [Maffei et al., 2000]. RhGH therapy should be considered still investigational [Marshall et al. 2007a]. Several studies are needed to prove that this therapy is cost-effective and without risk in patients with ALMS and severe insulin resistance.

4.5 Cardiomyopathy
Patients diagnosed with ALMS should be regularly monitored for cardiac function by echocardiography, even if asymptomatic [Makaryus et al., 2002, Zubrow et al., 2006]. Several authors [Loudon et al., 2009, Makaryus et al., 2007] stated the importance of serial cardiac magnetic resonance scanning in diagnosis of the underlying disease progression and responses to treatment. Long-term angiotensin-converting enzyme inhibition is indicated for the patient with cardiomyopathy. Many patients respond to other medications, which favorably affect heart function, such as diuretics, digitalis, beta-blockers, and spironolactone. Whether cardiac transplantation is a viable option is yet to be determined, due to the multisystemic involvement, particularly pulmonary, endocrine, and renal function. There has been one successful heart-lung transplantation reported in an adolescent patient with Alström Syndrome, but with no T2DM or significant renal failure [Görler et al., 2007]. A second successful heart transplant has been achieved in an infant prior to the onset of the endocrinological and renal disturbances [JD Marshall, Personal communication].

4.6 Thyroid
Replacement therapy with L-thyroxin, when needed, is very effective and well-tolerated in the majority of patients.
Thyroid function should be monitored closely in critical hospital settings [Marshall et al., 2007].

4.7 Urologic
Lack of coordination between bladder and urine outflow (detrusor-urethral dyssynergia) can be helped by intermittent self-catheterization of the bladder. Ileal diversion may be necessary in rare patients [Marshall et al., 2007; Charles, et al. 1990].

4.8 Hypogonadotropic hypogonadism
If abnormalities in pubertal development or menstrual abnormalities are present, the affected individual should be referred to an endocrinologist with expertise in sexual developmental abnormalities. Primary hypogonadism in ALMS males result in low levels of testosterone, treated with weekly or twice monthly injections of testosterone from puberty onwards. Treatment with cyclical oestrogen and progesterone is important and effective to regulate menstrual cycle and development.

4.9 Hepatic disease
Liver function parameters should be routinely monitored, beginning in childhood. Portal hypertension and varices may be aggressively treated with beta-blockers and sclerotherapy of the esophageal veins. Variceal banding could be useful to prevent upper gastro-intestinal hemorrhage. A transjugular intrahepatic portosystemic shunt (TIPS) is used to treat the complications of portal hypertension, when the patient has failed to respond to previous therapeutic measures. Patients with significant portal hypertension should be evaluated early for liver transplantation [Marshall et al., 2007].

4.10 Renal disease

Because renal insufficiency develops slowly as the patient ages, regular testing of renal function (plasma electrolytes, blood urea nitrogen, creatinine, and urea) is important, particularly in the older patient. Baseline values should be taken in children. Management of hypertension, a low-sodium and low-protein diet, avoidance of nephrotoxic drugs are very important in the preservation of renal function, as well as angiotensin-converting enzyme inhibitors prescribed according to general guidelines. Fibrosis and glomerulosclerosis in the kidneys may lead to eventual renal failure, requiring dialysis. Renal transplantation has been successful in several patients, although can be contraindicated in the presence of other complications including morbid obesity, uncontrolled diabetes, and cardiomyopathy [Marshall et al., 2007].

4.11 Pulmonary disease

Pulmonary fibrosis, dilated cardiomyopathy, and scoliosis can compromise cardio-respiratory function, particularly with concomitant respiratory infection or anesthesia in routine surgical procedures. Monitoring cardiac status and oxygenation during acute illness and postoperatively are mandatory, considering that ALMS patients can suddenly, without warning become critically hypoxic [Lynch et al., 2007, Tiwari et al., 2010]. Chronic obstructive airway disease and associated infection should be managed in line with appropriate national guidelines.

4.12 Other
4.12.1 Gastrointestinal

Reflux esophagitis should be diagnosed by barium swallow or upper gastrointestinal endoscopy, in the presence of suggestive symptoms and treated accordingly to the guidelines.

4.12.2 Orthopedic abnormalities

In the presence of flat feet, scoliosis, barrel chest, kyphoscoliosis the referral to an orthopedist is appropriate. Some patients have had surgical intervention for scoliosis, but care should be taken when undertaking surgical procedures, as previously mentioned.

4.12.3 Neurologic manifestations

ALMS patients should be examined for: absence seizures, autistic-spectrum behavioral abnormalities, excessive startle, unexplained joint or muscle pain, muscle dystonia, or hyporeflexia.

4.13 Prevention of secondary complications

There should be routine pediatric immunizations, especially against flu and hepatitis B virus infections.
Families should be encouraged to seek contact with good sources of support and information, such as Alström Syndrome International (www.alstrom.org) or other groups assisting families with this rare disorder.

5. Conclusion

Full understanding of the phenotypic characteristics, particularly with the help of existing mouse models [Collin et al., 2005, Arsov et al., 2006a, 2006b] will lead to better insight into the pathophysiology of *ALMS1*. By developing targeted therapies, certain debilitating aspects of ALMS could be prevented or treated earlier, improving the overall outcome in this complex disorder [Marshall et al., 2007]. Also, careful clinical and genetic studies can contribute to a better understanding of the disease evolution after different therapeutic attempts in Alström Syndrome.

6. References

Alström, C.H., Hallgren, B., Nilsson, L.B., & Åsander H. (1959). Retinal degeneration combined with obesity, diabetes mellitus and neurogenous deafness: a specific syndrome (not hitherto described) distinct from the Laurence-Moon-Bardet-Biedl syndrome: a clinical, endocrinological and genetic examination based on a large pedigree. *Acta psychiatrica et neurologica Scandinavica Supplementum*, Vol. 129, pp. 1-35, ISSN: 0365-5067.

Arsov, T., Larter, C.Z., Nolan, C.J., Petrovsky, N., Goodnow, C.C., Teoh, N..C, Yeh, M.M. & Farrell, G.C. (2006). Adaptive failure to high-fat diet characterizes steatohepatitis in Alms1 mutant mice. *Biochemichal and Biophysical Research Communications*. Vol. 342, No. 4 (April 2006), pp. 1152–1159. (a)

Arsov, T., Silva, D.G., O'Bryan, M.K., Sainsbury, A., Lee, N.J., Kennedy, C., Manji, S.S., Nelms, K., Liu, C., Vinuesa, C.G., de Kretser, D.M., Goodnow, C.C.& Petrovsky, N. (2006). Fat Aussie—a new Alström Syndrome mouse showing a critical role for Alms1 in obesity, diabetes and spermatogenesis. *Molecular Endocrinology*. Vol. 20, No. 7 (July 2006), pp. 1610–1622. (b)

Atabek, M.E. (2007). Re: "Effect of metformin and rosiglitazone in a prepubertal boy with Alström syndrome". *Pediatric Endocrinology & Metabolism*, Vol. 21, No. 1 (January 2008): 100; author reply 100-101.

Awazu, M., Tanaka, T., Yamazaki, K., Kato, S., Higuchi, M. & Matsuo, N. (1995). A 27-year-old woman with Alström syndrome who had liver cirrhosis. *The Keio Journal of Medicine*. Vol. 44, No. 2 (June 1995), pp. 67–73.

Awazu, M., Tanaka, T., Sato, S., Anzo, M., Higuchi, M., Yamazaki, K., & Matsuo, N. (1997). Hepatic dysfunction in two sibs with Alström syndrome: case report and review of the literature. *American journal of medical genetics*. Vol. 69, No. 1 (March 1997), pp. 13–16.

Badano, J.L., Mitsuma, N., Beales, P.L. & Katsanis, N. (2006). The ciliopathies: an emerging class of human genetic disorders. *Annual Review of Genomics and Human Genetics*, Vol.7, (September 2006), pp.125-148, ISSN: 1527-8204.

Bell,C.J., Dinwiddie, D.L., Miller, N.A., Hateley, S.L., Ganusova, E.E., Mudge, J., Langley, R.J., Zhang, L., Lee, C.C., Schilkey, F.D., Sheth, V., Woodward, J.E., Peckham, H.E., Schroth, G.P., Kim &R.W.,Kingsmore, S.F. (2011). Carrier testing for severe childhood recessive diseases by next-generation sequencing. *Science. Translational . Medicine.*, *3*, 65ra4.

Benso, C., Hadjadj, E., Conrath, J. & Denis, D. (2002). Three new cases of Alström syndrome. *Graefe's Archive for Clinical and Experimental Ophthalmology*. Vol. 240, No. 8 (August 2002), pp. 622-627.

Boor, R., Herwig, J., Schrezenmeir, J., Pontz, B.F. & Schönberger, W. (1993). Familial Insulin Resistant Diabetes Associated With Acanthosis Nigricans, Polycystic Ovaries, Hypogonadism, Pigmentary Retinopathy, Labyrinthine Deafness, and Mental

Retardation. *American Journal of Medical Genetics.* Vol. 45, No. 5 (March 1993), pp. 649-653.

Charles, S., Moore, A., Yates, J., Green, T. & Clark, P. (1990). Alström 's syndrome: further evidence of autosomal recessive inheritance and endocrinological dysfunction. *Journal of Medical Genetics.* Vol. 27, No. 9 (September 1990), pp. 590-592.

Collin, G.B., Marshall, J.D., Ikeda, A., W., So, V., Russell-Eggitt, I., Maffei, P., Beck, S., Boerkoel, C.F., Sicolo, N., Martin, M., Nishina, P.M. & Naggert, J.K. (2002). Mutations in ALMS1 cause obesity, type 2 diabetes and neurosensory degeneration in Alström syndrome. *Nature Genetics.* Vol. 31, (May 2002), pp. 74-78.

Collin, G.B., Cyr, E., Bronson, R., Marshall, J.D., Gifford, E.J., Hicks, W., Murray,. SA., Zheng, Q.Y., Smith, R.S., Nishina, P.M. & Naggert, J.K. (2005). Alms1-disrupted mice recapitulate human Alström syndrome. *Human Molecular Genetics.* Vol. 14, No. 16 (August 2005), pp. 2323-2333.

Connolly, M.B., Jan, J.E., Couch, R.M., Wong, L.T., Dimmick, J.E. & Rigg, J.M. (1991). Hepatic dysfunction in Alström disease. *American Journal of Medical Genetics.* Vol. 40, No. 4 (September 1991), pp. 421-424.

Deeble, V.J., Roberts, E., Jackson, A., Lench, N., Karbani, G. & Woods, C.G. (2000). The continuing failure to recognise Alström syndrome and further evidence of genetic homogeneity. *Journal of Medical Genetics.* Vol.37, No.3 (March 2000), pp. 219.

Florentzson, R., Hallén, K. & Möller, C. (2010). Alström syndrome and cochlear implantation. The first clinical experience. *10th International CI-conference June 27-July 1, 2010, Stockholm.*

Girard D. & Petrovsky, N. (2010). Alström syndrome: insights into the pathogenesis of metabolic disorders. *Nature Reviews. Endocrinology.* Vol. 7, No. 2 (February 2011), pp. 77-88.

Gogi, D., Bond, J., Long, V., Sheridan, E. & Woods, C.G. (2007). Exudative retinopathy in a girl with Alström syndrome due to a novel mutation. *The British Journal of Ophthalmology.* Vol. 91, No. 7 (July 2007), pp. 983-984.

Goldstein, J.L.& Fialkow, P.J. (1973). The Alström syndrome. Report of three cases with further delineation of the clinical, pathophysiological, and genetic aspects of the disorder. *Medicine.* Vol. 52, No. 1 (January 1973), pp. 53-71.

Goerler, H., Warnecke, G., Winterhalter, M., Müller, C., Ballmann, M., Wessel, A., Haverich, A., Strüber, M. & Simon, A. (2007). Heart-lung transplantation in a 14-year-old boy with Alström syndrome. *The Journal of Heart and Lung Transplantation.* Vol. 26, No. 11, pp: 1217-8

Hearn, T., Renforth, G.L., Spalluto, C., Hanley, N.A., Piper, K., Brickwood, S., White, C., Connolly, V., Taylor, J.F.N., Russell-Eggitt, I., Bonneau, D., Walker, M. & Wilson, D.I. (2002). Mutation of *ALMS1*, a large gene with a tandem repeat encoding 47 amino acids, causes Alström syndrome. *Nature Genetics.* Vol. 31, No. 1 (May 2002), pp. 79-83.

Hearn, T., Spalluto, C., Phillips, V.J., Renforth, G.L., Copin, N., Hanley, N.A. & Wilson, D.I.(2005). Subcellular localization of ALMS1 supports involvement of centrosome and basal body dysfunction in the pathogenesis of obesity, insulin resistance, and type 2 diabetes. *Diabetes.* Vol. 54, No. 5 (May 2005), pp. 1581-1587.

Hoffman, J.D., Jacobson, Z., Young, T.L., Marshall, J.D. & Kaplan, P. (2005). Familial variable expression of dilated cardiomyopathy in Alström syndrome: a report of four sibs. *American Journal of Medical Genetics*. Vol. 135A, No. 1 (May 2005), pp. 96–98.

Holder, M., Hecker, W. & Gilli, G. Impaired Glucose Tolerance Leads to Delayed Diagnosis of Alström Syndrome. *Diabetes Care*. Vol. 18, No. 5 (May 1995), pp. 698-700.

Joy, T., Cao, H., Black, G., Malik, R., Charlton-Menys, V., Hegele, R.A. & Durrington, P.N. (2007). Alström syndrome (OMIM 203800): a case report and literature review. *Orphanet Journal of Rare Diseases*. Vol. 2, No. 1 (December 2007): 49, Available from http://www.ojrd.com/content/2/1/49.

Khoo, E.Y., Risley, J., Zaitoun, A.M., El-Sheikh, M., Paisey, R.B., Acheson, A.G. & Mansell P.(2009): Alström syndrome and cecal volvulus in 2 siblings. *American Journal of Medical Sciences*. Vol. 337, No. 5 (May 2009), pp: 383-385.

Kinoshita, T., Hanaki, K., Kawashima, Y., Nagaishi, J., Hayashi, A., Okada, S., Murakami, J., Nanba, E., Tomonaga, R. & Kanzaki, S. (2003). A novel non-sense mutation in Alström syndrome: subcellular localization of its truncated protein. *Clinical Pediatric Endocrinology*. Vol. 12, No. 2, pp. 114.

Knorz, V.J., Spalluto, C., Lessard, M., Purvis, T.L., Adigun, F.F., Collin, G.B., Hanley, N.A., Wilson, D. &, Hearn, T.(2010). Centriolar association of ALMS1 and likelycentrosomal functions of the ALMS motif-containing proteins C10orf90 and KIAA1731. *Molecular biology of the cell*. Vol. 1, No. 21 (November 2010), pp:: 3617-3629.

Kocova, M., Sukarova-Angelovska, E., Kacarska, R., Maffei, P., Milan, G. & Marshall, J.D. (2010). The Unique Combination of Dermatological and Ocular Phenotypes in Alström Syndrome: Severe Presentation, Early Onset, and Two Novel *ALMS1* Mutations. *British Journal of Dermatology*. (December 2010) doi: 10.1111/j.1365-2133.2010.10157.x. [Epub ahead of print].

Koray, F., Dorter, C., Benderli, Y., Satman, I., Yilmaz, T., Dinccag, N. & Karsidag, K. (2001). Alström syndrome: a case report. *Journal of Oral Science*. Vol. 43, No. 3 (September 2001), pp. 221–224.

Lee, N., Marshall, J.D., Collin, G.B., Naggert, J.K., Chien, Y.H., Tsai, W.Y.& Hwu, W.L. (2009). Caloric restriction in Alström syndrome prevents hyperinsulinemia. *American Journal of Medical Genetics Part A*. Vol. 149A, No. 4 (February 2009), pp. 666-668.

Li, G., Vega, R., Nelms, K., Gekakis, N., Goodnow, C., McNamara, P., Wu, H., Hong, N. & Glynne, R. (2007). A Role for Alström Syndrome Protein, Alms1, in Kidney Ciliogenesis and Cellular Quiescence. *PLoS Genetics*. Vol. 3, No. 1 (January 2007): e8. doi:10.1371/journal.pgen.0030008.

Loudon, M.A., Bellenger, N.G., Carey, C.M. & Paisey, R.B. (2009). Cardiac magnetic resonance imaging in Alström syndrome. *Orphanet Journal of Rare Diseases*. Vol. 4 (June 2009):14. http://www.ojrd.com/content/4/1/14

Lynch, G., Clinton, S. & Siotia, A. (2007). Anaesthesia and Alström's Syndrome. *Anaesthesia and Intensive Care*. Vol. 35, No. 2 (April 2007), pp. 305-306.

Maffei, P., Munno, V., Marshall, J.D., Milanesi, A., Martini, C., De Carlo, E., Mioni, R., Pontoni, E., Menegazzo, C. & Sicolo, N. (2000). GH and IGF-I Axis in Alström Syndrome. *Journal of Endocrinological Investigation*. Vol. 23 (Suppl. to No. 6), pp. 29.

Maffei, P., Boschetti, M., Orsi, I., Marshall, J.D., Paisey, R.B., Beck, S., Munno, V., Minuto, F., Barreca, A.M. & Sicolo, N. (2002). The IGF system in Alström Syndrome. *Growth Hormone and IGF Research.* Vol. 12, No. 4, pp. 291.

Maffei, P., Munno, V., Marshall, J.D., Scandellari, C. & Sicolo, N. (2002). The Alström syndrome: is it a rare or unknown disease? *Annali Italiani di Medicina Interna.* Vol. 17, No. 4 (October-December 2002), pp. 221–228.

Maffei, P., Boschetti, M., Marshall, J.D., Paisey, R.B., Beck, S., Resmini, E., Collin, G.B., Naggert, J.K., Milan, G., Vettor, R., Minuto, F., Sicolo, N. & Barreca, A. (2007). Characterization of the IGF system in 15 patients with Alström syndrome. *Clinical endocrinology.* Vol. 66, No. 2 (February 2007), pp. 269–275.

Makaryus, A.N., Popowski, B., Kort, S., Paris, Y. & Mangion, J. (2003). A rare case of Alström syndrome presenting with rapidly progressive severe dilated cardiomyopathy diagnosed by echocardiography. *Journal of the American Society of Echocardiogr.aphy.* Vol. 16, No. 2 (February 2003), pp. 194–196.

Markaryus, A.N., Zubrow, M.E., Marshall, J.D., Gillam, L.D. &Mangion, J.R. (2007). Cardiac manifestations of Alström syndrome: echocardiographic findings. *Journal of American Society of Echocardiography.* Vol.20, No. 12, (December 2007), pp.1359-1363.

Malm, E., Ponjavic, V., Nishina, P.M., Naggert, J.K., Hinman, E.G., Andréasson, S., Marshall, J.D. & Möller, C. (2008). Full-field electroretinography and marked variability in clinical phenotype of Alström syndrome. *Archives of Ophthalmology.* Vol. 126, No. 1 (January 2008), pp. 51-57.

Marshall, J.D., Ludman, M.D., Shea, S.E., Salisbury, S.R., Willi, S.M., LaRoche, R.G. & Nishina, P.M. (1997). Genealogy, natural history, and phenotype of Alström syndrome in a large Acadian kindred and three additional families. *American Journal of Medical Genetics.*Vol.73, No.2 (December 1997), pp. 150–161.

Marshall, J.D., Bronson, R.T., Collin, G.B., Nordstrom, A.D., Maffei, P., Paisey, R.B., Carey, C., Macdermott, S., Russell-Eggitt, I., Shea, S.E., Davis, J., Beck, S., Shatirishvili, G., Mihai, C.M., Hoeltzenbein, M., Pozzan, G.B., Hopkinson, I., Sicolo, N., Naggert, J.K. & Nishina, P.M. (2005). *New Alström syndrome phenotypes based on the evaluation of 182 cases.* Archives of internal medicine. Vol. 165, No. 6 (March 2005), pp. 675–683.

Marshall, J.D., Beck, S., Maffei, P.& Naggert, J.K. 2007(a). Alström syndrome. *European Journal of Human Genetics.* Vol. 15, No.12 (December 2007), pp. 1193–1202.

Marshall, J.D., Hinman, E.G., Collin, G.B., Beck, S., Cerqueira, R., Maffei, P., Milan, G., Zhang, W., Wilson, D.I., Hearn, T., Tavares, P., Vettor, R., Veronese, C., Martin, M., So, W.V., Nishina, P.M. & Naggert, J.K. (2007). Spectrum of ALMS1 variants and evaluation of genotype–phenotype correlations in Alström syndrome. *Human Mutation.* Vol. 28, No. 11 (November 2007), pp. 1113-1123 (b).

Marshall, J.D., Paisey, R.B., Carey, C. & Macdermott, S. (Last update June 2010). *Alström Syndrome.* GeneReviews. NCBI Bookshelf. Available from http://www.ncbi.nlm.nih.gov/books/NBK1267/

Michaud, J.L., Héon, E., Guilbert, F., Weill, J., Puech, B., Benson, L., Smallhorn, J.F., Shuman, C.T., Buncic, J.R., Levin, A.V., Weksberg, R. & Brevière, G.M. (1996). Natural history of Alström syndrome in early childhood: Onset with dilated cardiomyopathy. *The Journal of Pediatrics.* Vol. 128, No. 2 (February 1996), pp. 225-229.

Mihai, C.M., Catrinoiu, D., Marshall, J.D., Stoicescu, R. & Tofolean, J.T. (2008). Cilia, Alström Syndrome - molecular concept, mechanisms and therapeutic perspectives. *Journal of Medicine and Life*. Vol. 1, No. 3 (July-September 2008), pp. 254-261.

Mihai, C.M., Catrinoiu, D., Toringhibel, M., Stoicescu, R.M., Negreanu-Pirjol, T. & Hancu, A. (2009). Impaired IGF1-GH axis and new therapeutic options in Alström Syndrome patients: a case series. *Cases Journal*. Vol. 2, No. 1 (January 2009): 19. http://www.casesjournal.com/content/2/1/19.

Minton, J.A., Owen, K.R., Ricketts, C.J., Crabtree, N., Shaikh, G., Ehtisham, S., Porter, J.R., Carey, C., Hodge, D., Paisey, R., Walker, M. & Barrett, T.G. (2006). Syndromic obesity and diabetes: changes in body composition with age and mutation analysis of ALMS1 in 12 United Kingdom kindreds with Alström syndrome. The Journal of Clinical Endocrinology and Metabolism.*Vol. 91, No. 8 (August* 2006), pp. 3110-3116.

Möller, C. (2005). Alström syndrome. *The National Swedish Board of Health and Welfare*. Nov 2005, *Available from http//www.sos.se*

Nag, S., Kelly, W.F., Walker, M. & Connolly, V. (2003). Type 2 diabetes in Alström syndrome: Targeting insulin resistance with a thiazolidinedione.*Endocrine Abstracts*. Vol. 5, pp. 104. British Endocrine Society, March 2003.

Paisey, R.B., Carey, C.M., Bower, L., Marshall, J., Taylor, P., Maffei, P. & Mansell, P. (2004). Hypertriglyceridaemia in Alström's syndrome: causes and associations in 37 cases. *Clinical Endocrinology*. Vol. 60, No. 2 (February 2004), pp. 228-231.

Paisey, R. B., Hodge, D. & Williams, K. (2008). Body fat distribution, serum glucose, lipid and insulin response to meals in Alström syndrome. *Journal of Human Nutrition and Dietetics*. Vol. 21, No. 3 (June 2008), pp. 268-274.

Paisey, R.B., Paisey, R.M., Thomson, M.P., Bower, L., Maffei, P., Shield, J.P., Barnett, S. & Marshall, J.D. (2009). Protection From Clinical Peripheral Sensory Neuropathy in Alström Syndrome in Contrast to Early-Onset Type 2 Diabetes. *Diabetes Care*. Vol. 32, No. 3 (March 2009b), pp. 462-464.

Paisey, R.B. (2009). New insights and therapies for the metabolic consequences of Alström syndrome. *Current Opinion in Lipidology*. Vol. 20, No. 4 (August 2009), pp. 315-230.

Quiros-Tejeira, R.E., Vargas, J. & Ament, M.E. (2001). Early-onset liver disease complicated with acute liver failure in Alström syndrome. *American Journal of Medical Genetics*. Vol. 101, No. 1 (June 2001), pp. 9-11.

Ozgül, R.K., Satman. I., Collin, G.B., Hinman, E.G., Marshall, J.D., Kocaman, O., Tütüncü, Y., Yilmaz, T. & Naggert, J.K. (2007). Molecular analysis and long-term clinical evaluation of three siblings with Alström syndrome. *Clinical Genetics*. Vol. 72, No.4 (October 2007), pp. 351-356.

Pagano, C., Romano, S., Maffei, P., Sicolo, N. & Vettor, R.(2008). Insulin resistance and diabetes in Alstrom syndrome. *5th International Scientific Congress. ALSTRÖM SYNDROME*. Padua – Venice , Italy, October 17-18, 2008.

Patel, S., Minton, J.A., Weedon, M.N., Frayling, T.M., Ricketts, C., Hitman, G.A., McCarthy, M.I., Hattersley, A.T., Walker, M. & Barrett, T.G. (2006). Common variations in the ALMS1 gene do not contribute to susceptibility to type 2 diabetes in a large white UK population. *Diabetologia*, Vol. 49, No. 6 (June 2006), pp. 1209-1213.

Russell-Eggitt, I.M., Clayton, P.T., Coffey, R., Kriss, A., Taylor, D.S. & Taylor, J.F. (1998). Alström syndrome. Report of 22 cases and literature review. *Ophthalmology*. Vol. 105, No. 7, pp. 1274-1280.

Satman, I., Yilmaz, M.T., Gursoy, N., Karsidag, K., Dinccag, N., Ovali, T., Karadeniz, S., Uysal, V., Bugra, Z., Okten, A., & Devrim, S. (2002). Evaluation of insulin resistant diabetes mellitus in Alström syndrome: a long-term prospective follow-up of three siblings. Diabetes Research and Clinical Practice. *Vol. 56, No. 3 (June* 2002), pp. 189-196.

Sebag J, Albert DM & Craft JL (1984): The Alström syndrome: ophthalmic histopathology and renal ultrastructure. *British Journal of Ophthalmology* Vol. 68 No. 7, (July 1984) pp. 494-501.

Sinha, S.K., Bhangoo, A., Anhalt, H., Maclaren, N., Marshall, J.D., Collin, G.B., Naggert, J.K. & Ten, S. (2007). Effect of metformin and rosiglitazone in a prepubertal boy with Alström syndrome. *Journal of Pediatric Endocrinology & Metabolism*, Vol. 21, No. 1 (September 2007), pp. 1045-1052.

Smith, J.C., McDonnell, B., Retallick, C., McEniery, C., Carey, C., Davies, J.S., Barrett, T., Cockcroft, J.R. & Paisey, R (2007). Is arterial stiffening in Alström syndrome linked to the development of cardiomyopathy? *European Journal of Clinical Investigation.* Vol. 37, No. 2, (February 2007), pp. 99-105.

Tai, T.S., Lin, S.Y. & Sheu, W.H.H. (2003). Metabolic Effects of Growth Hormone Therapy in an Alström Syndrome Patient. *Hormone Research.* Vol. 60, No. 6, pp. 297-301.

Titomanlio, L., De Brasi, D., Buoninconti, A., Sperandeo, M.P., Pepe, A. & Andria, G. (2004). Alström syndrome: intrafamilial phenotypic variability in sibs with a novel nonsense mutation of the ALMS1 gene. *Clinical Genetics 2004.* Vol. 65, No. 2 (February 2004), pp. 156-157.

Tiwari, A., Awasthi, D., Tayal, S. & Ganguly, S, (2010). Alström syndrome: A rare genetic disorder and its anaesthetic significance. *Indian Journal of Anesthesiology.* Vol. 54, No. 2 (March 2010), pp. 154-156.

Van den Abeele, K., Craen, M., Schuil, J. & Meire, F.M. (2001). Ophthalmologic and systemic features of the Alström syndrome: report of 9 cases. *Bulletin de la Société Belge d'Ophtalmologie.* Vol. 281 (2001), pp. 67-72.

Vingolo, E.M., Salvatore, S., Grenga, P.L., Maffei, P., Milan, G. & Marshall J (2010). High-resolution spectral domain optical coherence tomography images of alström syndrome. *Journal pediatric ophthalmology strabismus* Vol. 47: e1-e3 (May 2010)Welsh, L. W. Alström Syndrome: Progressive Deafness and Blindness (2007). *The Annals of Otology, Rhinology & Laryngology.* Vol. 116, Vol. 4 (April 2007), pp. 281-285.

Worthley, M.I. & Zeitz, C.J. (2001). Case of Alström syndrome with late presentation dilated cardiomyopathy. *Internal Medicine Journal.* Vol. 31, No. 9 (December 2001), pp. 569-570.

Wu, W.C., Chen, S.C., Dia, C.Y., Yu, M.L., Hsieh, M.Y., Lin, Z.Y., Wang, L.Y., Tsai, J.F. & Chang, W.Y. (2002). Alström Syndrome with Acute Pancreatitis: A Case Report. *The Kaohsiung Journal of Medical Sciences.* Vol. 19, No. 7 (July 2003), pp. 358-360.

Zubrow, M.E., Makaryus, A., Marshall, J.D., Horowitz, S., Gillam, L.D. & Mangion, J.R. (2006). Echocardiographic Features of the Cardiomyopathy Associated With Alström Syndrome: A Retrospective Review. *American Society for Echocardiology Scientific Sessions*, Baltimore, MD, June, 2006.

7

Alpha One Antitrypsin Deficiency: A Pulmonary Genetic Disorder

Michael Sjoding and D. Kyle Hogarth
University of Chicago
U.S.A

1. Introduction

Alpha one antitrypsin protein (A1AT), is encoded on the SERPINA1 (serpin peptidase inhibitor, claude A, member 1 gene), (OMIM 107400), located on chromosome 14q32.1 and functions as inhibitor of the enzyme neutrophil elastase. People with a low serum level of this protein are described as having the alpha-1-antrypsin deficiency (A1ATD), (OMIM #613490), one of the most common heritable disorders. Having this disorder can predispose an individual to a variety of clinical diseases, with the lungs and the liver being the two organs most commonly affected. The A1AT protein is synthesized mainly in the liver by hepatocytes, secreted into the blood stream, and acts as an inhibitor of neutrophil elastase released primarily in the lung during inflammation. The most common allele for the SERPINA1 gene is named M (Middle), which encodes a normal A1AT protein identified in the middle on an isoelectric focusing gel. Over 120 allelic variants have been discovered and are named based on their position and movement on isoelectric gels, A-L if they exhibit faster migration than M, and N-Z if the proteins migrate more slowly. Rare mutations are often named after the discoverer or location of discover (Mmalton, Lowell, etc). A patient's genotype is notated as PI*Allele-Allele, and so patient homozygous for the wild-type A1AT protein is noted as being PI*M-M.

The most common allelic variation causing clinical disease is the Z protein, manifesting most often in the setting of the genotype PI*Z-Z. This mutated protein spontaneously misfolds and then polymerizes with other misfolded A1AT proteins, becoming trapped in large quantities in the endoplasmic reticulum of liver hepatocytes. This results in liver inflammation and fibrosis, and can lead to clinically significant cholestasis and cirrhosis. Not all allelic variants of A1ATD cause liver damage, however, as some encode truncated proteins which do not misfold or polymerize. Rare null mutations have also been discovered due to point mutations that introduce a premature stop codon within the DNA sequence. Patients with the genotype PI*Null-Null do not develop liver disease because they do not synthesize mutated protein, but are at extremely high risk for the development of lung disease because of their inability to inhibit neutrophil elastase.

In the case of the Z allele, the trapped protein is ineffectively secreted into the blood stream, resulting in a low serum concentration of A1AT. The mutated protein also has a reduced functional activity, making it a less effective inhibitor of neutrophil elastase. Without an appropriate level of functional A1AT in lung tissue, neutrophil elastase is free to break down elastin, a critical component of lung structure, which is thought to be the major mechanism leading to lung damage and the development of emphysema. The lung injury is worsened in the setting of chronic tobacco use, making smoking cessation paramount in the management of people with the deficiency.

Clinical disease associated with the A1AT deficiency is highly variable, suggesting that many genetic modifiers and environmental exposures play a role in the disease expression. The typical symptoms of pulmonary disease include exertional shortness of breath, wheezing, and chronic cough. The cornerstone of disease management is ensuring total smoking abstinence in all patients, as smoking is associated with a much higher rate of decline in lung function in patients with A1AT deficiency. Replacement therapy with purified A1AT protein given intravenously has been approved in several countries as treatment of the deficiency state, and can prevent decline in lung function. Though many studies support its use and clinical benefit, true randomized placebo controlled studies have been limited in size and scope.

2. History of the disorder

In 1962 at the University of Lund, Sweden, Dr. Carl-Bertil Laurell (1919-2001) was examining the serum protein electrophoresis strips of patients with chronic obstructive pulmonary disease, when he noted an absence of the alpha-one band in a small group of patients. Dr. Sten Eriksson was a resident at the University hospital at the time and assisted Laurell in the study because of his previous experience with protein chemistry. Together, they discovered five cases that formed the basis of their first report of alpha one- antitrypsin deficiency. Three of the five patients in their report developed emphysema at an early age, leading to the conclusion that there must be an association between pulmonary disease and the alpha-one band deficiency (Laurell & Eriksson 1963).

It was later discovered that the major function of the alpha 1-antitrypsin protein was to inhibit the enzyme neutrophil elastase, a protease released by neutrophils in the lungs during inflammation. Neutrophil elastase was shown to induce experimental emphysema in animals. (Senior, et al. 1977). These findings lead to the first hypothesis describing the pathogenesis of lung disease, that an imbalance of proteases and anti-proteases could result in an unregulated destruction of critical components of lung structure, namely elastin, leading to the development of clinical lung disease. This hypothesis continues to be central to the understanding of lung disease pathogenesis to this day, and helps explain why patient deficient in A1AT, which could not regulate neutrophil elastase, would be predisposed to emphysema development.

Work by Dr. H. L. Sharp described the association between alpha one antitrypsin deficiency and liver disease in 10 children in 1969 (Sharp et al., 1969). Sharp discovered intracellular inclusions in the liver hepatocytes of A1ATD individuals, and further work found these inclusions to be polymers of the mutant Z allele of the A1AT protein. Evidence for A1ATD was also supported from the results of a large epidemiologic study published in 1976 by Sveger in Sweden (Sveger, 1976). After screening 200,000 infants for A1ATD he identified 127 infants and found that 14 developed cholestatic jaundice in infancy. These studies established the role of A1AT in liver disease pathogenesis.

3. Genetics

Alpha-1-antitrypsin deficiency has been described as an autosomal co-dominant disorder or as an autosomal recessive disorder. Patients who are heterozygote for the enzyme deficiency have roughly half the serum concentration of A1AT compared with normal individuals, and homozygote have a very low serum concentration of enzyme. This pattern of enzyme levels has lead many authors to describe the inheritance pattern as autosomal co-dominant, (see DeMeo's review on the genetics of A1ATD as one example (DeMeo & Silverman, 2004)). Heterozygotes have only a small increased risk for developing clinically significant disease, while homozygotes are at a much higher risk for developing disease, leading other authors to describe the deficiency as having autosomal recessive inheritance (see Alpha-1 antitrypsin deficiency page on the National Center for Biotechnology Information website as an example). We prefer to describe the inheritance pattern as autosomal co-dominant, as this highlights the fact that heterozygotes for the deficiency are at an increased risk for clinical disease when compared with the general population, especially in the setting of external risk factors for lung disease (e.g. smoking). Another important characteristic of the deficiency is its variable clinical expressivity. Some homozygotes for the deficiency do not develop impairment in the lung function and never develop symptoms related to the disease (Seersholm & Kok-Jensen 1998). Incomplete penetrance and variable clinical phenotype (expressivity) is one of the reasons why population studies estimating the number of individuals with the deficiency are much higher than the actual number of people who have been diagnosed. For unclear reasons, A1ATD is rarely tested for despite guidelines that recommend otherwise for clear patient types. Complicating A1ATD diagnosis is the continued low rate of diagnosis and management of Chronic Obstructive Pulmonary Disease (COPD).

More than 120 mutations in the SERPINA1 gene have been identified, although many do not cause a defect in the serum protein or function or relevant clinical disease (US National Library of Medicine August 2009). The allele most common to the general population is the M allele, and the most clinically relevant variants are the S and Z alleles. People with the PI*Z-Z genotype make up at least 95% of deficient individuals who present with clinical disease, and PI*M-Z heterozygotes on very rare occasion have any symptoms. The Z allele is caused by a glutamic acid to lysine substitution at position 342. A more common allelic variant is the S protein, caused by a glutamic acid to valine substitution at position 264. This protein is successfully degraded before accumulating in the liver and does not cause liver disease. PI*S-S individuals are not thought to be at risk for pulmonary disease, however the compound heterozygotes PI*S-Z or PI*S-null are at an increased risk for developing pulmonary symptoms. Null alleles are due to mutations that introduce an early stop codon, which prevents complete transcription of the gene. Patients who are homozygote for the null mutation (PI*null-null), or heterozygote with Z (PI*null-Z) are at the highest risk for developing severe pulmonary symptoms (Stoller & Aboussouan, 2005).

The Z allele occurs mainly within one haplotype, meaning that other genetic material surrounding the allele is similar, and suggests a single relatively recent origin in Caucasians (Cox et al., 1985). Its high frequency in southern Scandinavia and estimated origination date of approximately 2000 years ago suggests that the mutation originated in the Viking population and was spread across Europe by Viking raiders. Using the pooled epidemiological data on 75,390 individuals, researchers estimated the prevalence of both the Z and S mutation in 21 countries. With this information, they created a topographic map of the mutation prevalence, depicting how the mutation may have spread. The ZZ phenotype shows highest prevalence in the southern Scandinavian Peninsula, Latvia, and Denmark, and progressively decreases towards the South and the East of Europe. The S allele has its highest prevalence in the Iberian Peninsula, which includes modern day Portugal, and Spain, as well as Southern France and gradually decreases towards the North, South and

East of the continent. The S mutation appears to have originated within the Portuguese population, but its date of origin is unknown. It is assumed that both mutations were introduced to North America by mass migration.

Most Common Phenotypes and likely Pulmonary Consequences of A1AT alleles

Allele	Concentration of A1AT (micromoles/L)	COPD risk
Pi-MM	20-53	General population
Pi-MS	20-48	Very low/ gen population
Pi-SS	15-33	Low
Pi-MZ	12-35	Low
Pi-SZ	9-19	Variable
Pi-ZZ	2.5-7	High
Pi-Z-null	<2.5	Very high
Pi-null-null	none	Very high

Fig. 1. Common alleles of the SERPINA1 gene (adapted from Hogarth & Rachelefsky, 2008)

4. Epidemiology

There is an estimated 1.1 million people with severe A1ATD and 116 million carriers in the world (Luisetti & Seersholm, 2004). Although previously consider a disease of Caucasians, recent data shows that A1ATD exists in all racial subgroups worldwide including African blacks, Arabs and Jews in the Middle East, as well as people from central, far east and south east Asia (de Serres, 2002). Determining the number of people in the United States with emphysema primarily due to A1ATD can made by taking the estimate of the number of Americans with COPD (3.1 million), and the estimate that about 1.9% of patients with emphysema are likely due to A1ATD (Lieberman et al., 1986). This results in an estimate that at least 59000 individuals in the United States have severe symptomatic COPD due to A1ATD. Large screening studies have also been undertaken, including the classic prevalence study done by Sveger, where 200,000 neonates were screened at birth in Sweden (Sveger 1974). The results demonstrated 1 in 1575 live births were homozygous for the Z mutation (PI*ZZ). A similar study undertaken in Oregon, USA screened 107,038 newborns and found the prevalence of the ZZ phenotype in that population to be 1 in 5097 (O'Brien et al., 1978). Among 20,000 healthy blood donors tested in St. Louis, Missouri in the United States, 1 in 2857 were homozygous for the Z mutation. With this information, the researchers estimated a total prevalence of 700 individuals in St. Louis with the deficiency, however they were only to locate 28 (4%) after contacting local doctors (Silverman, et al., 1989). Estimates from Central and Southern Africa based on limited data from screening studies estimated that 1 in 15 Africans are S carriers. Our own data on carrier rate in Americans of African Descent demonstrate 1 in 18 are S carriers. Epidemiologic data not only highlight that prevalence of the deficiency is high, but reinforce that the disease is significantly under diagnosed in most populations.

5. Pathophysiology

The SERPINA1 gene, previously known as the PI (proteasome inhibitor) gene, is located between 14q31.1-32.3 on the human genome, and encodes A1AT, which is a 52-kD glycoprotein composed of 394 amino acids. The active site is a single peptide bond, Met358-

Ser359. The protein is primarily synthesized and secreted by hepatocytes, but also in mononuclear cells, intestinal and lung epithelial cells. A1AT is an acute phase reactant with a normal concentration in serum of 20-53 micromole/L. Alpha one antitrypsin is a member of the serpin family of protease inhibitors, which regulate important proteolytic enzyme cascades including the coagulation cascade, complement cascade, and plasmin inhibition (Crowther et al., 2004). Serpins not only inhibit proteases but cause a conformational change in their structure readying them for destruction. A1AT's mechanism of inhibition has been likened to a mouse-trap. When neutrophil elastase attacks A1AT enzyme, it binds and then cleaves its reactive center loop, which causes a spring-like movement within the A1AT molecule to fling the elastase molecule across itself, inhibiting its function and altering its structure so it can be destroyed (Huntington et al., 2000).

5.1 Pulmonary pathophysiology

The prevailing theory describing the pathogenesis of emphysema in A1AT deficient individuals is of an imbalance in protease and anti-protease enzymes in lung tissue. Neutrophil elastase is released during inflammation and leads to an uncontrolled proteolytic attack on elastin, which is left unchecked by the low concentration of alpha one antitrypsin (Gadek et al., 1981). Furthermore, the circulating Z allele of A1AT has been shown to have a less functional active site, making the small amount of mutant protein a functionally ineffective inhibitor of neutrophil elastase (Ogushi et al., 1987). Elastin is the backbone of lung structure, and a critical component of the lungs ability to recoil. It is thought that elastin's destruction leads to lung hyperinflation and obstruction, leading to development of emphysema.

More recently, studies have shown that the mutated protein can form polymers within the lungs, similar to the polymerization occurring in the liver, and become chemoattractants for neutrophils resulting in excessive inflammation. Polymers of the mutated A1AT protein have been identified in the bronchial alveolar lavage fluid of individuals with the PiZZ phenotype (Mulgrew et al., 2004). These findings have lead to a possible evolutionary explanation for why alpha-one anti-trypsin deficiency became so prevalent in many populations. The argument for the selective advantage of being a carrier is that a less regulated pulmonary inflammatory response to an external noxious stimulus (e.g. infection) would lead to higher chances of recovery. Prior to the discovery of antibiotics for respiratory infections, the mortality rate from these illnesses was high. A more robust and unregulated inflammatory response in the lungs could have provided a survival advantage to the carriers (Lomas, 2006). In the modern antibiotic era, and the advent of mass-produced external noxious stimuli (smoking, pollution), this mutation does not appear to have a theoretical selective advantage anymore.

How cigarette smoke accelerates the decline of lung function in A1ATD has also been studied. When the methionine amino acid in the active site of A1AT protein is oxidized by cigarette smoke, the kinetics of neutrophil elastase inhibition is reduced (Ogushi et al., 1991). Newer experimental data shows A1AT may have other roles in the lung epithelium besides inhibiting neutrophil elastase. A1AT has recently been found to block the cigarette smoke mediated release of TNF-alpha and MMP-12 in alveolar macrophages (Churg at al., 2007). In cellular studies, A1AT has also been found to inhibit apoptosis through direct inhibition of activated Caspase-3 (Petrache et al., 2006). The link between A1AT and apoptosis has lead to new theories of emphysema development as both an inflammatory disorder and accelerated lung aging process.

5.2 Liver pathophysiology

People with the alpha one antitrypsin deficiency develop liver damage by a completely different mechanism. After being synthesized in hepatocytes, the mutated A1AT alleles bind together to form large polymers that result in inflammation and fibrosis. Liver disease caused by A1ATD has become the prototypical disease in a new category of diseases, termed the conformational diseases. Also included in this category of diseases are Alzheimer's and other forms of neurodegenerative dementias, which are caused by the aggregation of proteins in neurons (Carrell & Lomas, 2002). People with the PI*ZZ mutation of A1AT have a high concentration of the mutated alpha-one antitrypsin allele in the endoplasmic reticulum of liver cells. The Z mutation allows the protein to undergo a spontaneous structural change, which opens up the main sheets of the molecule and bind to the reactive center in the next molecule. These interactions can result in the formation of long polymers of mutated proteins (Lomas et al., 1992). The large protein structures aggregate in liver cells, which is thought to lead to inflammation, fibrosis and cirrhosis by a still unclear mechanism. The reason why some people with ZZ allele genotype do not develop clinically relevant liver disease is also not clear.

6. Clinical manifestations

A1ATD is often unrecognized despite the high prevalence of lung disease in the United States and the world. Alpha-1–related lung disease presents with common respiratory symptoms including dyspnea, decreased exercise tolerance, wheezing, cough, excess sputum production, frequent lower respiratory tract infections, and a history of suspected allergies and/or asthma (Needham & Stockley, 2004). These symptoms are often ascribed to other diseases for years prior to the correct diagnosis of alpha one antitrypsin deficiency. A 1994 mail survey found that on average it took 7.2 years after symptom onset before the diagnosis was made, and 44% of people saw three different physicians before a diagnosis was made (Stoller et al., 1994). A similar survey repeated in 2003 found the mean time to diagnosis was 5.6 years, however, the delay was more pronounced in older and female patients (Stoller et al., 2005). Since the diagnosis of A1ATD requires one simple blood test, clearly more effort needs to be made to educate both physicians and the public of the disease and the importance of a diagnosis.

There is significant variability in the age of symptom onset in people with A1ATD, and some smokers and non-smokers may never develop symptoms. This highlights the variability in disease penetrance among deficient individuals, and makes accurate descriptions of the common symptoms and other clinical characteristics of deficient individuals difficult to obtain. Most of the clinical characteristics and other features of the deficiency are obtained by studying large registries of patients with the disease. These data sets are often flawed by ascertainment bias. Most of the patients in the large A1ATD registries presented initially to a doctor with concerning pulmonary symptoms, eventually leading to a diagnosis of A1ATD. These patients are then referred to a specialist who will enroll them into the registry, and are termed index cases. Less often, asymptomatic individuals who are diagnosed after a family screening are enrolled (non-index cases). This was true of the large group of 1129 A1AT deficient individuals in the National Heart, Lung and Blood Institute Registry (McElvaney et al., 1997). 72% of the enrollees were index cases, receiving a diagnosis of the A1ATD after developing concerning pulmonary symptoms, and 20% were non-index cases, diagnosed by screening following an investigation of family members of individuals with A1ATD. In that registry, the remaining smaller percentage of people were diagnosed after they were discovered to have abnormal chest radiograph findings, abnormal pulmonary function tests, liver abnormalities, or other blood testing. therapy with the purified A1AT protein.

6.1 Pulmonary clinical manifestations

The NHLBI registry data provides the best clinical picture of the typical patients diagnosed with this deficiency. 97% of them had the PI*ZZ mutation, and most were diagnosed in the third or fourth decade of life. The most common symptom in this group was shortness of breath on exertion (83%). Other common symptoms included wheezing during an upper respiratory illness (75%), wheezing without upper respiratory illness (65%), recent lung infection (67%), and chronic productive cough (49%). Pulmonary function testing of individuals in the NHLBI registry demonstrated a pattern consistent with emphysema: the median Forced Expiratory Volume in one second (FEV1) was 47% of predicted, the ratio of the FEV1/FVC (Forced Vital Capacity) was 43% of predicted, and the DLCO (which represents the amount of destruction in alveoli-capillary units) was 50% of predicted. These numbers highlight a common feature of people with A1ATD: the airflow obstruction (represented by low FEV1 and low FEV1/FVC) seen on pulmonary function testing seems to be out of proportion to the lifetime quantity of cigarettes they have smoked. Also in the NHLBI registry, 28% of people showed significant bronchodilator responsiveness (i.e., reversibility) of their airflow obstruction on pulmonary function tests during their initial visit, which is a characteristic of people with asthma (Eden et al., 2003). With these common symptoms and pulmonary function test characteristics, it is easy to see why patients with A1ATD are often misdiagnosed as having only uncomplicated asthma, emphysema or COPD.

In contrast to the above registry data, a study with high level of non-index cases (e.g. siblings of affected individuals) found that far fewer of this population had typical pulmonary symptoms of A1ATD (Seersholm & Kok-Jensen, 1998). After a mean follow-up of 8 years, only 46% of the non-index case patients reported symptoms of shortness of breath, 27% reported wheezing, and 14% reported a chronic cough. Also in this group, their average FEV1 was 100% of predicted, and their FEV1/FVC = 0.79, essentially normal pulmonary function tests.

Classically, severe A1ATD causes panlobar emphysema with lower lobe predominance on radiologic imagining studies (Guenter et al., 1968). However, with high-resolution chest CT scanning, bronchiectasis has also been found to be a common feature of patients with A1ATD. In a study of 74 people with the P*ZZ phenotype, 70 subjects had bronchiectasis changes on CT scan. 27% of the study participates were felt to have clinically significant bronchiectasis, which was described as 4 or more airway segments with bronchiectasis plus symptoms of regular sputum production (the most common symptom of people with bronchiectasis) (Parr et al., 2007).

Multiple studies have measured the rate of decline in lung function among patients with A1ATD using the forced expiratory volume in one second (FEV1) as a marker of lung disease progression. This measure is used regularly to quantify the severity and progression of patients with COPD and asthma. For non-smokers with normal levels of A1AT, the rate of FEV1 decline is around 20-30 mL/year. The decline in the FEV1 among a group of A1ATD patients who never smoked was 67 mL/year, was 54 mL/year in ex-smokers, and was 109 mL/year in current smokers (Alpha-1-antitrypsin deficiency study group, 1998). The first two numbers are not statistically significantly different, however the third is significant, which highlights the extreme importance of smoking cessation in all people with A1ATD. The difference in the rate of decline of FEV1 between A1ATD and normal patients highlights the principle of augmentation therapy with replacement alpha-one protein. Mortality in people with A1ATD is most frequently due to respiratory failure, followed by liver cirrhosis. The observed yearly mortality rate ranges between 1.7-3.5%. Factors associated with increased mortality include older age, lower education, lower FEV1, history of lung transplant, and people who were not receiving augmentation therapy with the purified A1AT protein (Stoller et al., 2005).

6.2 Liver clinical manifestations

A1ATD has a strong association with liver disease, leading to a recommendation that all individuals of any age with unexplained liver dysfunction should undergo testing for the deficiency. In the Swedish population screening study by Sveger, of 200,000 people, 18% of the 120 people found to be homozygote for the Z mutation had some evidence of liver dysfunction (Sveger, 1974). This included obstructive jaundice in 12%, and minor abnormalities in others. Among those with liver dysfunction, the risk of developing cirrhosis is high. It is possible that younger individuals more often have liver dysfunction because their hepatocytes are less well equipped to handle the polymerized A1AT proteins. In a small autopsy series of patients with A1AT disease, cirrhosis was observed in 34% of patients, and hepatocellular carcinoma was observed in 34% of those with cirrhosis (Eriksson, 1987).

6.3 Necrotizing panniculitis

Panniculitis is an uncommon skin disorder with a strong association with A1ATD. It is characterized by painful, cutaneous nodules at the sites of trauma, often on the trunk, back and thighs. On biopsy, areas of fat necrosis are interspersed with areas of normal tissue. The skin necrosis is felt to develop because of unopposed proteolysis, and augmentation therapy has been described as causing a rapid resolution of the disease (Dowd et al., 1995).

7. Testing for disease

Guidelines published by the American Thoracic Society and European Respiratory Society in 2003 have helped clarify who should undergo testing for A1ATD (American Thoracic Society, 2003). The guidelines divided people into categories for whom testing is recommended, those for whom testing could be discussed and considered, and those for whom testing was discouraged. For the following group of people testing should be recommended. These include: adults with emphysema, chronic obstructive pulmonary disease, or asthma with incompletely reversible airflow obstruction, people of all ages with otherwise unexplained liver disease, or adults with necrotizing panniculitis. In the following group of people testing could be considered and discussed: adults with bronchiectasis without an obvious etiology, adults with anti-proteinase 3-positive vasculitis (C-ANCA [anti-neutrophil cytoplasmic antibody]-positive vasculitis, formerly known as "Wegener's Granulomatosis"), adolescents with airflow obstruction on pulmonary function tests.

When family history is considered, the following recommendations were made. There is a strong recommendation for testing all siblings of an individual with A1ATD. There is also a recommendation to consider testing in the following situations: individuals with a family history of emphysema or liver disease, or anyone with a family history of A1ATD or A1ATD heterozygote. The 2003 guidelines recommended against routine population screening except in the following circumstances - if the prevalence of A1ATD is greater than 1 in 1500 the population, smoking is prevalent, and adequate genetics counseling services are available. Nephelometry or Rocket Immunodiffusion can measure serum levels of A1AT and is a reasonable screening test for the deficiency. However, this method is subject to errors because the protein is an acute phase reactant and rise with inflammation. The gold standard for diagnosis is "Phenotyping" of the protein is done via isoelectric focus gel analysis, which can only be performed at a few specialized laboratories within the United States. DNA Analysis of genotype is done to probe for the common S and Z genes. A1ATD testing can be done via serum and whole blood draw from the vein, but can also be done via a single finger-stick of blood placed onto a card that is mailed into a central lab for testing. A combination of measuring the serum A1AT concentration and performing a PCR based assay to identify S and Z alleles will accurately identify 96% of individuals as compared to the more difficult gold standard isoelectric focusing (Snyder, 2006).

8. Treatment

The corner stone of alpha one antitrypsin management is smoking cessation and smoke avoidance in all individuals with the deficiency. Guidelines for the management of the chronic airflow obstruction (COPD) have been published elsewhere (GOLD guidelines, ATS guidelines, etc.) Augmentation therapy is utilized to increase serum and lung epithelial lining fluid (ELF) levels of A1AT through the weekly intravenous infusion of purified human A1AT protein (Wewers et al., 1987).

It is FDA approved to treat for adult patients with A1ATD (protein concentration < 11 micromoles/dL) and evidence of air flow obstruction. The treatment can be very costly because it involves life-long regular infusions of a blood product, and it is not available worldwide. The treatment was approved based on two factors, that there is biochemical equivalence between exogenous replacement protein and protein found in normal human serum, and there is normalization of serum protein levels in deficient individuals who are receiving replacement. Many non-randomized prospective studies have demonstrated the effectiveness of augmentation via reduction in the annual rate of decline of lung function. Well-designed and adequately powered randomized trials have been limited to date. A recent meta-analysis of published human studies demonstrated augmentation therapy does reduce the annual rate of lung function decline (as measured by FEV_1) in A1ATD individuals (Chapman et al., 2009).

8.1 Future therapies

Ongoing work in areas of inhaled therapy, longer half-life protein, recombinant forms, small molecule chaperone inhibitors to increase liver secretion and gene transfer therapy continue. These studies and fields are all in various stages of development.

9. Conclusion

Alpha1- antitrypsin deficiency is a not uncommon disease, which is not limited to the European and Caucasian American population, but now affects all ethnic groups. Effective treatments for this disease, including smoking cessation, management of COPD/emphysema and other complications, and augmentation therapy with purified A1AT protein is well established. However, the disease remains under-diagnosed, and many times patients are diagnosed years after symptoms have developed. Future work to improve education among healthcare professionals to improve rates of diagnosis, as well as improved disease specific treatments are important steps in making this disease a more treatable illness.

10. References

Alpha-1-antitrypsin deficiency study group. (1998). Survival and FEV1 decline in individuals with severe deficiency of alpha1-antitrypsin. *Am J Respir Crit Care Med*, Vol. 158, No. 1, (July 1998). pp. 49-59.

American Thoracic Society/European Respiratory Society statement: standards for the diagnosis and management of individuals with alpha-1 antitrypsin deficiency. *Am J Respir Crit Care Med*, Vol. 168, No. 7, (October 2003). pp. 818-900.

Blanco, I., de Serres, FJ., Fernandex-Bustillo, E., Lara, B., & Miravitlles, M. (2006). Estimated numbers and prevalence of PI*S and PI*Z alleles of alpha 1-antitrypsin deficiency in European countries. *Eur Resp J*, Vol. 27, No. 1, (January 2006). pp. 77-84.

Carrell, RW. & Lomas, DA. (2002) Alpha 1-antitrypsin deficiency - a model for conformational disease. *NEJM* Vol. 346, No. 1 (January 2002), pp. 45-53.

Chapman, KR., Stockley, RA., Dawkins, C. Wilkes, MM., Navickis, RJ. (2009). Augmentation therapy for alpha1-antitrypsin deficiency: a meta analysis. *COPD*, Vol. 6, No. 3, (June 2009). pp. 177-18

Churg, A., Wang, X., Wang, RD., Meixner, SC. Pryzdial, EL., & Wright, JL. (2007) Alpha1-antitrypsin suppresses TNF-alpha and MMP-12 production by cigarette smoke-stimulated macrophages. *Am J Resp Cell Mol Bio*, Vol. 37, No. 2 (August 2007), pp. 144-151

Cox, DW., Woo, SL., & Mansfield, T. (1985). DNA restriction fragments associated with alpha 1-antitrypsin indicate a single origin for deficiency allele PI Z. *Nature*, Vol. 316, No. 6023, (July 1985). pp. 79-81

Crowther, DC., Belorgery, D., Miranda, E., Kinghorn, KJ., Sharp, LK., & Lomas, DA. (2004) Practical genetics: alpha1-antitrypsin deficiency and the serpinopathies. *Eur J of Human Gen*, Vol. 12, No. 3 (March 2004). pp. 167-172

de Serres, FJ. (2002). Worldwide racial and ethinic distribution of alpha1-antitrypsin deficiency. *Chest*, Vol. 122, No. 5 (November 2002). pp. 1818-1829.

DeMeo, DL, & Silverman, EK. (2004). Alpha1-Antitrypsin deficiency - 2: Genetic aspects of of alpha1-antitrypsin deficiency: phenotypes and genetic modifiers of emphysema risk. *Thorax*, Vol. 59, No. 3, (March 2004). pp. 259-264

Dowd, SK., Rodgers, GC., & Callen, JP. (1995). Effective treatment with alpha-protease inhibitor of chronic cutaneous vasculitis associated with alpha1-antitrypsin deficiency. *J Am Acad Dermatol*, Vol. 33, No. 5 pt 2, (November 1995). pp. 913-916.

Eden, E., Hammel, J., Rouhani, FN., Brantly, ML., Barker, AF., Buist, AS., Fallat, RJ., Stoller, JK., Crystal, RG., & Turino, GM. (2003). Asthma features in severe alpha1 antitrypsin deficiency: experience of the National heart , Lung, and Blood Institute Resistry. *Chest*, Vol. 123, No. 3, (March 2003). pp. 765-771.

Eriksson, S. (1987). Alpha 1-antitrypsin deficiecny and liver cirrhosis in adults: an analysis of 35 Swedish autopsied cases. *Act Med Scand*, Vol. 221, No. 5, pp. 461-67

Gadek, JE., Fells, GA., Zimmeran, RL. Rennard, SI., & Crystal, RG. (1981). Anti-elastase of the human alveolar structures: implications for the protease-antiprotease theory of emphysema. *J Clin Invest*, Vol. 68, No. 4 (October 1981), pp.889-898

Guenter, CA., Welch, MH., Russell TR, Hyde, RM., & Hammarsten, JF. (1968). The pattern of lung disease associated with alpha1-antitrypsin deficiency. *Arch Int Med*, Vol. 122, No. 3 (September 1968). pp. 254-257

Hogarth, KD., & Rachelefsky, G. (2008). Screening and Familial Testing of Patients for Alpha1 Antitrypsin Deficiency. *Chest*, Vol. 133, No. 4 (April 2008). pp. 981-988

Huntington, JA., Read, RJ., Carrell RW. (2000). Structure of a serpin-protease complex shows inhibition by deformation. *Nature*, Vol. 407, No. 6806 (October 2000). pp. 923-926

Laurell, CV., & Eriksson A. (1963) The electrophoretic alpha 1-globulin pattern of serum in alpha 1-antitrypsin deficiency. *Scandinavian Journal of Clinical Laboratory Investigation*, Vol. 15, pp. 132-40

Lieberman, J., Winter, B., & Sastre, A. (1986). Alpha1-antitrypsin Pi-types in 965 COPD patients. *Chest*, Vol. 89, No. 3 (March 1986). pp. 370-73.

Lomas, DA. (2006). The selective advantage of alpha 1-antitrypsin deficiency. *Am J Respir Crit Care Med*, Vol. 173, No. 10 (May 2006), pp. 1072-1077

Lomas, DA., Evans, DL., Finch, JT., & Carrell, RW. (1992). The mechanism of Z alpha1-antitrypsin accumulation in the liver. *Nature*, Vol. 357, No. 6379, (June 1992), pp. 605-607.

Luisetti, M., & Seersholm, N. (2004). Alpha1 antitrypsin deficiency: 1. Epidemiology of alpha1 antitrypsin deficiency. *Thorax*, Vol. 59, No. 2, (Febuary 2004). pp. 164-169.

McElvaney, NG., Stoller, JK., Buist, AS., Prakash, UB., Brantly, ML., Schluchter, MD., & Crystal, RD. (1997). Baseline Characteristics of Enrollees in the National Heart, Lung and Blood Institute Registry of Alpha-1 Antitripysin Deficiency. *Chest*, Vol. 111, No. 2, (Febuary 1997). pp. 394-403.

Mulgrew, AT., Taggart, CC., Lawless, MW., Greene, CM., Brantly, ML., O'Neill, SJ., McElvaney, NG. (2004). Z alpha1-antitrypsin polymerizes in the lung and acts as a neutrophil chemoattractant. *Chest*, Vol. 125, No. 5 (May 2004), pp. 1952-57

Needham, M. & Stockley, RA. (2004). Alpha1-antitrypsin deficiency - 3: clinical manifestations and natural history. *Thorax*, Vol. 59, No. 5, (May 2004), pp. 441-445

O'Brien, ML., Buist, NR., & Murphey (1978), WH. Neonatal screening for alpha 1-antitrypsin deficiency. *J Pediatr*, Vol. 92, No. 6 (June 1978). pp. 1006-1010.

Ogushi, F., Fells, GA., Hubbard, RC., Straus, SD., & Crystal, RG. (1987). Z-type alpha1-antitrypsin is less competent than M1-type alpha1-proteinase inhibitor as an inhibitor of neutrophil elastase. *J Clin Invest*, Vol. 80, No. 5 (November 1987), pp.1366-1374

Ogushi, F., Hubbard, RC., Vogelmeier, C., Fells, GA., & Crystal, RG. (1991) Risk factors for emphysema. Cigarette smoking is associated with a reduction in the association rate constant of alpha1 antitrypsin for neutrophil elastase. *J Clin Invest*, Vol. 87, No. 3 (March 1991), pp. 1060-1065.

Online Mendelian Inheritance in Man (July 2010). "MIM ID #613490: Alpha-1-Antitrypsin Deficiency. Available from http://www.ncbi.nlm.nih.gov/omim/613490, created 7/20/2010, accessed 3/14/2011

Online Mendelian Inheritance in Man (September 2010). MIM ID *107400: Serpin Peptidase Inhibitor, Clade A, Member 1; Serpina1. 3.14.2011. Available from http://www.ncbi.nlm.nih.gov/omim/613490. Accessed 3/14/2011

Parr, DG., Guest, PG., Reynolds, JH. Dowson, LJ. & Stockley, RA. (2007). Prevalence and Impact of Bronchiectasis in alpha 1-antitrypsin deficiency. *Am J Respir Crit Care Med*, Vol. 176, No. 12, (December 2007). pp. 1215-1221.

Petrache, I., Fijalkowska, I., Medler, TR., Skirball, J., Cruz, P., Zhen, L., Petrache, HI., Flotte, TR., & Tuder, RM. (2008). Alpha1-anti-trypsin Inhibits Caspase-3 Activity, Preventing Lung Endothelial Cell Apoptosis. *Am J of Path*, Vol. 169, No. 4 (October 2006), pp. 1155-1166.

Seersholm, N. & Kok-Jensen, A. (1998). Clinical features and prognosis of life time non-smokers with severe alpha1 antitrypsin deficiency. *Thorax*, Vol. 53, No. 4 (April 1998). pp. 265-268.

Seersholm, N., & Kok-Jensen A. (1998). Clinical features and prognosis of life time non-smokers with severe alpha1 antitrypsin deficiency. *Thorax*, Vol. 53, No. 4, (April 1998). pp. 265-268.

Senior, RM., Tegner, H., Kuhn, C., Ohlsson, K., Starcher, BC., & Pierce, JA. (1977). The induction of pulmonary emphysema with human leukocyte elastase. *Am Rev Respir Dis*, Vol. 166, No. 3, (September 1977). pp. (469-475)

Sharp, HL., Bridges, RA., Krivit, W., & Freier, ER. (1969). Cirrhosis associated with alpha1-antitrypsin deficiency: a previously unrecognized inherited disorder. *J Lab Clin Med*, Vol. 73, No. 6, (June 1969). pp. 934-939

Silverman, EK., Miletich, JP, Pierce, JA. Sherman, LA., Endicott, SK., Broze, GJ. & Campbell, EJ. (1989). Alpha1-antitrypsin deficiency: high prevalence in the St. Louis area determine by direct population screening. *Am Rev Respir Dis*, Vol. 140, No. 4 (October 1989). pp. 961-66

Snyder, MR., Katzmann, JA., Butz, ML., Wiley, C., Yang, P., Dawson, DB., Halling, KC., Highsmith, WE., & Thibodeau, SN. (2006). Diagnosis of alpha1-antitrypsin deficiency: an algorithm of quantitation, genotyping and phenotyping. *Clin Chem*, Vol. 52, No. 12, (December, 2006). pp. 2236-2242

Stoller, JK., & Aboussouan, LS. (2005). Alpha1-antitrypsin deficiency. *Lancet*, Vol. 365, No. 9478, (June 2005). pp. 2225-2236

Stoller, JK., Sandhaus, RA., Turino, G., Dickson, R., Rodgers, K. & Strange, C. (2005). Delay in diagnosis of alpha 1-antitrypsin deficiency: a continuing problem. *Chest*, Vol. 128, No. 4, (October 2005). pp. 1989-94.

Stoller, JK., Smith, P., Yang, P. & Spray, J. (1994). Physical and social impact of alpha 1-antitrypsin deficiency: results of a mail survey of the readership of a national newsletter. *Cleve Clin J Med*, Vol. 61, No. 6, (Nov-Dec 1994). pp. 461-467.

Stoller, JK., Tomashefski, J., Crystal, RG., Arroliga, A., Strange, C., Killian, DN., Schluchter, MD., & Wiedemann, HP., (2005). Mortality in individuals with severe deficiency of alpha1-antitrypsin. *Chest*, Vol. 127, No. 4, (April 2005). pp. 1196-1204.

Sveger, T. (1976). Liver disease in alpha 1-antitrypsin deficiency detected by screening of 200,000 infants. *N Enl J Med*, Vol. 294, No. 24, (June 1976). pp. 1316-1321

US National Library of Medicine, (August 2009) Genetics Home Reference, "SERPINA1" Available at http://ghr.nlm.nih.gov/gene/SERPINA1, Accessed 3/14/2011

Wewers, MD., Casolaro, MA., Sellers, SE., Swayze, SC., McPhaul, KM., Wittes, JT., & Crystal, RG. (1987). Replacement therapy for alpha1-antitrypsin deficiency associated with emphysema. *NEJM*, Vol. 316, No. 17, (April 1987). pp. 1055-1062

8

Fabry Disease:
A Metabolic Proteinuric Nephropathy

Jonay Poveda Nuñez[1], Alberto Ortiz[1], Ana Belen Sanz[2]
and Maria Dolores Sanchez Niño[2]
[1]*IIS-Fundacion Jimenez Diaz and Universidad Autonoma de Madrid, Madrid,*
[2]*IdiPaz, Madrid*
Spain

1. Introduction

Fabry disease is a rare disease. However, Fabry disease is more common than other inherited lysosomal storage disorders, affecting 1 in 40,000 to 1 in 117,000 worldwide (Mehta et al., 2004, Germain, 2010). Fabry disease is the caused by an inherited deficiency of galactosylgalactosylglucosylceramidase" (EC 3.2.1.14), commonly referred to as α-galactosidase A (α-Gal A). As a result, there is progressive cellular accumulation of glycosphingolipids, leading to organ failure and premature death. For decades, only symptomatic therapy was available, that did not prevent the fatal evolution of the disease. In the last decade, two forms of Enzyme Replacement Therapy (ERT), that prevent disease progression as well as potentially reverse symptoms, have been developed. However, these drugs are expensive and do not cure the disease.

2. Fabry disease: concept

Fabry disease is an X-linked lysosomal storage disorder caused by mutations in the gene encoding the lysosomal enzyme α-galactosidase A (α-Gal A). α-galactosidase A catalyzes the hydrolytic cleavage of the terminal alpha-galactosyl moieties from globotriaosylceramide (Gb3) and glycoproteins. The deficiency of α-galactosidase leads to accumulation of Gb3 and other glycosphingolipids in plasma and different cell types throughout the body (Nance et al., 2006) (Figure 1). Glycosphingolipid storage may interfere with cellular membrane proteins, such as ion channels, become cytotoxic, or lead to accumulation of soluble cytotoxic metabolites (Schiffmann et al., 2002, Aerts et al., 2008, Sanchez-Niño et al., 2010), although the precise molecular link between lipid storage and disease manifestations is unclear. Progressive accumulation of Glycosphingolipid is associated with systemic disease, with a wide spectrum of clinical manifestations that reduce the life expectancy of patients.

3. Genetics

The α-galactosidase A gene (*GLA*) is located on the minus strand of the chromosome X on the locus Xq22.1. The *GLA* gene is 10,223 base pairs long and contains 7 exons. *GLA* gene may give rise to 7 different processed transcripts by alternative splicing. However, just one of these encodes the 429-aminoacid lysosomal α-Gal A with a molecular mass of 48.7 kD.

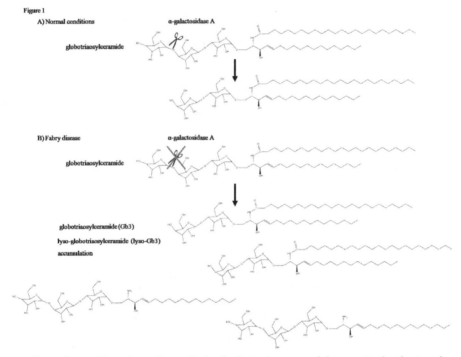

Figure 1

A) Normal conditions   α-galactosidase A

globotriaosylceramide

B) Fabry disease   α-galactosidase A

globotriaosylceramide

globotriaosylceramide (Gb3)
lyso-globotriaosylceramide (lyso-Gb3)
accumulation

Fig. 1. A) α-galactosidase A catalyzes the hydrolytic cleavage of the terminal galactose from globotriaosylceramide (Gb3). B) The deficiency of α-galactosidase leads to accumulation of Gb3 and other glycosphingolipids, such as lyso-globotriaosylceramide (lyso-Gb3)

Within the coding region, 239 single nucleotide polymorphisms present in the general population and more than 400 *GLA* mutations that lead to Fabry disease have been found. Exons 5, 6 and 3 comprise the majority of point mutations respectively. Missense mutations may be classified in 3 groups in accordance with the effect they have on the protein function (Garman & Garboczi, 2004). First, mutations that alter the active site of the enzyme; second, mutation that interfere with the correct folding and stability of the protein; and finally, the remaining mutations that negatively affect the function of the enzyme. The nature of the mutation may influence therapeutic approaches. Most mutations are family-specific, which explains the marked variability in the residual enzyme activity and precludes the use of a single, fast genetic testing technique. Rather, the whole gene should be sequenced.

4. Clinical manifestations of Fabry disease

4.1 Early clinical features
Although glycolipid accumulation begins in the prenatal period, symptoms of the classic form of Fabry disease do not arise until childhood (Vedder et al., 2006). Symptoms include

episodes of extremity pain or acroparesthesia, gastrointestinal symptoms, hypohidrosis and associated heat sensitivity (Cable et al., 1982; Ries et al., 2005; Rowe et al., 1974) (Table 1). Pain has been linked with small fiber neuropathy (Attal & Bouhassira, 1999) and is thought to be caused by either reduced perfusion of peripheral nerves or glycosphingolipid accumulation in neural or perineural cells (Gadoth & Sandbank, 1983; Gemignani et al., 1984). Pain has been described as burning and starts in the hands and feet but can radiate proximally. It may be present throughout the life of the patient, but frequently peaks in childhood or adolescence and then decreases. This has been attributed to end-stage nerve injury. Pain may be continuous or episodic, but is triggered by extreme temperature changes, fever, stress or physical exercise (MacDermot et al., 2001). Both, acute and chronic pains are difficult to deal with medically, requiring the use of narcotic or neuroleptic drugs respectively (Schiffmann & Scott, 2002).

Organ system	Sign/Symptom
Nervous system	Acroparesthesias
	Nerve deafness
	Heat intolerance, hypohidrosis
	Hearing loss, tinnitus
Gastrointestinal tract	Nausea, vomiting, diarrhea
	Postprandial bloating and pain, early satiety
Skin	Angiokeratomas
Eyes	Corneal and lenticular opacities
	Vasculopathy (retina conjunctiva)
Kidneys	Microalbuminuria, proteinuria
	Impaired concentration ability
Heart	Impaired heart rate variability
	ECG abnormalities (shortened PR interval)
	Mild valvular insufficiency
	Left ventricular hypertrophy

Table 1. Early signs and symptoms of Fabry disease

Gastrointestinal manifestations include nausea, vomiting, abdominal pain, early satiety, diarrhea and constipation (Hoffmann & Keshav, 2007). It has been proposed that delayed gastric emptying, in conjunction with lipid accumulation within ganglion cells of the autonomic nervous system, are responsible for the early satiety, whereas diarrhea has been linked to bacterial overgrowth (O'Brien et al., 1982).

Decreased sweating or hypohidrosis is another common feature of Fabry disease. It causes heat intolerance and inability to physical exercise. Hypohidrosis has also been attributed to autonomic neuropathy (Zarate & Hopkin, 2008). Less frequent than hypohidrosis is hyperhidrosis (excessive sweating), which is especially noticeable in the palms of the hands and soles of the feet (Zarate & Hopkin, 2008).

These symptoms highly reduce the quality of life of patients. However, the lack of physical findings frequently preclude the correct diagnosis in the absence of family history (Ries et al., 2005).

More characteristic disease manifestations arise in adolescence, such as angiokeratomas and corneal opacities. Angiokeratomas are reddish-purple vascular skin lesions, usually clustered around the swimming trunk region, which tend to increase in size and number with age (Zarate & Hopkin, 2008).

Corneal opacity (cornea verticillata) is the most characteristic ophthalmological abnormality observed in Fabry patients. They are the result of glycosphingolipids deposition between the basal membrane of the corneal epithelium and Bowman's membrane (Rodríguez-González-Herrero et al., 2008). Corneal opacities usually do not interfere with visual acuity. Other ophthalmological manifestations include conjunctival and retinal vascular tortuosity (Nguyen et al., 2005) and occlusion of retinal vessels (Utsumi et al., 1997).

Later in life many patients develop life-threatening complications including end-stage renal disease, heart and cerebrovascular diseases that may cause death (Table 2).

Organ system	Sign/Symptom
Central nervous system	Stroke
Kidneys	End-stage renal disease
Heart	Arrythmia, sudden death
	Ischemis
	Heart failure
	Heart fibrosis

Table 2. Life threatening signs and symptoms of Fabry disease

4.2 Life-threatening complications

Classical Fabry disease progresses to irreversible tissue damage and organ dysfunction, limiting life-expectancy in middle-age patients (Zarate & Hopkin, 2008). The main cause leading to death in men suffering from classic Fabry disease was renal failure before the widespread availability of renal replacement therapies, while now cardiac causes predominate (Mehta et al., 2006.).

Renal abnormalities include proteinuria, nephrotic range proteinuria, rarely nephrotic syndrome and chronic renal failure, requiring dialysis or kidney transplantation (Branton et al., 2002; Tsakiris et al., 1996, Ortiz et al., 2008, Ortiz et al., 2010)

Some patients develop end-stage renal disease at the same age as those with the classic form but lack other characteristic signs of the classical phenotype such as angiokeratomas, acroparesthesias or hypohidrosis, thus hindering the diagnosis of the condition (Nakao et al., 2003).

Cardiac disease may have several clinical manifestations. (Patel et al, 2011) The most frequent cardiac abnormality is progressive hypertrophic cardiomyopathy, although diastolic dysfunction, arrhythmia, myocardial fibrosis and short P-R are also seen (Linhart & Elliott, 2007). Fabry patients are frequently hypotensive. However, Fabry patients may have blood pressure that may be above recommended targets for chronic kidney disease patients (which are below 130 mmHg systolic and below 80 mmHg diastolic) (Ortiz et al., 2008). Cardiac symptoms may include palpitations, angina, shortness of breath and sudden death (Shah & Elliott, 2005).

The mechanisms leading to myocardial hypertrophy are not completely understood. The fact that only 1-2% of heart hypertrophy is attributable to actual storage of glycosphingolipids within the cardiac cells suggests that activation of signaling pathways leading to fibrosis play an important role (Linhart & Elliott, 2007). In this regard, much of the heart volume consists of fibrosis. Actual promoters of fibrosis are unknown. However, if we take a clue from the kidney, both death of myocardial cells and the presence of fibrogenic soluble mediators, such as lyso-gb3, that promote release of transforming growth factor beta 1 (TGFβ1), a fibrogenic cytokine, may be contributors (Sanchez-Niño et al, 2010).

A cardiac variant of Fabry disease has been described. In these patients, clinical manifestations and Gb3 storage are almost restricted to the heart (Ogawa et al., 1990). This is associated with residual α-galactosidase A activity or certain mutations. There is no clinical evidence of classical Fabry disease in other organs, although mild proteinuria has been observed (Ishii et al., 2002). Clinical manifestations appear later in life than in classical Fabry disease.

Cerebrovascular complications, mainly ischemic episodes, occur in Fabry disease (Sims et al. 2009). This is thought to be due to the accumulation of Gb3 in the cerebral blood vessels (Altarescu et al., 2001). However, the effect of sphingolipid storage is different depending on vessels' diameter. Thus, Gb3 deposition leads to progressive stenosis in small blood vessels, whereas in larger vessels weakened walls dilate, causing hyper-perfusion and tortuosity (Mitsias P, 1996). Clinical consequences of cerebrovascular injury include stroke, transient ischemic attacks, epilepsy, vertigo and headache (Mehta & Ginsberg, 2005).

Arterial remodeling and intima-media thickening have been described and may explain ischemic events. By contrast, classical atherosclerotic lesions are uncommon. It is unclear whether this is due to the relative young age of most patients or to a specific change in the vascular response to injury brought about the glycolipid accumulation or the metabolic consequences of the disease. In this regard, high HDL cholesterol levels have been described in Fabry patients (Cartwright et al., 2004). In at least in some Fabry patients HDL particles contribute disproportionately to carry glycosphingolipids (Clarke et al., 1976).

4.3 Other clinical manifestations

Additional clinical manifestations may include anemia, azoospermia, depression, facial dysmorphism, hypothyroidism, lymphoedema, parapelvic kidney cysts and priapism (Ries et al., 2004, Sunder-Plassmann, 2006), although there is discussion whether some of these, such as hypothyroidism, are real Fabry disease manifestations.

Tinnitus and substantial hearing loss have been described, especially in men (Hegemann et al., 2006). Hearing loss seems to be directly related to neuropathy (Ries et al., 2007).

Significant airflow reduction is common in Fabry patients. Respiratory involvement manifests as shortness of breath and dyspnea with exercise, chronic cough, and less frequently asthma (Rosenberg et al., 1980).

4.4 Fabry disease in women

Traditionally females were considered to be at low risk of clinical manifestations of Fabry disease. However, there is accumulating evidence that some females may suffer symptoms as severe as males (Wilcox et al., 2008). In this regard, Fabry disease may be considered as an X-linked disease with a high penetrance in females. Terms such as "recessive X-linked disease" are no longer used. It has been estimated that only 70% of women with *GLA* mutations develop clinical manifestations of the disease, which tend to be less severe and more variable than in men (Dobyns, 2006, Schiffmann R, 2009). As a result, it is likely that a large number of affected women remain undiagnosed. Women are affected because of the lack of cross-correction between cells with normal α-Gal A activity and cells with deficient α-Gal A (Romeo et al., 1975). Female cells have two X chromosomes, but one of them is randomly inactivated (lyonization). It is thought that the percentage of disease-carrying X chromosomes that are inactivated is a key factor contributing to disease expression variability in females (Dobrovolny et al., 2005).

5. Fabry nephropathy

5.1 Natural course

Fabry nephropathy is one of the most severe manifestations of Fabry disease and was the cause of death before the widespread availability of dialysis and kidney transplantation. Like most aspects of Fabry disease, kidney disease is thought to result from Gb3 accumulation in glomerular endothelial, mesangial and intersticial cells, podocytes and renal vasculature. Progressive intracellular accumulation of Gb3 is thought to cause glomerulosclerosis and interstitial fibrosis (Alroy J, 2002) as well as its urinary excretion together with other lipids (Branton MH, 2002). More recently a role of soluble glycolipid metabolites in the pathogenesis of podocyte injury has been suggested (Sanchez-Niño et al, 2010). As a result of lipid storage, kidneys may increase in size, although, as is the case with other renal disease characterized by enlarged kidney, such as diabetic nephropathy, in advanced renal failure the kidneys eventually shrink (Torra R, 2008).

Manifestations of kidney injury in Fabry disease include urinary concentrating defect, proteinuria, renal insufficiency and eventually renal failure requiring renal replacement therapy. The severity of kidney manifestations increases with age.

5.1.1 Renal function

Progressive loss of kidney function is characterized by elevated serum creatinine levels and decreasing glomerular filtration rates (GFR) (Ortiz et al, 2008). There is some debate as to the existence of an early hyperfiltration period, analogous to that observed in diabetic nephropathy, since assessment with of GFR by precise, research-grade technique is lacking. Early reports indicated that the loss of GFR was similar to that observed in diabetic nephropathy, around 10 ml/min/year (Branton et al., 2002). Lower rates have been described in recent times, that may be partially attributed to an overall better symptomatic control of chronic kidney disease aimed at proteinuria and blood pressure targets. Urinary protein excretion is the main predictor of GFR loss. Males with urinary protein/creatinine > 1.5 had a mean eGFR slope -5.6 ml/min per 1.73 m(2) per year, while this value was -1.3 ml/min per 1.73 m(2) per year for women with the highest urinary protein/creatinine (> 1.2) (Wanner et al., 2010).

Men with classical Fabry disease reach end-stage renal disease requiring dialysis or transplantation at a mean age of 40 years (Ortiz et al, 2010). Females reaching end-stage renal disease do so at the same mean age as males. However, there are ten-fold less females than males in both United States and European end-stage renal disease registries (Tsakiris et al., 1996, Thadhani et al, 2002). This suggests that in most females, Fabry nephropathy does not progress to reach end-stage renal disease, but in those in whom progression occurs, the time-course is similar to males.

5.1.2 Proteinuria

Early kidney injury is manifested as microalbuminuria which progresses to overt proteinuria (Schiffmann, 2009, Ortiz et al, 2008). Microalbuminuria is a misnomer that only indicates that pathological abnormalities may be detected by methods not available when the first tests to study albuminuria were commercialized. The term microalbuminuria indicates a urinary albumin excretion of > 30 mg/24h or >30 mg/g creatinine. In this regard, Fabry nephropathy usually recapitulates the sequence of events observed in diabetic nephropathy, another proteinuric nephropathy also consequence of a metabolic derangement. Overt proteinuria (>300 mg/24 h) was present in 43 and 26% of males and with early Fabry disease, respectively, and the proportions were higher with more severe kidney involvement (Ortiz et al, 2008). Established proteinuria (Albuminuria > 300 mg/day) is a sign of irreversible damage to the kidney (Zarate & Hopkin, 2008). Numerous experimental studies have shown a direct relationship between the degree of proteinuria and the rate of decline of renal functions (Tryggvason & Pettersson, 2003). Proteinuria is a consequence of glomerular damage but itself causes tubulointerstitial injury. Reabsorption of excess specific proteins filtered at the glomerulus by the proximal tubule activates these cells to release inflammatory factors and undergo apoptosis (Thomas ME, 1999). Thus, the magnitude of proteinuria could be used as a marker of glomerular damage. Interestingly, morphological studies, not specifically performed in Fabry disease, have confirmed a stronger correlation between tubulo-interstitial damage and renal function than between glomerular injury and renal function (Nath, 1992). Little is known about the factors that may speed up the process of Fabry nephropathy. Proteinuria is clearly a risk factor (Wanner et al., 2010). Thus, controlling proteinuria is thought to be important to for the progression of Fabry disease and evidence for this approach is discussed below.

5.1.3 Blood pressure

Hypertension is rarely found as an early symptom in Fabry disease but becomes more prevalent with the progression of the condition, indicating kidney declining function (Branton et al., 2002). Higher blood pressure values favor glomerular hyperperfusion as a compensatory response to nephron loss (Schieppati & Remuzzi, 2003). However, glomerular hypertension promotes kidney disease progression. Although not specifically tested in Fabry disease, lowering blood pressure to below 130 mmHg systolic AND 80 mmHg diastolic is recommended in patients with chronic kidney disease in order to slow the progression of nephropathy (K/DOQI clinical practice guidelines, 2004).

5.2 Heterogeneity

There is a great variability both in disease manifestations and the timing of kidney disease progression within and between families. Thus, the age at initiation of renal replacement therapy in the Fabry Registry data had a range of 15 to 79 years in males and 17 to 78 years in females (Ortiz A et al., 2010). The genetic or environmental factors that influence disease heterogeneity are unknown. However, unraveling them is a key priority since it will lead to a better understanding of the disease and potentially to novel therapeutic approaches.

5.3 Women

Most heterozygous women with Fabry disease used to be considered asymptomatic carriers. However, they may be as severely affected as men with the classic phenotype (Desnick et al., 2001, Wang et al., 2007, Wilcox et al., 2008). The clinical manifestation of Fabry disease in females tend to be less severe and to arise later than in males (Schiffmann. 2009). In this regard they may develop albuminuria and progressive renal dysfunction leading to the need of renal replacement therapy (Ortiz et al., 2008; Ortiz et al; 2010). If this occurs the mean age at initiation of renal replacemebt therapy is similar to men (Ortiz et al, 2010).

5.4 Diagnosis

In spite of the early onset of Fabry disease in some cases, the absence of family history, the variety of clinical manifestations and their similarity with those of other conditions may delay the diagnosis of Fabry disease, in some cases for years. Due to the availability of specific therapy, an early diagnosis would be desirable.

5.4.1 Diagnosis of Fabry disease

Diagnosis involves measuring residual enzyme activity in plasma, leukocytes or whole blood as well as sequencing of the gene to characterize the genetic defect (Ortiz et al., 2010b). Confirming the genetic defect may be important for the eligibility for treatment with novel approaches, such as chaperones. In the absence of family history, confirmation of the genetic defect by gene sequencing is mandatory in females when Fabry disease is suspected, since enzymatic assays may be normal even in the presence of Fabry disease due to random chromosome X inactivation. Genetic confirmation is also highly recommended in males.

A key, often forgotten aspect of Fabry disease, is the need to take a careful family history which allows the diagnosis of individuals in early stages of the disease.

5.4.2 Screening for Fabry disease

Screening by means of rapid and low-cost strategies to detect Fabry disease is indicated in high-risk populations (Oqvist et al., 2009). These include patients with unexplained left ventricular hypertrophy, younger patients with unexplained stroke and patients with chronic kidney disease of unknown etiology. However, neonatal screening has not yet been incorporated into routine clinical practice. Current screening methods are based on quantification of enzyme activity in dry blood spots. Performance for males is adequate. However, given the mosaicisms of females regarding X chromosome inactivation, Fabry women may have near normal whole blood enzyme activity and still have the disease. Thus, dried blood spot analysis is unable to detect about a 33% of heterozygous females leads to the need for more efficient strategies (Linthorst GE, 2005). Novel screening methods, such as proteomic analysis of urine, and quantification of urinary Gb3 or lyso-Gb3 are under study.

5.4.3 Renal biopsy for diagnosis of Fabry nephropathy

Kidney biopsy is recommended in Fabry patients exhibiting reduced GFR or proteinuria to confirm the diagnosis of Fabry kidney involvement (Ortiz et al., 2008b). In addition, renal biopsy for kidney disease of unknown origin may reveal unsuspected Fabry disease. Biopsies reveal typical Gb3 accumulation in tubular epithelial cells, glomerular and endothelial cells, and provide information on the extent of renal damage. In patients with Fabry disease, glomeruli present a striking white color under illumination in a stereomicroscope as a result of lipid-laden podocytes in contrast to the usual red color of normal glomeruli (Svarstad et al., 2004).

5.5 Pathogenesis and pathology

Fabry disease manifestations had traditionally been ascribed to intracellular accumulation of Gb3 and related glycosphingolipids (Figure 1). However, the precise pathways leading to tissue injury were unknown. Recent evidence suggests a role for more soluble molecules, such as lyso-Gb3, that may activate target tissue cells, such as podocytes, to release secondary mediators of injury that would be responsible for tissue injury and disease manifestations (Figure 2). This model (accumulation of a soluble metabolite with cytotoxic properties) would be analogous to the diabetes situation, where high glucose concentrations as a result of the metabolic derangement promote activation of target tissue cells to release mediators that cause tissue injury. If correct, this paradigm would greatly enhance research into novel therapeutic approaches to Fabry nephropathy by allowing the extrapolation of concepts from diabetic nephropathy, a better understood and more common disease (Sanchez- Niño et al., 2010b).

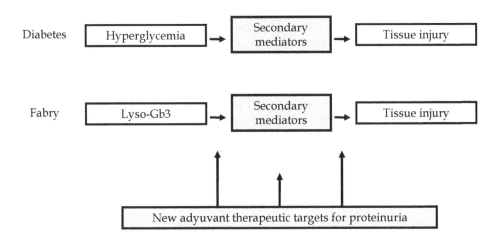

Fig. 2. Hypothetical similarities between the pathogenesis of diabetic nephropathy and Fabry disease nephropathy and potential therapeutic implications

Detailed descriptions of kidney pathology in children and adults with Fabry disease have recently been published (Tondel et al., 2008, Fogo et al., 2010, Najafian et al., 2010). There is widespread glycolipid accumulation in glomerular podocytes, mesangial and endothelial cells, as well as proximal and distal tubular cells, interstitial endothelial cells and other endothelial cells. While early pathogenic theories were centered in endothelial cell glycolipid accumulation, that was thought to lead to ischemic injury, the total early clearance of endothelial deposits by ERT, but persistence of proteinuria and chronic kidney disease progression despite this endothelial clearance have focused the attention to podocytes. In this regard, podocytes are the cells with a worse response to ERT in terms of glycolipid clearance (Germain et al, 2007). Only after 5 years of ERT a mild decrease in podocytes glycolipid deposition was noted. Furthermore, podocyte injury is a key feature of other proteinuric kidney diseases (Moreno et al., 2008). In addition, in children with early Fabry nephropathy the best pathological correlate of albuminuria was the presence and amount of podocytes glycolipid accumulation (Najafian et al., 2010). Thus, recent research into the pathogenesis of Fabry nephropathy has focused on the cell biology of the podocyte (Sanchez-Niño et al., 2010). The other key pathology feature of Fabry nephropathy is glomerular (glomerulosclerosis) and interstitial fibrosis, which is associated with loss of parenchymal renal cells (podocytes and tubular cells)(Fogo et al., 2010). Thus, there is renewed interest in the link between metabolites accumulated in Fabry disease and the synthesis and deposition of extracellular matrix components.

5.5.1 Metabolic initiators: Gb3 and lyso-Gb3

In Fabry disease, Gb3 is widely distributed in lysosomes and other cellular compartments such as the cell membrane, the ER or the nucleus (Askari et al., 2007). It was hypothesized that Gb3 may disrupt intracellular trafficking (Pagano RE, 2003) or alter the composition of membrane lipid rafts. Lipid rafts interact with other lipids and proteins that signal from cell surface receptors (Galbiati et al., 2001), such as endothelial nitric oxide synthase (eNOS) (Mogami et al., 2005). It was further hypothesized that cell stress due to Gb3 accumulation could promote the production of reactive oxygen species (ROS) that induce cell death (Shen et al., 2008).

Although Gb3 accumulation is widespread, serum Gb3 or Gb3 deposits do not necessarily correlate with clinical manifestations (Aerts et al., 2008). Instead, a new biologically active soluble glycolipid metabolite, globotriaosylsphingosine (lyso-Gb3), has been found in high serum, kidney and urinary concentrations in Fabry patients (Aerts et al., 2008, Auray-Blais et al., 2010, Togawa et al.2010b). Lyso-Gb3 is involved in vascular smooth muscle cell proliferation and induces in podocytes the production of mediators of glomerular injury such as TGF-β1, a critical mediator of extracellular matrix (ECM) production, fibrosis and podocyte injury (Alsaad & Herzenberg, 2007; Mason & Wahab, 2003; Pantsulaia. 2006; Park et al., 1997) (Sharma et al, 1997) and CD74, a MIF receptor that regulates the expression of lethal cytokines (Sanchez-Niño et al., 2009), suggesting a role in the pathogenesis of Fabry disease (Sanchez-Niño et al., 2010).

Lyso-Gb3 seems to be involved in glomerular injury in Fabry disease by triggering the release of TGF-beta1 and CD74, both secondary mediators of glomerular injury common to diabetic nephropathy (Sanchez-Niño et al., 2010). TGF-beta1, in turn, leads to release of excess ECM components, including type IV collagen and fibronectin, by podocytes, contributing to the characteristic glomerulosclerosis of Fabry nephropathy. Further unpublished data suggest a more widespread release of inflammatory mediators by podocytes exposed to lyso-Gb3.

5.6 Therapy of Fabry nephropathy

The first therapies for Fabry disease were oriented to deal with the symptomatic effects of the disorder, such as pain, cardiac and cerebrovascular complications. However, most patients would die for ESRD unless kidney transplantation or renal dialysis was applied. Guidelines for the management of Fabry nephropathy have recently been published (Ortiz et al., 2008b).

5.6.1 Enzyme replacement therapy (ERT)

Until 2000, recognition of Fabry disease did not change the patient management or prognosis, since no specific treatment was available. However, in the last decade enzyme replacement therapy (ERT) is available and addresses the metabolic defect, although it does not cure the disease. ERT provides the chance to modify the natural history of Fabry disease. Two companies commercialize human recombinant α-galactosidase synthesized by genetically engineered cell lines.

Indications: ERT is indicated in every male with classical Fabry disease. In this population ERT should be initiated as early as possible. In addition, ERT should be prescribed to females with any evidence of injury to the heart, central nervous system or kidney and considered in females with symptoms in other organs and systems (Germain DP, 2010, Ortiz et al., 2010b). In case of a transitory limitation in ERT supplies, prioritization guidelines have been published (Linthorst et al., 2011). These guidelines should not be considered compelling indications in the absence of limited availability of treatment. Furthermore, these guidelines do not apply to a chronic limitation of resources since they take into account both the indication of ERT as well as the urgency of the need of ERT. Thus, they do not answer the question who should and should not be treated. They answer the question, if therapy is indicated but ERT availability is limited, who should be treated first, implying that not prioritized patients will also be treated but later, as soon as supplies are available.

There are currently two commercially available enzyme preparations for the treatment of Fabry disease: (1) Replagal® (agalsidase alfa; Shire Human Genetic Therapies, Inc., Cambridge, MA) and (2) Fabrazyme® (agalsidase beta; Genzyme Corporation, Inc., Cambridge, MA). Algasidase alfa is produced by cultured human fibroblasts, whereas agalsidase beta produced by the expression of human a-galactosidase cDNA in Chinese Hamster Ovary (CHO) cells. In the USA, only agalsidase β has been approved by the US Food and Drug Administration, while in Europe both enzymes are available for clinical use.

The approved doses of agalsidase-alfa and agalsidase-beta are 0.2 mg/kg and 1.0 mg/kg, given intravenously every 2 weeks, respectively. There is evidence that agalsidase-beta may be used at 0.3 mg/kg every two weeks for certain patients. This difference in dose remains unexplained by the molecular nature of the preparations and there is an ongoing debate whether they are similarly effective. The only published head-to-head clinical trial concluded that disease progression occurred when both enzymes where used at a dose of 0.2 mg/kg every two weeks (Vedder et al, 2007). We must emphasize that this dose is the approved one for agalsidase-alfa, but was 5-fold lower than the approved dose for agalsidase-beta. There is some indication, although the evidence is not strong, for a superiority of the higher dose in patients who develop anti-agalsidase antibodies. Furthermore a doubling of the approved agalsidase alfa dose provided further benefit in terms of nephroprotection for patients whose disease was progressing despite treatment with the approved dose. In addition, only agalsidase beta has shown a benefit on hard end-points in a phase IV randomized clinical trial (Banikazemi et al., 2007). Despite these considerations, a number of publications have documented that both enzymes at approved doses have proved effective in reducing glycolipid deposits and disease manifestations at least if used early (Eng et al, 2001, Schiffmann et al., 2001; Schiffmann et al., 2006; Germain et al., 2007; Mehta et al., 2009; Schaefer et al., 2009).

5.6.2 Benefits and unmet needs of ERT

ERT addresses the underlying metabolic cause of Fabry disease. ERT slows the loss of kidney function in patients with relatively preserved renal function and low proteinuria (Schiffmann et al., 2006) (Germain et al., 2007). However, progression occurs despite ERT in patients with more advanced renal disease, including those with proteinuria> 1g/d or glomeruloscerotic lesions in renal biopsyl, as ERT does not reduce proteinuria and may be unable to avoid its development in treated pediatric patients (Tøndel et al., 2008). Thus, since proteinuria is a major risk factor for progression of Fabry disease, it is advisable to combine antiproteinuric therapy with early institution of ERT.

5.6.3 Antiproteinuric approaches

ACEI/ARBs: the lesser efficacy of ERT once Fabry nephropathy has caused proteinuria or glomerulosclerosis (Germain et al., 2007) raises the need for adjuvant therapies that cooperate with ERT in improving outcomes. Co-treatment with angiotensin-converting enzyme (ACE) inhibitors and angiotensin-receptor blockers (ARB) decreases proteinuria (Tahir et al., 2007). These agents help to control hypertension when present, although in some case a low blood pressure may limit their use. To prevent unwanted blood pressure lowering effects initiation of therapy with low, fractionated doses is recommended.

Active vitamin D has pleiotropic effects that go well beyond the regulation of bone metabolism (Rojas-Rivera et al., 2010). Vitamin D receptor (VDR) activators such as calcitriol and paricalcitol prevent podocyte activation by lyso-Gb3 in podocytes (Sanchez-Niño et al., 2010). In this regard, there is some evidence that paricalcitol, a selective VDR activator, reduces proteinuria in diabetic nephropathy, even in patients treated with ACEIs or ARBs (Agarwal et al., 2005; Lambers Heerspink et al., 2009; de Zeeuw et al., 2010). Interestingly, patients suffering from chronic kidney disease frequently have deficiencies of both 25(OH) vitamin D and calcitriol. Vitamin D deficiencies should be corrected in these patients and VDR agonists are indicated for the prevention and treatment of secondary hyperparathyroidism in chronic kidney disease (Kidney Disease: Improving Global Outcomes (KDIGO) CKD-MBD Work Group. 2009) (National Kidney Foundation. 2003). Thus, VDR agonist therapy used to treat vitamin D deficiency or secondary hyperparathyroidism might be beneficial for proteinuria in Fabry disease.

5.6.4 Novel therapies in the horizon

The search for an ideal treatment of the underlying enzymatic defect is still ongoing. Current ERT is expensive, inconvenient and may not reach certain key cells such as the podocytes. Additional therapeutic approaches are being explored.

Substrate reduction therapy by small molecules may be associated with ERT to improve efficacy or reduce ERT dose. Gene therapy is also being explored. In addition certain mutations may benefit from novel therapeutic strategies. Thus, individuals carrying mutation that interfere with the correct folding and stability of the protein may benefit from small molecule chaperone therapy. In addition, an orally active small molecule, ataluren, might be useful in individuals carrying premature stop codons (Torra et al. 2010). Although never tested in Fabry disease, clinical trials in other genetic diseases are underway or have been completed (Kerem et al., 2008).

5.6.5 Monitoring therapy and disease progression

We lack reliable biomarkers that enable assessing disease progression, monitoring treatment response and individualizing ERT dose in Fabry disease. Biomarkers may represent lipid storage burden or target organ injury or response to therapy. Potential biomarkers of glycolipid storage include plasma or urine Gb3 and lyso-Gb3. Lyso-Gb$_3$ plasma and urinary levels are elevated in Fabry disease. Plasma lyso-Gb3 was found to be useful to diagnose Fabry disease (Rombach et al., 2010). Furthermore, while multiple regression analysis did not demonstrate correlation between plasma lyso-Gb3 concentration and total disease severity score in Fabry males, plasma lysoGb3 concentration did correlate with white matter lesions. In addition, in females, plasma lyso-Gb3 concentration correlated with overall disease severity (Rombach et al., 2010). In Fabry patients plasma lyso-Gb3 falls on ERT, and even more dramatically than Gb3 levels (Togawa et al., 2010, Van Breemen et al., 2011). Urinary lysoGb3 was also correlated with type of mutations, enzyme replacement therapy status and with a number of indicators of disease severity (Auray-Blais et al, 2010). Decreased urinary lyso-Gb3 may reflect decreased kidney lyso-Gb3 burden, since renal tissue lyso-Gb3 was decreased in Fabry mice upon ERT (Togawa et al., 2010b). Despite these promising observations, studies approaching the potential value of lyso-Gb3 concentrations to make clinical decisions regarding ERT dose have not been performed and, thus, it cannot be considered a biomarker for such purpose.

Albuminuria is a biomarker of kidney injury. Both in Fabry and non-Fabry kidney injury the magnitude of albuminuria predicts renal disease progression. In this regard there is solid evidence supporting targeting albuminuria as a therapeutic objective in non-Fabry disease. Anecdotal evidence suggests that this is the case too in Fabry disease, where lowering albuminuria is considered a target to be pursued through adjunctive antiproteinuric therapy (Tahir et al., 2007). A clinical trial (FAACET) is underway to test this hypothesis. Unfortunately, since albuminuria does not improve on ERT in adults, it cannot guide ERT dosing.

Finally promising preliminary data are available of the use of urinary protemics for the diagnosis and eventual monitoring of Fabry disease. The most promising technique is capillary electrophoresis coupled to mass spectrometry (CE-MS) (Mischak H et al., 2010).

6. Conclusions

Research in Fabry disease is very active in recent times and has led to a paradigm shift in our understanding of the disease and its management (Table 3). The advent of ERT has changed the prospects for Fabry disease patients. However, there are, still unsolved problems:

1. ERT does not modify proteinuria, a key risk factor for renal disease progression (Wanner et al., 2010), in adults and does not stop renal disease progression once a certain degree of renal injury, manifested as histological injury, decreased eGFR or proteinuria (>1g/d), has been reached (Germain DG et al., 2007).
2. Despite adequate endothelial cell clearance, ERT does not clear deposits in podocytes, key cells responsible for avoiding proteinuria (Germain DG et al., 2007). This and the correlation of early podocyte injury with proteinuria (Najafian et al., 2010) support a more central role of podocytes in the pathogenesis of renal disease than previously thought.

3. The lack of biomarkers of tissue injury activity and response to therapy hinders dose individualization, the follow-up of the therapeutic response and early identification of females most at risk for progressive disease.

4. The molecular link between the metabolic defect and tissue injury is still poorly characterized. This hinders the development of adjuvant therapies.

The full scope of these gaps in knowledge became evident during the global shortage on ERT availability, which took place in 2009-2010 (Linthorst et al, 2011). Hopefully this realization, as well as recent advances in the pathogenesis and treatment approaches for the disease will further improve the outcome of Fabry patients.

Classical concepts	New paradigms
Endothelium as key target cell	Podocyte as key target cell
Intracellular deposits cause injury	Soluble metabolites cause injury
Deposits injure cells containing them	Injury of distant or adjacent cells
Unknown tissue injury mechanisms	Recruitment of secondary mediators
ERT as only therapy	Need for adjuvant therapies
Same dose fits all	Individualize dose: biomarkers need
Therapeutic nihilism for advanced tissue injury	Target secondary mediators of injury in advanced tissue injury

Table 3. Classical concepts and new paradigms in Fabry nephropathy

7. Acknowledgements

Work by the authors was supported by FEDER funds FIS PS09/00447. JPN was supported by Fundacion Conchita Rabago and AO, MDSN and ABS by FIS.

8. References

Aerts, JM.; Groener, JE.; Kuiper, S.; Donker-Koopman, WE.; Strijland, A.; Ottenhoff, R.; van Roomen, C.; Mirzaian, M.; Wijburg, FA.; Linthorst, GE.; Vedder, AC.; Rombach, SM.; Cox-Brinkman, J.; Somerharju, P.; Boot, RG.; Hollak, CE.; Brady, RO. & Poorthuis, BJ. (2008). Elevated globotriaosylsphingosine is a hallmark of Fabry disease. *Proc Natl Acad Sci USA.*, Vol. 8, No. 105, (February 2008), pp. 2812-2817, ISSN 1091-6490

Agarwal, R.; Acharya, M.; Tian, J.; Hippensteel, RL.; Melnick, JZ.; Qiu, P.; Williams, L. & Batlle, D. (2005). Antiproteinuric effect of oral paricalcitol in chronic kidney disease. *Kidney Int.*, Vol. 6, No. 68, (December 2005), pp.2823-2828, ISSN 0085-2538

Alroy, J.; Sabnis, S. & Kopp, JB. (2002). Renal pathology in Fabry disease. *J Am Soc Nephro,.* Suppl. 2, No. 13, (June 2002), pp. 134-138, ISSN 1046-6673

Alsaad, KO. & Herzenberg, AM. (2007). Distinguishing diabetic nephropathy from other causes of glomerulosclerosis: an update. *J Clin Pathol.*, Vol. 1, No. 60, (January 2007), pp. 18-26, ISSN 1046-6673

Altarescu, G.; Moore, DF.; Pursley, R.; Campia, U.; Goldstein, S.; Bryant, M.; Panza, JA. & Schiffmann, R. (2001). Enhanced endothelium-dependent vasodilation in Fabry disease. *Stroke,* Vol. 7, No. 32, (July 2001), pp. 1559-1562, ISSN 1524-4628

Askari, H.; Kaneski, CR.; Semino-Mora, C.; Desai, P.; Ang, A.; Kleiner, DE.; Perlee, LT.; Quezado, M.; Spollen, LE.; Wustman, BA. & Schiffmann, R. (2007). Cellular and tissue localization of globotriaosylceramide in Fabry disease. *Virchows Arch.*, Vol. 4, No. 451, (October 2007), pp. 823-834, ISSN 0945-6317

Attal, N. & Bouhassira, D. (1999). Mechanisms of pain in peripheral neuropathy. *Acta Neurol Scand.*, No. 173, (1999), pp. 12-24, ISSN 0945-6317

Banikazemi, M.; Bultas, J.; Waldek, S.; Wilcox, WR.; Whitley, CB.; McDonald, M.; Finkel, R.; Packman, S.; Bichet, DG.; Warnock, DG. & Desnick, RJ.; Fabry Disease Clinical Trial Study Group. (2007). Agalsidase-beta therapy for advanced Fabry disease: a randomized trial. *Ann Intern Med.*, Vol. 2, No. 146, (January 2007), pp. 77-86, ISSN 1539-3704

Branton, MH.; Schiffmann, R.; Sabnis, SG.; Murray, GJ.; Quirk, JM.; Altarescu, G.; Goldfarb, L.; Brady, RO.; Balow, JE.; Austin Iii, HA. & Kopp, JB. (2002). Natural history of Fabry renal disease: influence of alpha-galactosidase A activity and genetic mutations on clinical course. *Medicine (Baltimore)*, Vol. 2, No. 81, (March 2002), pp. 122-138, ISSN 0025-7974

Branton, M.; Schiffmann, R. & Kopp, JB. (2002). Natural history and treatment of renal involvement in Fabry disease. *J Am Soc Nephrol.*, Suppl. 2, No. 13, (June 2002), pp. 139-143, ISSN 1046-6673

Cable, WJ.; Kolodny, EH. & Adams, RD. (1982) Fabry disease: impaired autonomic function. *Neurology*, Vol. 5, No. 32, (May 1982), pp. 498-502, ISSN 0028-3878

Cartwright, DJ.; Cole, AL.; Cousins, AJ. & Lee, PJ. (2004). Raised HDL cholesterol in Fabry disease: response to enzyme replacement therapy. *J Inherit Metab Dis.*, Vol. 6, No. 27, (2004), pp. 791-793, ISSN 0141-8955

Clarke JT; Stoltz JM & Mulcahey MR. (1976).Neutral glycosphingolipids of serum lipoproteins in Fabry's disease. *Biochim Biophys Acta.*, Vol. 2, No. 431, (May 1976), pp. 317-325, ISSN 0006-3002

de Zeeuw, D.; Agarwal, R.; Amdahl, M.; Audhya, P.; Coyne, D.; Garimella, T.; Parving, HH.; Pritchett, Y.; Remuzzi, G.; Ritz, E. & Andress, D. (2010). Selective vitamin D receptor activation with paricalcitol for reduction of albuminuria in patients with type 2 diabetes (VITAL study): a randomised controlled trial. *Lancet*, Vol. 9752, No. 376, (Novemer 2010), pp. 1543-1551, ISSN 1474-547X

Desnick, RJ.; Ioannou, YA. & Eng, CM. (2001) Alpha-Galactosidase A deficiency: Fabry disease. In: *The Metabolic Bases of Inherited Disease*, Scriver CR., pp. 3733-3774 McGraw-Hill, ISBN 0071163360, New York

Dobrovolny, R.; Dvorakova, L.; Ledvinova, J.; Magage, S.; Bultas, J.; Lubanda, JC.; Elleder, M.; Karetova, D.; Pavlikova, M. & Hrebicek, M. (2005) Relationship between X-inactivation and clinical involvement in Fabry heterozygotes. Eleven novel mutations in the alpha-galactosidase A gene in the Czech and Slovak population. *J Mol Med.*, Vol. 8, No. 83, (August 2005), pp. 647-654, ISSN 0946-2716

Dobyns, WB. (2006) The pattern of inheritance of X-linked traits is not dominant or recessive, just X-linked. *Acta Paediatr* , Vol 451, No. 95, (April 2006), pp. 11-15, ISSN 0803-5326

Eng, CM.; Guffon, N.; Wilcox, WR.; Germain, DP.; Lee, P.; Waldek, S.; Caplan, L.; Linthorst, GE. & Desnick, RJ.; International Collaborative Fabry Disease Study Group. (2001). Safety and efficacy of recombinant human alpha-galactosidase A--replacement therapy in Fabry's disease. *N Engl J Med.*, Vol. 1, No. 345, (July 2001), pp. 9-16, ISSN 0028-4793

Fogo, AB.; Bostad, L.; Svarstad, E.; Cook, WJ.; Moll, S.; Barbey, F.; Geldenhuys, L.; West, M.; Ferluga, D.; Vujkovac, B.; Howie, AJ.; Burns, A.; Reeve, R.; Waldek, S.; Noël, LH.; Grünfeld, JP.; Valbuena, C.; Oliveira, JP.; Müller, J.; Breunig, F.; Zhang, X. & Warnock, DG; all members of the International Study Group of Fabry Nephropathy (ISGFN). (2010). Scoring system for renal pathology in Fabry disease: report of the International Study Group of Fabry Nephropathy (ISGFN). *Nephrol Dial Transplant.*, Vol. 7, No. 25, (July 2010), pp. 2168-2177, ISSN 1460-2385

Gadoth, N. & Sandbank, U. (1983) Involvement of dorsal root ganglia in Fabry's disease. *J Med Genet.*, Vol. 4, No. 20, (August 1983), pp. 309-312, ISSN 0022-2593

Galbiati, F. ; Razani, B. & Lisanti, MP. (2001) Emerging themes in lipid rafts and caveolae. *Cell*, Vol. 4, No. 16 (August 2001), pp. 403-411, ISSN 0092-8674

Garman, SC. & Garboczi, DN. (2004) The molecular defect leading to Fabry disease: structure of human α-galactosidase. *J Mol Biol.*,Vol. 2, No. 337, (March 2004), pp. 319-335, ISSN 0022-2836

Gemignani, F.; Marbini, A.; Bragaglia, MM. & Govoni, E. (1984) Pathological study of the sural nerve in Fabry's disease. *Eur Neurol.*, Vol. 3, No. 23, (1984), pp. 173-181, ISSN 0014-3022

Germain, DP.; Waldek, S.; Banikazemi, M.; Bushinsky, DA.; Charrow, J.; Desnick, RJ.; Lee, P.; Loew, T.; Vedder, AC.; Abichandani, R.; Wilcox, WR. & Guffon, N. (2007) Sustained, long-term renal stabilization after 54 months of agalsidase beta therapy in patients with Fabry disease. *J Am Soc Nephrol.*, Vol. 5, No. 18, (May 2007), pp. 1547-1557, ISSN 1046-6673

Germain, DP. (2010). Fabry disease. *Orphanet J Rare Dis.*, No. 5, (Novemer 2010), pp. 30, ISSN 1750-1172

Hegemann, S.; Hajioff, D.; Conti, G.; Beck, M.; Sunder-Plassmann, G.; Widmer, U.; Mehta, A. & Keilmann, A. (2006) Hearing loss in Fabry disease: data from the Fabry Outcome Survey. Eur *J Clin. Invest.*,Vol. 9, No, 36, (September 2006), pp. 654-662, ISSN 0014-2972

Hoffmann, B. & Keshav S. (2007) Gastrointestinal symptoms in Fabry disease: everything is possible, including treatment. *Acta Paediatr.*, Vol. 455, No. 96, (April 2007), pp. 84-86, ISSN 0803-5326

Ishii, S.; Nakao, S.; Minamikawa-Tachino, R.; Desnick, RJ. & Fan, JQ. (2002) Alternative splicing in the α-galactosidase A gene: increased exon inclusion results in the Fabry cardiac phenotype. *Am J Hum Genet.*,Vol.4, No. 70, (April 2002), pp. 994-1002, ISSN 0002-9297

Kerem, E.; Hirawat, S.; Armoni, S.; Yaakov, Y.; Shoseyov, D.; Cohen, M.; Nissim-Rafinia, M.; Blau, H.; Rivlin, J.; Aviram, M.; Elfring, GL.; Northcutt, VJ.; Miller, LL.; Kerem, B. & Wilschanski, M. (2008). Effectiveness of PTC124 treatment of cystic fibrosis caused by nonsense mutations: a prospective phase II trial. *Lancet*, Vol. 9640, No. 372, (August 2008), pp. 719-727, ISSN 1474-547X

Kidney Disease: Improving Global Outcomes (KDIGO) CKD-MBD Work Group. (2009) KDIGO clinical practice guideline for the diagnosis, evaluation, prevention, and treatment of Chronic Kidney Disease-Mineral and Bone Disorder (CKD-MBD). *Kidney Int Suppl.*, No. 113, (August 2009), pp. 1-130, ISSN 0098-6577

Kidney Disease Outcomes Quality Initiative (K/DOQI). (2004). K/DOQI clinical practice guidelines on hypertension and antihypertensive agents in chronic kidney disease. *Am J Kidney Dis.*, Vol. 5, No. 53, (May 2004), pp. 1-290, ISSN 1523-6838

Lambers Heerspink, HJ.; Agarwal, R.; Coyne, DW.; Parving, HH.; Ritz, E.; Remuzzi, G.; Audhya, P.; Amdahl, MJ.; Andress, DL. & de Zeeuw, D. (2009) The selective vitamin D receptor activator for albuminuria lowering (VITAL) study: study design and baseline characteristics. *Am J Nephrol.*, Vol. 3, No. 30, (June 2009), pp. 280-286, ISSN 1421-9670

Linhart, A. & Elliott, PM. (2007) The heart in Anderson-Fabry disease and other lysosomal storage disorders. *Heart*, Vol. 4, No. 93, (April 2007), pp. 528-535, ISSN 1468-201X

Linthorst, GE.; Vedder, AC.; Aerts, JM. & Hollak, CE. (2005) Screening for Fabry disease using whole blood spots fails to identify one-third of female carriers. *Clin Chim Acta.*, Vol 1-2, No. 353, (March 2005), pp. 201-203, ISSN 0009-8981

Linthorst, GE.; Germain, DP.; Hollak, CE.; Hughes, D.; Rolfs, A.; Wanner, C. & Mehta, A. (2011). Expert opinion on temporary treatment recommendations for Fabry disease during the shortage of enzyme replacement therapy (ERT). *Mol Genet Metab.*, Vol. 1, No. 102, (January 2011), pp. 99-102, ISSN 1096-7206

MacDermot, KD.; Holmes, A. & Miners, AH. (2001) Anderson–Fabry disease: clinical manifestations and impact of disease in a cohort of 98 hemizygous males. *J Med Genet.*, Vol. 11, No. 38, (November 2001), pp. 750-760, ISSN 1468-6244

Mason, RM. & Wahab, NA. (2003) Extracellular matrix metabolism in diabetic nephropathy. *J Am Soc Nephrol.* Vol. 5, No. 14, (May 2003), pp. 1358-1373, ISSN 1046-6673

Mehta, A.; Ricci, R.; Widmer, U.; Dehout, F.; Garcia de Lorenzo, A.; Kampmann, C.; Linhart, A.; Sunder-Plassmann, G.; Ries, M. & Beck, M. (2004) Fabry disease defined: baseline clinical manifestations of 366 patients in the Fabry Outcome Survey. *Eur J Clin Invest.*, Vol. 3, No. 34, (March 2004), pp. 236-242, ISSN 0014-2972

Mehta, A.; Ginsberg, L.; FOS Investigators. (2005) Natural history of the cerebrovascular complications of Fabry disease. *Acta Paediatr.*, Vol. 447, No. 94, (March 2005), pp 24-27, ISSN 0803-5326

Mehta, A.; Beck, M. & Sunder-Plassmann, G. (2006). *Fabry Disease: Perspectives from 5 Years of FOS*. Oxford: Oxford PharmaGenesis, ISBN-10: 1-903539-03-X

Mehta, A.; Beck, M.; Elliott, P.; Giugliani, R.; Linhart, A.; Sunder-Plassmann, G.; Schiffmann, R.; Barbey, F.; Ries M & Clarke, JT.; Fabry Outcome Survey investigators. (2009). Enzyme replacement therapy with agalsidase alfa in patients with Fabry's disease: an analysis of registry data. *Lancet*, Vol. 9706, No. 374, (December 2009), pp. 1986-1996, ISSN 1474-547X

Mischak, H.; Delles, C.; Klein, J. & Schanstra, JP. (2010). Urinary proteomics based on capillary electrophoresis-coupled mass spectrometry in kidney disease: discovery and validation of biomarkers, and clinical application. *Adv Chronic Kidney Dis.*, Vol. 6, No. 17, (November 2010), pp. 493-506, ISSN 1548-5609

Mitsias, P. & Levine SR. (1996) Cerebrovascular complications of Fabry's disease. *Ann Neurol.*, Vol. 1, No. 40, (July 1996), pp. 8-17, ISSN 0364-5134

Mogami, K.; Kishi, H. & Kobayashi, S. (2005) Sphingomyelinase causes endothelium-dependent vasorelaxation through endothelial nitric oxide production without cytosolic Ca(2+) elevation. *FEBS Lett.*, Vol. 2, No. 579, (January 2005), pp. 393-397, ISSN 0014-5793

Moreno, JA.; Sanchez-Niño, MD.; Sanz, AB.; Lassila, M.; Holthofer, H.; Blanco-Colio, LM.; Egido, J.; Ruiz-Ortega, M. & Ortiz, A. (2008). A slit in podocyte death. *Curr Med Chem.*, Vol. 16, No. 15, (2008), pp. 1645-1654, ISSN 0929-8673

Najafian. B.; Svarstad, E.; Bostad, L.; Gubler, MC.; Tøndel, C.; Whitley, C.& Mauer, M. (2011). Progressive podocyte injury and globotriaosylceramide (GL-3) accumulation in young patients with Fabry disease. *Kidney Int.*, Vol. 6, No. 79, (March 2011), pp. 663-670, ISSN 1523-1755

Nakao, S.; Kodama, C.; Takenaka, T.; Tanaka, A.; Yasumoto, Y.; Yoshida, A.; Kanzaki, T.; Enriquez, AL.; Eng, CM.; Tanaka, H.; Tei, C. & Desnick RJ. (2003). Fabry disease: detection of undiagnosed hemodialysis patients and identification of a "renal variant" phenotype. *Kidney Int.*, Vol. 3, No. 64, (September 2003), pp. 801-807, ISSN 0085-2538

Nance, CS.; Klein, CJ.; Banikazemi, M.; Dikman, SH.; Phelps, RG.; McArthur, JC.; Rodriguez, M. & Desnick, RJ. (2006) Later-onset Fabry disease: an adult variant presenting with the cramp-fasciculation syndrome. *Arch Neurol.*, Vol. 3, No. 63, (March 2006), pp. 453-457, ISSN 0003-9942

Nath, KA. (1992) Tubulointerstitial changes as a major determinant in the progression of renal damage. *Am J Kidney Dis.*, Vol. 1, No. 20, (July1992), pp. 1-17, ISSN 0272-6386

National Kidney Foundation. (2003) K/DOQI clinical practice guidelines for bone metabolism and disease in chronic kidney disease. *Am J Kidney Dis.*,Vol. 4, No. 42, (October 2003), pp. 1-201, ISSN 1523-6838

Nguyen, TT.; Gin, T.; Nicholls, K.; Low, M.; Galanos, J. & Crawford, A. (2005) Ophthalmological manifestations of Fabry disease: a survey of patients at the Royal Melbourne Fabry Disease Treatment Centre. *Clin Experiment Ophthalmol.*, Vol. 2, No. 33, (April 2005), pp. 164-168, ISSN 1442-6404

O'Brien, BD.; Shnitka, TK.; McDougall, R.; Walker, K.; Costopoulos, L.; Lentle, B.; Anholt, L.; Freeman, H. & Thomsom, AB. (1982) Pathophysiologic and ultrastructural basis for intestinal symptoms in Fabry's disease. *Gastroenterology.* Vol. 5, No. 82, (May 1982), pp. 957-962, ISSN 0016-5085

Ogawa, K.; Sugamata, K.; Funamoto, N.; Abe, T.; Sato, T.; Nagashima, K. & Ohkawa, S. (1990). Restricted accumulation of globotriaosylceramide in the hearts of atypical cases of Fabry's disease. *Hum Pathol.*, Vol. 10, No. 21, (October 1990), pp. 1067-1073, ISSN 0046-8177

Oqvist, B.; Brenner, BM.; Oliveira, JP.; Ortiz, A.; Schaefer, R.; Svarstad, E.; Wanner, C.; Zhang, K. & Warnock, DG. (2009). Nephropathy in Fabry disease: the importance of early diagnosis and testing in high-risk populations. *Nephrol Dial Transplant.*, Vol. 6, No. 24, (June 2009), pp. 1736-1743, ISSN 1460-2385

Ortiz, A.; Oliveira, JP.; Waldek, S.; Warnock, DG.; Cianciaruso, B. & Wanner, C.; Fabry Registry. (2008). Nephropathy in males and females with Fabry disease: cross-sectional description of patients before treatment with enzyme replacement therapy. *Nephrol Dial Transplant.*, Vol. 5, No. 23, (May 2008), pp. 1600-1167, ISSN 1460-2385

Ortiz, A.; Oliveira, JP.; Wanner, C.; Brenner, BM.; Waldek, S. & Warnock, DG. (2008). Recommendations and guidelines for the diagnosis and treatment of Fabry nephropathy in adults. *Nat Clin Pract Nephrol.*, Vol. 6, No. 4, (June 2008), pp. 327-336, ISSN 1745-8331

Ortiz, A.; Cianciaruso, B.; Cizmarik, M.; Germain, DP.; Mignani, R.; Oliveira, JP.; Villalobos, J.; Vujkovac, B.; Waldek, S.; Wanner, C. & Warnock, DG. (2010). End-stage renal disease in patients with Fabry disease: natural history data from the Fabry Registry. *Nephrol Dial Transplant.*, Vol. 3, No. 25, (March 2010), pp. 769-775, ISSN 1460-2385

Pagano, RE. (2003) Endocytic trafficking of glycosphingolipids in sphingolipid storage diseases. *Philos Trans R Soc Lond B Biol Sci.*, Vol. 1433, No. 358, (May 2003), pp. 885-891, ISSN 0962-8436

Pantsulaia, T. (2006) Role of TGF-beta in pathogenesis of diabetic nephropathy. *Georgian Med News.*, No.131, (February 2006), pp. 13-18, ISSN 1512-0112

Park, IS.; Kiyomoto, H.; Abboud, SL. & Abboud, HE. (1997) Expression of transforming growth factor-beta and type IV collagen in early streptozotocin-induced diabetes. *Diabetes*, Vol. 3, No. 46, (March 1997), pp. 473-480, ISSN 0012-1797

Patel, MR.; Cecchi, F.; Cizmarik, M.; Kantola, I.; Linhart, A.; Nicholls, K.; Strotmann, J.; Tallaj, J.; Tran, TC.; West, ML.; Beitner-Johnson, D. & Abiose, A. (2011).Cardiovascular events in patients with fabry disease natural history data from the fabry registry. *J Am Coll Cardiol.*, Vol. 9, No. 57, (March 2011), pp. 1093-1099, ISSN 1558-3597

Ries, M.; Bettis, KE.; Choyke, P.; Kopp, JB.; Austin, HA 3rd.; Brady, RO. & Schiffmann, R. (2004). Parapelvic kidney cysts: a distinguishing feature with high prevalence in Fabry disease. *Kidney Int.*, Vol. 3, No. 66, (September 2004), pp. 978-982, ISSN 0085-2538

Ries, M.; Gupta, S.; Moore, DF.; Sachdev, V.; Quirk, JM.; Murray, GJ.; Rosing, DR.; Robinson, C.; Schaefer, E.; Gal, A.; Dambrosia, JM.; Garman, SC.; Brady, RO. & Schiffmann, R. (2005). Pediatric Fabry disease. *Pediatrics*, Vol. 3, No. 115, (March 2005), pp. 344-355, ISSN 1098-4275

Ries, M.; Kim, HJ.; Zalewski, CK.; Mastroianni, MA.; Moore, DF.; Brady, RO.; Dambrosia, JM.; Schiffmann, R. & Brewer. CC. (2007). Neuropathic and cerebrovascular correlates of hearing loss in Fabry disease. *Brain*, Vol. 1, No. 130, (January 2007), pp. 143-150, ISSN 1460-2156

Rodríguez-González-Herrero, ME.; Marín-Sánchez, JM.; Gimeno, JR.; Molero-Izquierdo, C.; De-Casas-Fernández, A.; Rodríguez-González-Herrero, B.; San-Román, I.; Lozano, J.; De-la-Morena, G. & Llovet-Osuna, F. (2008). Ophthalmological manifestations in Fabry's disease. Four clinical cases showing deficient alpha-galactosidase-A activity. *Arch Soc Esp Oftalmol.*, Vol. 12, No. 83, (December 2008), pp. 713-717, ISSN 1989-7286

Rojas-Rivera, J.; De La Piedra, C.; Ramos, A.; Ortiz, A. & Egido, J. (2010). The expanding spectrum of biological actions of vitamin D. *Nephrol Dial Transplant.*, Vol. 9, No. 25, (September 2010), pp. 2850-2865, ISSN 1460-2385

Rombach, SM.; Dekker, N.; Bouwman, MG.; Linthorst, GE.; Zwinderman, AH.; Wijburg, FA.; Kuiper, S.; Vd Bergh Weerman, MA.; Groener, JE.; Poorthuis, BJ.; Hollak, CE. & Aerts, JM. (2010). Plasma globotriaosylsphingosine: diagnostic value and relation to clinical manifestations of Fabry disease. *Biochim Biophys Acta.*, Vol. 9, No. 1802, (Septemer 2010), pp. 741-748, ISSN 0006-3002

Romeo, G.; D'Urso, M.; Pisacane, A.; Blum, E.; De Falco, A. & Ruffilli, A. (1975). Residual activity of alpha-galactosidase A in Fabry's disease. *Biochem Genet.*, Vol. 9-10, No. 13, (October 1975), pp.615-628, ISSN 0002-9343

Rosenberg, DM.; Ferrans, VJ.; Fulmer, JD.; Line, BR.; Barranger, JA.; Brady, RO. & Crystal, RG. (1980). Chronic airflow obstruction in Fabry's disease. *Am J Med.*, Vol. 6, No. 68, (June 1980), pp. 898-905, ISSN 0002-9343

Rowe, JW.; Gilliam, JI. & Warthin, TA. (1974). Intestinal manifestations of Fabry's disease. *Ann Intern Med.*, Vol. 5, No. 81, (November 1974), pp. 628-631, ISSN 0003-4819

Sanchez-Niño, MD.; Sanz, AB.; Ihalmo, P.; Lassila, M.; Holthofer, H.; Mezzano, S.; Aros, C.; Groop, PH.; Saleem, MA.; Mathieson, PW.; Langham, R.; Kretzler, M.; Nair, V.; Lemley, KV.; Nelson, RG.; Mervaala, E.; Mattinzoli, D.; Rastaldi, MP.; Ruiz-Ortega, M.; Martin-Ventura, JL.; Egido, J. & Ortiz, A. (2009). The MIF receptor CD74 in diabetic podocyte injury. *J Am Soc Nephrol.*, Vol. 2, No. 20, (February 2009), pp. 353-362, ISSN 1533-3450

Sanchez-Niño, MD.; Sanz, AB.; Carrasco, S.; Saleem, MA.; Mathieson, PW.; Valdivielso, JM.; Ruiz-Ortega, M.; Egido, J. & Ortiz, A. (2010). Globotriaosylsphingosine actions on human glomerular podocytes: implications for Fabry nephropathy. *Nephrol Dial Transplant.*, (May 2010) [Epub ahead of print], ISSN 1460-2385

Sanchez-Niño, MD.; Benito-Martin, A. & Ortiz, A. (2010). New paradigms in cell death in human diabetic nephropathy. *Kidney Int.*, Vol. 8, No. 78, (October 2010), pp. 737-744, ISSN 1523-1755

Schaefer, RM.; Tylki-Szymańska, A. & Hilz, MJ. (2009). Enzyme replacement therapy for Fabry disease: a systematic review of available evidence. *Drugs*, Vol. 16, No. 69, (November 2009), pp. 2179-2205, ISSN 0012-6667

Schieppati, A. & Remuzzi, G. (2003). Proteinuria and its consequences in renal disease. *Acta Paediatr Suppl.*, Vol. 443, No. 92, (December 2003), pp. 9-13, ISSN 0803-5326

Schiffmann, R.; Kopp, JB.; Austin, HA 3rd.; Sabnis, S.; Moore, DF.; Weibel, T.; Balow, JE. & Brady, RO. (2001). Enzyme replacement therapy in Fabry disease: a randomized controlled trial. *JAMA.*, Vol. 21, No. 285, (June 2001), pp. 2743-2749, ISSN 0098-7484

Schiffmann, R. & Scott, LJ. (2002) Pathophysiology and assessment of neuropathic pain in Fabry disease. *Acta Paediatr Suppl.*, Vol. 439, No. 91, (2002), pp. 48-52, ISSN 0803-5326

Schiffmann, R.; Ries, M.; Timmons, M.; Flaherty, JT. & Brady, RO. (2006). Long-term therapy with agalsidase alfa for Fabry disease: safety and effects on renal function in a home infusion setting. *Nephrol Dial Transplant.*, Vol. 2, No. 21, (February 2006), pp. 345-354, ISSN 0931-0509

Schiffmann, R.; Rapkiewicz, A.; Abu-Asab, M.; Ries, M.; Askari, H.; Tsokos, M. & Quezado, M. (2006). Pathological findings in a patient with Fabry disease who died after 2.5 years of enzyme replacement. *Virchows Arch.*, Vol. 3, No. 448, (March 2006), pp. 337-343, ISSN 0945-6317

Schiffmann, R. (2009). Fabry disease. *Pharmacol Ther.*, Vol. 1, No. 122, (April 2009), pp. 65-77, ISSN 1879-016X

Schiffmann, R.; Warnock, DG.; Banikazemi, M.; Bultas, J.; Linthorst, GE.; Packman, S.; Sorensen, SA.; Wilcox, WR. & Desnick, RJ. (2009). Fabry disease: progression of nephropathy, and prevalence of cardiac and cerebrovascular events before enzyme replacement therapy. *Nephrol Dial Transplant.*, Vol. 7, No. 24, (July 2009), pp. 2102-2111, ISSN 1460-2385

Shah, JS. & Elliott, PM. (2005). Fabry disease and the heart: an overview of the natural history and the effect of enzyme replacement therapy. *Acta Paediatr Suppl.*, Vol. 447, No. 94, (March 2005), pp. 11-14, ISSN 0803-5326

Sharma, K.; Ziyadeh, FN.; Alzahabi, B.; McGowan, TA.; Kapoor, S.; Kurnik, BR.; Kurnik, PB. & Weisberg, LS. (1997). Increased renal production of transforming growth factor-beta1 in patients with type II diabetes. *Diabetes*. Vol. 5, No. 46, (May 1997), pp. 854-859, ISSN 0012-1797

Shen, JS., Meng, XL., Moore, DF., Quirk, JM., Shayman, JA., Schiffmann, R. & Kaneski, CR. (2008) Globotriaosylceramide induces oxidative stress and up-regulates cell adhesion molecule expression in Fabry disease endothelial cells. *Mol Genet Metab.*, Vol. 3, No. 95, (November 2008), pp. 163-168, ISSN 1096-7206

Sims, K.; Politei, J.; Banikazemi, M. & Lee, P. (2009). Stroke in Fabry disease frequently occurs before diagnosis and in the absence of other clinical events: natural history data from the Fabry Registry. *Stroke*, Vol. 3, No. 40, (March 2009), pp. 788-794, ISSN 1524-4628

Sunder-Plassmann, G. (2006). Renal manifestations of Fabry disease, In: *Fabry Disease: Perspectives from 5 Years of FOS*, Mehta, A.; Beck M. & Sunder-Plassmann G., Oxford: Oxford PharmaGenesis, ISN 190353903X, Oxford

Svarstad, E., Iversen, BM. & Bostad, L. (2004). Bedside stereomicroscopy of renal biopsies may lead to a rapid diagnosis of Fabry's disease. *Nephrol Dial Transplant.*, Vol. 12, No. 19, (December 2004), pp. 3202-3203.

Tahir, H.; Jackson, LL. & Warnock, DG. (2007). Antiproteinuric therapy and fabry nephropathy: sustained reduction of proteinuria in patients receiving enzyme replacement therapy with agalsidase-beta. *J Am Soc Nephrol.*, Vol. 9, No. 18, (September 2007), pp. 2609-2617, ISSN 1046-6673

Thadhani, R.; Wolf, M.; West, ML.; Tonelli, M.; Ruthazer, R.; Pastores, GM. & Obrador, GT. (2002). Patients with Fabry disease on dialysis in the United States. *Kidney Int.*, Vol. 1, No. 61, (January 2002), pp. 249-255, ISSN 0085-2538

Thomas, ME.; Brunskill, NJ.; Harris, KP.; Bailey, E.; Pringle, JH.; Furness, PN. & Walls, J. (1999). Proteinuria induces tubular cell turnover: A potential mechanism for tubular atrophy. *Kidney Int.*, Vol. 3, No. 55, (March 1999), pp. 890-898, ISSN 0085-2538

Togawa, T.; Kodama, T.; Suzuki, T.; Sugawara, K.; Tsukimura, T.; Ohashi, T.; Ishige, N.; Suzuki, K.; Kitagawa, T. & Sakuraba, H. (2010). Plasma globotriaosylsphingosine as a biomarker of Fabry disease. *Mol Genet Metab.*, Vol. 3, No. 100, (July 2010), pp. 257-261, ISSN 1096-7206

Togawa, T.; Kawashima, I.; Kodama, T.; Tsukimura, T.; Suzuki, T.; Fukushige, T.; Kanekura, T. & Sakuraba, H. (2010). Tissue and plasma globotriaosylsphingosine could be a biomarker for assessing enzyme replacement therapy for Fabry disease. *Biochem Biophys Res Commun.*, Vol. 4, No. 399, (September 2010), pp. 716-720, ISSN 1090-2104

Tøndel, C.; Bostad, L.; Hirth, A. & Svarstad, E. (2008). Renal biopsy findings in children and adolescents with Fabry disease and minimal albuminuria. *Am J Kidney Dis.*, Vol. 5, No. 51, (May 2008), pp. 767-776, ISSN 1523-6838

Torra, R. (2008). Renal manifestations in Fabry disease and therapeutic options. *Kidney Int.*, No. 111, (December 2008), pp. 23-32, ISSN 0098-6577

Torra, R.; Oliveira, JP. & Ortiz, A. (2010). UGA hopping: a sport for nephrologists too? *Nephrol Dial Transplant.*, Vol. 8, No. 25, (August 2010), pp. 2391-2395, ISSN 1460-2385

Tryggvason, K. & Pettersson, E. (2003) Causes and consequences of proteinuria: the kidney filtration barrier and progressive renal failure. *J Intern Med.*, Vol. 3, No. 254, (September 2003), pp. 216-224, ISSN 0954-6820

Tsakiris, D.; Simpson, HK.; Jones, EH.; Briggs, JD.; Elinder, CG.; Mendel, S.; Piccoli, G.; dos Santos, JP.; Tognoni, G.; Vanrenterghem, Y. & Valderrabano, F. (1996). Report on management of renal failure in Europe, XXVI, 1995. Rare diseases in renal replacement therapy in the ERA-EDTA Registry. *Nephrol Dial Transplant.*, Suppl. 7, No. 11, (1996), pp. 4-20, ISSN 0931-0509

Utsumi, K.; Yamamoto, N.; Kase, R.; Takata, T.; Okumiya, T.; Saito, H.; Suzuki, T.; Uyama, E. & Sakuraba, H. (1997). High incidence of thrombosis in Fabry's disease. *Intern Med.*, Vol. 5, No. 36, (May 1997), pp. 327-329, ISSN 0918-2918

van Breemen, MJ.; Rombach, SM.; Dekker, N.; Poorthuis, BJ.; Linthorst, GE.; Zwinderman, AH.; Breunig, F.; Wanner, C.; Aerts, JM. & Hollak, CE. (2011). Reduction of elevated plasma globotriaosylsphingosine in patients with classic Fabry disease following enzyme replacement therapy. *Biochim Biophys Acta.*, Vol. 1, No. 1812, (January 2011), pp. 70-76, ISSN 0006-3002

Vedder, AC.; Strijland, A.; vd Bergh Weerman, MA.; Florquin, S.; Aerts, JM. & Hollak, CE. (2006). Manifestations of Fabry disease in placental tissue. *J Inherit Metab Dis.*, Vol. 1, No. 29, (February 2006), pp. 106-111, ISSN 0141-8955

Vedder, AC.; Linthorst, GE.; Houge, G.; Groener, JE.; Ormel, EE.; Bouma, BJ.; Aerts, JM.; Hirth, A. & Hollak, CE. (2007). Treatment of Fabry disease: outcome of a comparative trial with agalsidase alfa or beta at a dose of 0.2 mg/kg. *PLoS One*, Vol. 7, No. 2, (July 2007), pp. 598, ISSN 1932-6203

Wang, RY.; Lelis, A.; Mirocha, J. & Wilcox, WR. (2007). Heterozygous Fabry women are not just carriers, but have a significant burden of disease and impaired quality of life. *Genet Med.*, Vol. 1, No. 9, (January 2007), pp. 34-45, ISSN 1098-3600

Wanner, C., Oliveira, JP., Ortiz, A., Mauer, M., Germain, DP., Linthorst, GE., Serra, AL., Maródi, L., Mignani, R., Cianciaruso, B., Vujkovac, B., Lemay, R., Beitner-Johnson, D., Waldek, S. & Warnock, DG. (2010). Prognostic indicators of renal disease progression in adults with Fabry disease: natural history data from the Fabry Registry. *Clin J Am Soc Nephrol.*, Vol. 12, No. 5, (December 2010), pp. 2220-2228, ISSN 1555-905X

Wilcox, WR.; Oliveira, JP.; Hopkin, RJ.; Ortiz, A.; Banikazemi, M.; Feldt-Rasmussen, U.; Sims, K.; Waldek, S.; Pastores, GM.; Lee, P.; Eng, CM.; Marodi, L.; Stanford, KE.; Breunig, F.; Wanner, C.; Warnock, DG.; Lemay, RM. & Germain, DP; Fabry Registry. (2008). Females with Fabry disease frequently have major organ involvement: lessons from the Fabry Registry. *Mol Genet Metab.*, Vol. 2, No. 93, (February 2008), pp. 112-128, ISSN 1096-7206

Zarate, YA. & Hopkin, R J. (2008). Fabry's disease. *Lancet.* Vol. 9647, No. 372, (October 2008), pp. 1427-1435, ISSN 1474-547X

9

Fabry Cardiomyopathy: A Global View

Rocio Toro Cebada, Alipio Magnas and Jose Luis Zamorano
Departamento de Medicina de la Universidad de Cadiz, c/DR Marañon S/N, Cadiz
Spain

1. Introduction

Fabry disease (FD) is a lysosomal storage disease (LSD). It has been stated that the second most common LSD after Gaucher disease is Fabry disease; its worldwide incidence is from approximately 1 in 40 000 to 1 in 117 000 live newborns for the classic form of the disease, but the precise prevalence is unknown. Wide variations in the prevalence of FD have been reported in different countries and, with increasing awareness and screening, it is likely that the actual prevalence may be higher than previously recorded, particularly when late-onset phenotypes are taken into account. An accurate estimation of its epidemiology is difficult to make because FD is clinically very heterogeneous and its early classic manifestations tend to be non-specific and often unrecognized. Patients are therefore frequently mis-diagnosed, or not diagnosed until late in life. Recently a newborn screening showed an incidence of one in 3100 live-newborns, and according to this study, the later-onset forms of FD present a surprisingly high incidence [1].

Lysosomal biogenesis involves ongoing synthesis of lysosomal hydrolases, membrane constitutive proteins, and new membranes. Lysosomes originate in the fusion of trans-Golgi network vesicles (TGN) with late endosomes. Progressive vesicular acidification accompanies the maturation of the TGN vesicles and this gradient facilitates the pH-dependent dissociation of receptors and ligands, as well as activation of lysosomal hydrolases.

Abnormalities at any stage of the biosynthesis can impair enzyme activation and lead to lysosomal storage disorder. Lysosomal integral or associated membrane proteins are sorted to the membrane or interior of the lysosome by several different signals. Phosphorylation, sulfation, additional proteolytic processing, and macromolecular assembly of heteromers occur concurrently. These are critical to enzyme function, and defects can result in multiple enzyme/protein deficiencies.

The common pathway for LSD is the accumulation of specific macromolecules within tissues and cells that normally have a high flux of these substrates. The majority of lysosomal enzyme deficiencies result from point mutations or genetic arrangements at a locus that encodes a single lysosomal hydrolase[3-5].

Most LSDs are inherited as autosomal recessive disorders, except Hunter and FD. The latter is an X-linked inherited lysosomal storage disorder that results from mutations in the α-galactosidase gene. The gene encoding human α-galactosidase A enzyme (α-Gal A), located at Xq22.1, spans genomic sequences of approximately 13 kb, containing seven exons, which have been isolated and characterized [6,7].

Alpha-galactosidase A is a lysosomal exoglycohydrolase. The mature α-Gal A enzyme polypeptide is 398 amino acids and contains three functional N-glycosylation sites. The active enzyme is a homodimer of approximately 101 kd. This mutation has significant consequences in glycosphingolipid catabolism resulting from deficient or absent activity of the lysosomal enzyme α-gal A. This enzyme helps to break down and remove glycolipids. The enzymatic defect leads to progressive accumulation of the glycolipid globotriaosyl ceramide (Gb3 or Gl3), or ceramide trihexoside, in the lysosomes in the cells of most organs. Substrate accumulation leads to lysosomal distortion, which has significant pathologic consequences [8-9].

Up to now, more than 300 mutations that cause FD have been identified, including missense, nonsense, small deletions and insertions, large gene rearrangements, and splice mutations. Most mutations are private and unique, occurring in one or a few affected families. In the cardiac variant of FD all individuals to date have missense or splicing mutations that express residual α-Gal A activity. All renal variants identified to date have been associated with missense mutations. Three mutations (p.Arg112His, p.Arg301Gln, and p.Gly328Arg) have been identified in individuals with the classic phenotype and the cardiac variant phenotype, suggesting that other modifying factors are involved in disease expression. Therefore it is necessary to sequence the entire α-gal A gene and adjacent regions to identify the FD mutation in a family [10-14].

FD is considered highly penetrating in males, although variable in its expression. In affected males, the clinical diagnosis is confirmed by α-gal A deficiency. The majority of males with FD have absent or very low enzyme activity (1–2% of normal level) and classical phenotype with multiple disease manifestations. Males who show higher residual enzyme activity, approximately 3–10% of normal level, appear to have milder expression of FD. These individuals are diagnosed with FD later in life, after cardiomyopathy of unknown etiology (in most cases, hypertrophic cardiomyopathy - HMC) is discovered [4].

About 60–70% of females heterozygous for a Fabry disease mutation have some disease manifestations, and approximately 10% of these heterozygous females have severe manifestations, similar to the phenotype in males. Enzyme activity is not reliable for determining female carrier status because women who are obligate carriers have variable levels of α-gal A that can overlap with enzyme levels found in healthy controls. Therefore it is necessary to sequence the entire α-gal A gene and adjacent regions to identify the Fabry disease mutation in a family. The absence of family history suggestive of FD, or de novo mutations documented, does not rule out the diagnosis of FD. The rate of new mutations is unknown [8].

2. Cellular physiopathology

Many theories have been proposed with respect to the pathology of FD. It has been hypothesized that the overloading of lysosomes with Gb3 simply leads to the apoptosis of the cell [15]. Another theory argues that the inflammation process is related to the accumulation of Gb3. This theory has been defended based on the parallel structure between Gb3 and CD77, which is supposed to play an important role in apoptosis and necrosis [16]. Finally, Gb3-accumulation has been reported to induce oxidative stress and/or the formation reactive oxygen species (ROS). Another gateway into alteration of endothelial function may be given by the Nitric-Oxide-Synthase-3-genotypes. Endothelium-derived nitric oxide (eNO), produced by eNO synthase (eNOS), is a key regulator of vessel wall function and cardiovascular homeostasis[17]. Furthermore, the possible relationship between the relative thickness of the left posterior wall and endothelium-derived nitric oxide synthase has been demonstrated. These are the first data showing a significant association of non-GLA-derived sequence variants with the cardiac phenotype in Fabry disease that may, in part, explain the great phenotypic variability of the disease[18].

3. Clinical presentation

Clinically, FD may present as cardiomyopathy, renal disease or neurological small-vessels disease. The age range at which FD presents is quite broad and extends from childhood to the forties, depending on the enzyme residual activity.

Nephropathy is one of the major complications of FD: the nephropathy is progressive and is marked by a persistent insidious development. An analysis of the causes of death reported for 181 affected relatives and 42 patients (699 males and 754 females), enrolled in the Fabry outcome survey (FOS) indicates that the incidence of renal disease as a cause of death appears to be decreasing, while the incidence of cardiac disease is increasing; these trends probably reflect improvements in the management of renal disease in these patients. By adulthood, renal failure frequently becomes a major complication of FD, with more than 50% of male and more than 20% of female patients eventually developing advanced renal disease or end-stage renal disease (ESRD) [19-20].

Effects on the renal system in FD can and need to be detected in the earlier years of life. Renal involvement has previously been categorized as the second phase of the disease and, as stated by West et al.,[21] older patients are more likely to be diagnosed with severe Fabry nephropathy on their first consultation.

Microalbuminuria is one of the first signs of impairment of renal function, and overt proteinuria may start as early as 10 years of age. Biopsy studies have shown that glomerular and vascular changes are present before progression to overt proteinuria, although chronic kidney lesions may already be present. In young patients, glomerular hyperfiltration can mask the detection of early decline in the glomerular filtration rate (GFR) to the extent that a critical number of nephrons become damaged and cannot maintain adequate glomerular filtration.

The decline in GFR typically commences once proteinuria is established but may precede it. Overt proteinuria is more prominent in men than in women. Proteinuria is a risk factor for progression of nephropathy.

Progression to ESRD is common in hemizygous males (in the third to fifth decades of life), and this population group presents more rapid rates of FD progression than those who do not suffer ESRD. The survival of patients with FD in dialysis is better than that of diabetic patients, but it is clearly decreased compared with uremic patients with other nephropathies, despite a lower mean age of uremia. The outcome of kidney transplantation is similar to that found in other patients with ESRD, despite controversial issues published in the past. The use of a kidney donor with normal α-Gal-A activity in the control of the metabolic systemic disease is unproven. The recurrence of Gb3 deposits in the kidney graft has been documented only rarely [20].

Cardiac involvement is very common and is the most frequent cause of death not only in hemizygote males but also in female heterozygote carriers with α-Gal A deficiency, with a reduction of life expectancy of approximately 20 and 15 years respectively. The heart may be the only organ affected in the classic phenotype of FD, and this is designated the "cardiac variant". Within the heart, the myocites, vascular endothelium, conducting system and valves can all be affected. Abnormal storage of the lipid in the blood vessels, with eventual occlusion of the small arterioles, leads to most of the clinical manifestations. Although cardiac involvement of FD begins early, the average age for presenting clinically overt cardiac symptoms (including dyspnea, reduced exercise tolerance, angina, chest pain, palpitations, ventricular arrhythmias, syncope, transient ischemic attacks, stroke and heart failure) has been reported to be 32 years in men and 40 years in women. Cardiovascular manifestations include renovascular and systemic hypertension, aortic root dilatation, mitral prolapse and congestive heart failure [22].

Although angina is often reported, the incidence of epicardial coronary stenosis is not a dominant feature, and is probably related to coronary microvascular dysfunction. In respect of arrhythmias, a broad spectrum can be seen including shortened or prolonged PR-intervals, AV blocks of different degrees and, sometimes, malignant ventricular arrhythmias. The most frequent cardiac manifestations of the disease are permanent and paroxysmal atrial fibrillation and intermittent ventricular tachycardia. Moreover, an impairment of autonomic control of the heart in boys with FD increases heart variability and may be responsible for the increased cardiac morbidity [23].

LV hypertrophy is detected in more than 50% of patients. It is more frequent and has an earlier age of onset in males than in females. LVH is a hallmark of FD that can initially present with preserved ventricular function, as has been reported in 3% of men with LVH, and in up to 6% of men and 12% of women with late-onset hypertrophic cardiomyopathy (HCM). LVH is generally symmetrical, although asymmetric septal hypertrophy has been described, and the condition can mimic the phenotypical and clinical features of HCM.

FD is a relatively prevalent cause of HCM and is associated with significant morbidity and early death due to heart failure or ventricular arrhythmias. HCM, mainly characterized by LVH and conduction abnormalities, may in fact be the major presenting feature of the disease.

The electrocardiogram may show LV hypertrophy, P-wave abnormalities, conduction defects, and ventricular dysrhythmias. Typically the echocardiogram shows marked increases in wall thickness and ventricular dilatation later in the disease process. Leaflet and cuspid thickening can be seen, and this produces valve impairment that usually does not require surgical treatment [24].

Tissue Doppler Imaging (TDI) and strain rate echocardiography represent new echocardiographic tools. In particular, with TDI allow measuring myocardial contraction and relaxation velocities can be measured, thus providing an objective assessment of both diastolic and systolic ventricular function. In addition, it has been demonstrated that specific TDI parameters (E\Ea ratio) provide a good estimate of left ventricular and atrial filling pressure. The study of left ventricular hypertrophy and cardiomyopathies represents one of the most important fields of application for this imaging technique. TDI can detect the first sign of myocardial damage in a patient with FC and normal cardiac wall thickness. Furthermore, Tissue Doppler (TD) studies have been shown to be useful in detecting cardiac involvement in female carriers with no systemic manifestations of Fabry disease. TDI analysis in mutation-positive patients can enable professionals to recognize preclinical cardiac damage in Fabry disease: a reduction of TDI velocities may represent the first sign of initial intrinsic myocardial impairment.

The clinical usefulness of TD echocardiography includes a predictive role, in a proper clinical setting. TDI has demonstrated cardiac impairment in patients without LVH, and the correlation between hypertrophy and severity of baseline dysfunction as measured by TDI supports the specificity of this technique. In addition, an inverse relationship between LVH and myocardial systolic velocity (Sa) has been found. Data suggest that Sa correlates very closely with LV wall thickness. In studies, the IVCT was significantly shorter in the group without LVH, compared with the control group, but showed a tendency to be longer in the group with LVH. This may be attributable to the onset of compensating mechanisms as a result of myocardial impairment, due to the stored vacuolated material being mostly confined to the perinuclear zone, with no or only mild instances of fibrosis in this population [26,27].

Cardiac magnetic resonance imaging (c-MRI) with delayed enhancement may be useful in the non-invasive recognition of myocardial fibrosis, in the context of cardiac involvement of FD. With delayed gadolinium enhancement, c-MRI can identify areas of myocardial damage in HCM and in FD. The evaluation of the myocardial location and distribution patterns of delayed enhancement helps in the identification of the two causes of LV hypertrophy, HCM and LVH associated with Fabry cardiomyopathy.

Furthermore, the myocardial T2 relaxation time is prolonged in patients with Fabry's disease compared with that in hypertrophic patients, and its measurement could be complementary to the delayed enhancement technique [28,29].

Dermatological lesions usually appear in hemizygotous patients, but less frequently in children and women. The earliest clinical signs of Fabry disease often manifest as dermatological disturbances such as angiokeratomas, hypohidrosis, acroparesthesias, and impaired thermal and vibration detection. These disturbances are caused by accumulation of cellular globotriaosylceramide in the skin due to deficient lysosomal α-galactosidase A activity.

The simplest recognizable, but not pathognomonic, characteristics are angiokeratomas, described mostly (66%) in males but also (33%) in females. Angiokeratomas, which are another hallmark of FD, are red papulomatous lesions occurring in groups on the buttocks and in umbilical areas, the thighs and genital areas. Telangiectasias have been described, again mostly in men. Some authors have described the typical "FD rash" that includes angiokeratomas and telangiectasias. It has been established that there is an association between these dermatological lesions and other early signs such as proteinuria, paresthesias and cornea verticillata. Facial dysmorphism with a characteristic coarsening of the facial features is increasingly recognized[30, 31].

Xeroderma has also been described; reduced production of tears and saliva affect 50 % of this population. Although hypohidrosis/anhidrosis is a classic feature of FD, it has been detected in only 11.9% of females and 6.4% of males, and is also reported in childhood.

With respect to ocular and auditory symptoms, the most characteristic manifestation is increased vascular tortuosity. Located in the superficial layer of the cornea, using a slit lamp, a haze has been described as the most frequent cornea abnormality. Some authors have suggested that the haze is the natural evolution of cornea verticillata. This latter condition has been described in the majority of patients affected with FD (70%); it is termed cornea verticillata because the deposits are distributed in a vortex pattern. Two types of lens opacity have been described in FD: one type is anterior capsular and subcapsular cataracts, which are always bilateral, and the other type is posterior subcapsular cataracts, which have been described more rarely but specifically, hence these latter have been designated "Fabry cataracts". Vascular lesions are demonstrated using ocular fundus examination [32-34]

High frequency sensorineural hearing loss is common in FD, and affects males earlier in life. Hearing is worse in patients with FD than in the general population, but clinically relevant hearing impairment only affects16% of patients. Sensorineural hearing loss is less common in children than previously reported, although tinnitus appeared to correlate significantly with severity of clinical presentation in children

The earliest neurological manifestation is painful neuropathy observed in the majority of the patients, mean age of onset 9-14 years in males and 16-20 years in females. Most invalidating neuropathic pain is described as acroparesthesias, which can affect the whole body, but are reported mostly in the hands and feet. Fabry neuropathy has a typical neurophysiological pattern that enables it to be differentiated from other neuropathies. The incidence of carpal tunnel syndrome appears higher than in the general population. Gastrointestinal manifestations of autonomous nervous system involvement may range from abdominal pain to diarrhoea and, more rarely, constipation; in women, abdominal pain may be considered, erroneously, to be of gynecological origin. Altered sweating function is a frequent and classic feature. High temperature increases poor tolerance: fever, and high environmental temperature, as well as physical exercise, can trigger acute pain at the extremities with weakness, which is often intense, and generalized malaise. The central nervous system can be affected, and this contributes to earlier mortality, with a median age of 50 years. As happens with the heart, men will typically be affected in their forties, and women ten years later.

Cerebrovascular events (TIAs, stroke), are present in over 25% of FD cases; in FD they occur at a rather early age and increase progressively. The areas most affected are those supplied by posterior circulation. Renal and cardiac disease can co-exist with cerebrovascular disease, and may predispose patients with FD disease to neurological disability and stroke; however, recent data show that most patients (70.9% of males and 76.9% of females) had not experienced renal or cardiac disease before their first stroke. In addition, 50% of males and 38.3% of females had their first stroke before being diagnosed with FD. In female FD patients, who were for a long time considered to be merely "carriers", and so less affected, the prevalence of cerebrovascular events reported now seems to be as high as in male patients. Differences in cerebral blood velocity have been shown in these patients. These observations have been confirmed after the patients had been treated for a long period of time. Typically, MRI may show lesions attributable to small infarctions, and diffuse alteration of the white matter, especially in deeper sections, with images suggestive of arteriolar involvement of the perforating arteries (lacunar infarctions and leukoaraiosis). The 'pulvinar sign' is a characteristic MRI manifestation of FD; it is a symmetric hyperintensity image in both pulvinar nuclei [1, 35-36].

Fabry patients, even those with marked structural alterations of the brain, show only mild cognitive deficits.

Neuro-psychiatric symptoms have been demonstrated in patients affected with FD. Depression is a frequent and under- diagnosed problem. Depression can have a serious effect on quality of life in patients with FD. The high frequency of depression in FD is likely to be related to the general burden of this chronic multi-organic hereditary disease, but not to the structural brain alterations typical of FD.

Other symptoms associated with FD are gastrointestinal (GI) symptoms. Abdominal pain (often after eating) and diarrhoea are the most frequent manifestations, but other GI symptoms include constipation, nausea and vomiting. The median age of onset of many GI symptoms is before the age of 15 years. FD may be complicated by osteopenia of the lumbar spine and femoral neck.

4. Diagnosis of FD

Diagnosis of FD is often delayed by at least 3 years, and often by 20 years, after the onset of clinical instauration. Male patients with a family member affected need a biochemical analysis in order to measure the plasma or urinary Gb3(lys-Gb3), or α-galactosidase A activity. In addition, genetic analysis of the GLA gene can confirm the diagnosis.

For suspected heterozygotous females, demonstration of markedly decreased α-Gal A enzyme activity in plasma and/or isolated leukocytes confirms the carrier state in a female. In those women with normal α-Gal A enzyme activity, molecular genetic testing is necessary to clarify genetic status. Some studies have confirmed the need for direct sequencing in females, instead of other screening strategies.

Those patients with symptoms suggestive of FD require a screening based on the measurement of the accumulated substrate, Gb3, in the urine, especially male patients. Measurement of enzyme levels and assessment of mutational status using blood spots are increasingly utilized. Similarly, quantifying the enzyme in urine samples by enzyme-linked immunoabsorbent assay (ELISA) shows promise, although such diagnostic methods are only reliable in males[3].

Molecular prenatal diagnosis has become feasible in families with known mutations, or by analysis of intragenetic and closely-linked markers. The prenatal diagnosis of FD is performed using cultured amniocytes, direct and cultured chorionic villi, or blastomeres for preimplantation diagnosis. As soon as the fetal sex is known, the α-Gal A activity or mutation analyses are performed. Chorionic villus sampling is the optimal procedure, providing fresh fetal tissues after the first trimester[37] .

5. Treatment of FD

Specific pharmacologic therapy for FD with enzyme replacement therapy (ERT) is endorsed by health regulatory agencies. Two authorized drugs are available in Europe for ERT.

ERT supplies recombinant GLA to cells and reverses several of the metabolic and pathologic abnormalities. ERT has been available for the treatment of FD since 2001 with the introduction of two products, agalsidase-α (Repaglal@, ShireHGT Inc) and agalsidase β (Fabrazyme, Genzyme Corp).

Agalsidase-α is purified from a stably transfected human cell line 120 and is infused at a dose of 0.2 mg/kg over a period of 40 min, every two weeks. The extra efficacy of agalsidase alpha administered at 0.2 mg/kg in weekly infusions may be beneficial in some patients.

Agalsidase-β is produced in Chinese hamster ovary cells and is infused at a dose of 1.0 mg/kg over a period of up to 4 h, every 2 weeks. The use of a lower maintenance dose of agalsidase beta, 0.3 mg/kg, has been shown to maintain Gb3 clearance in the short term in some patients but not all.

Emerging treatment strategies for FD involve molecular chaperone therapy, and these are very promising for specific mutations. Pharmaceutical chaperones, currently in phase 3 clinical trials, are small molecular ligands that can be administered orally and which bind selectively to the mutant enzyme, promoting correct folding and delivery of the enzyme to the lysosome. In the case of FD, use of the chaperone 1-deoxygalactojirimycin hydrochloride has been shown to increase the activity of several a-galactosidase A-responsive mutants and to reduce urinary levels of Gb3 in those patients who have missense mutations. Recent studies have shown that chemical chaperones can improve the efficacy of ERT.

Substrate reduction therapy (SRT) circumvents enzyme replacement /modification by inhibiting synthesis of globotriaosyl ceramide. This approach involves the use of a glucosyl ceramide synthase inhibitor, which would slow the rate of Gb3 synthesis, and thus decrease lysosomal storage. Combinatorial therapy using ERT and SRT is being considered as a treatment strategy. Enzyme activators may increase the residual activity of mutant GLA in the lysosomes of patients with FD, thereby lessening lysosomal storage of the substrate and alleviating symptoms. However, these activators may not be beneficial if their efficacy is not high enough or if the residual activity of mutant GLA is inadequate.

Specific small molecule promoter activators may increase the amount of GLA in lysosomes by stimulating expression of the target protein. This would result in an increased amount of GLA in the lysosomes, as the enhancement of mutant enzyme expression may proportionally increase protein trafficking to the lysosome. Therefore, in Fabry patients with significant residual GLA enzyme activity, a small molecule promoter activator may correct lysosomal storage by amplifying the amount of enzyme in lysosomes.

Another future treatment strategy involves altering the proteostasis network in cells; this network consists of many highly-regulated biological pathways that influence protein synthesis, folding, trafficking, disaggregation and degradation In addition, the combination of proteostasis regulators with small molecule chaperones may further increase the amount of folded protein trafficked to lysosomes and thus enhance the therapy, although this hypothesis needs to be tested.

In addition to ERT, the standard treatment strategy, many symptoms of FD can be managed through supportive and palliative approaches. Daily prophylactic doses of neuropathic pain agents, such as phenytoin, carbamazepine, and gabapentin are effective in decreasing the frequency and severity of pain episodes in many patients.

Some patients need more potent analgesics, such as opioids, for pain management while avoiding potential dependency problems. For gastrointestinal disturbances, metoclopramide, H2 blockers, loperamide and hydrochloride can be beneficial. Therapeutic management primarily focuses on the control of blood pressure, lipids, and proteinuria. ACE inhibitors and ARA II /or blockers should be used in patients with proteinuria. Hypertension and hypercholesterolemia should be managed appropriately as usual. Prophylaxis with anti-aggregants is important in patients who have had ischemic attacks or stroke, and permanent cardiac pacing should be considered in high-risk patients. Furthermore, patients need to be encouraged to maintain a healthy lifestyle. While renal failure is the most frequent cause of death in classic FD, in patients with advanced renal disease, dialysis or transplantation can prolong life. However, in FD, even with the engrafted kidneys, other organ system damage continues, particularly vascular disease affecting the heart and brain. It is clear that, even with ERT, other treatments and preventative measures are necessary to manage Fabry disease [38-40].

6. Efficacy of ERT

Generally, ERT normalizes Gb3 levels in a wide variety of organs in most patients, and may be associated with symptomatic benefits. Overall measures of FD severity have shown a general reduction in disease severity after at least 1 year of ERT.

The efficacy of ERT in Fabry cardiomyopathy can be evaluated as the stabilization or decrease of the LV mass and regional myocardial function after 1 year of this treatment, and better exercise capacity at 3 years of therapy in those patients without fibrosis. In addition, clearance of Gb3 from cardiac interstitial capillary endothelial cells has been seen after ERT with agalsidase beta, although not in other cardiac cells such as cardiomyocites. The long-term effects of ERT on Fabry cardiomyopathy are related to the extent of myocardial fibrosis at baseline, when therapy is started. Fabry patients at an early stage of the disease have virtually no myocardial fibrosis. These patients with no detectable fibrosis and mild hypertrophy at baseline have shown a normalization of LV wall thickness and mass during ERT. Subsequently, the patients with no fibrosis have also improved in exercise capacity, which might be related, at least partly, to the positive effects of ERT on the Fabry cardiomyopathy

Concerning the optimal time for starting enzyme replacement therapy, prospective clinical trials in affected males and female carriers still in a preclinical phase using TDI and strain rate to assess non-invasively the efficacy of therapy are required to establish the benefits of starting treatment as soon as the diagnosis is reached. Strain-rate imaging based on tissue Doppler is superior to global parameters, like ejection fraction, in monitoring and quantifying LV function in patients with Fabry disease. The increase in peak systolic strain rate appears to be more specific for regional contractility and rather independent of wall thickness

In relation to renal function, the initiation of ERT before the development of significant proteinuria may be critical for preventing future kidney disease in these patients. Thus, creatinine clearance and eGFR have remained stable after ERT. Treatment with agalsidase alpha for 3 years has been shown to be effective in slowing the deterioration of renal function in patients with Fabry nephropathy. Even in patients with advanced renal disease or in kidney transplant recipients, ERT, by addressing the underlying metabolic deficiency, may slow the progression or development of extra-renal signs and symptoms of the disease.

Neither of the synthetic enzymes cross the blood brain barrier (BBB). Treatments can, therefore, only act on the endothelial cells of the cerebral arterial circulation, at least when the BBB is intact (in aggressive and aseptic meningitis-like forms of Fabry disease with lacunar infarcts, BBB may be seriously altered). More studies are necessary to provide evidence of the efficacy of ERT in preventing new cerebrovascular events.

7. References

[1] Germain DP. Fabry disease. *Orphanet J Rare Dis*. 2010; 22;5:30-36.

[2[Fuller M, Tucker JN, Lang DL, Dean CJ, Fietz MJ, Meikle PJ, Hopwood JJ. Screening patients referred to a metabolic clinic for lysosomal storage disorders. *J Med Genet*.

[3] Mehta A, Beck M, Eyskens F, Feliciani C, Kantola I, Ramaswami U, Rolfs A, Rivera A, Waldek S, Germain DP. Fabry disease: a review of current management strategies. QJM. 2010 ;103(9):641-59.

[4] Spada M, Pagliardini S, Yasuda M, Tukel T, Thiagarajan G, Sakuraba H, Ponzone A, Desnick RJ. High incidence of later-onset fabry disease revealed by newborn screening. *Am J Hum Genet.* 2006 ;79(1):31-40.

[5] Schiffmann R , Brady RO. New prospects for the treatment of lysosomal storage diseases. *Drugs* 2002; 62: 733-735.

[6] Froissart R, Guffon N, Vanier MT, Desnick RJ, Maire I. Fabry disease: D313Y is an alpha-galactosidase A sequence variant that causes pseudodeficient activity in plasma. *Mol Genet Metab.* 2003 ;80(3):307-14

[7] Desnick DP. Enzyme replacement and beyond. J Inherit Metab Dis. 2001;24(2):251-65.

[8] Desnick RJ, Wasserstein MP . Fabry disease: clinical features and recent advances in enzyme replacement therapy. *Adv Nephrol Necker Hosp.* 2001;31:317-39

[9] Germain DP. Fabry disease: recent advances in enzyme replacement therapy. *Expert Opin Investig Drugs.* 2002;11(10):1467-76.

[10] Rodríguez-Marí A, Coll MJ, Chabás A. Molecular analysis in Fabry disease in Spain: fifteen novel GLA mutations and identification of a homozygous female. *Hum Mutat.* 2003;22(3):258.

[11] Shabbeer J, Yasuda M, Benson SD, Desnick RJ. Fabry disease: identification of 50 novel alpha-galactosidase A mutations causing the classic phenotype and three-dimensional structural analysis of 29 missense mutations. *Hum Genomics.* 2006 ;2(5):297-30

[12] Nakao S, Kodama C, Takenaka T, Tanaka A, Yasumoto Y, Yoshida A, Kanzaki T, Enriquez AL, Eng CM, Tanaka H, Tei C, Desnick RJ. Fabry disease: detection of undiagnosed hemodialysis patients and identification of a "renal variant" phenotype. *Kidney Int.* 2003 ;64(3):801-7.

[13] Ashton-Prolla P, Tong B, Shabbeer J, Astrin KH, Eng CM, Desnick RJ. Fabry disease: twenty-two novel mutations in the alpha-galactosidase A gene and genotype/phenotype correlations in severely and mildly affected hemizygotes and heterozygotes. *J Investig Med.* 2000;48(4):227-35.

[14] MacDermot KD, Holmes A, Miners AH. Natural history of Fabry disease in affected males and obligate carrier females. *J Inherit Metab Dis.* 2001;24 Suppl 2:13-4; discussion 11-2.

[15] Valbuena C, Carvalho E, Bustorff M, Ganhão M, Relvas S, Nogueira R, Carneiro F,Oliveira JP. Kidney biopsy findings in heterozygous Fabry disease females with early nephropathy. *Virchows Arch.* 2008 ;453(4):329-38

[16] Safyan R, Whybra C, Beck M, Elstein D, Altarescu G. An association study of inflammatory cytokine gene polymorphisms in Fabry disease. *Eur Cytokine Netw.* 2006;17(4):271-5.

[17] Pastores GM, Hughes DA. To see a world in a grain of sand: elucidating the pathophysiology of Anderson-Fabry disease through investigations of a cellular model. *Kidney Int.* 2009;75(4):351-3

[18] Rombach SM, Twickler TB, Aerts JM, Linthorst GE, Wijburg FA, Hollak CE. Vasculopathy in patients with Fabry disease: current controversies and research directions. *Mol Genet Metab.* 2010;99(2):99-108.)

[19] Joosten H, Strunk AL, Meijer S, Boers JE, Ariës MJ, Abbes AP, Engel H, Beukhof JR. An aid to the diagnosis of genetic disorders underlying adult-onset renal failure: a literature review. *Clin Nephrol.* 2010;73(6):454-72.

[20] Feriozzi S, Schwarting A, Sunder-Plassmann G, West M, Cybulla M; International Fabry Outcome Survey Investigators. Agalsidase alpha slows the decline in renal function in patients with Fabry disease. *Am J Nephrol.* 2009;29(5):353-61.

[21] West M, Nicholls K, Mehta A, Clarke JT, Steiner R, Beck M, Barshop BA, Rhead W, Mensah R, Ries M, Schiffmann R. Agalsidase alpha and kidney dysfunction in Fabry disease. *J Am Soc Nephrol.* 2009;20(5):1132-9.

[22.] Gambarin FI, Disabella E, Narula J, Diegoli M, Grasso M, Serio A, Favalli BM, Agozzino M, Tavazzi L, Fraser AG, Arbustini E. When should cardiologists suspect Anderson-Fabry disease? *Am J Cardiol.* 2010 ;106(10):1492-9

[23] Perrot A, Osterziel KJ, Beck M, Dietz R, Kampmann C. Herz. Fabry disease: focus on cardiac manifestations and molecular mechanisms. 2002;27(7):699-702

[24] Hoigné P, Attenhofer Jost CH, Duru F, Oechslin EN, Seifert B, Widmer U, Frischknecht B, Jenni R. Simple criteria for differentiation of Fabry disease from amyloid heart disease and other causes of left ventricular hypertrophy. *Int J Cardiol.* 2006 ;111(3):413-22.

[25] Weidemann F, Linhart A, Monserrat L, Strotmann J. Cardiac challenges in patients with Fabry disease. *Int J Cardiol.* 2010 ;14:141(1):3-10.

[26] Pieroni M, Chimenti C, Russo A, Russo MA, Maseri A, Frustaci A. Tissue Doppler imaging in Fabry disease. *Curr Opin Cardiol.* 2004;19(5):452-7.

[27] Toro R, Perez-Isla L, Doxastaquis G, Barba MA, Gallego AR, Pintos G, Barbados FJ,Mangas A, Zamorano JL. Clinical usefulness of tissue Doppler imaging in predicting preclinical Fabry cardiomyopathy. *Int J Cardiol.* 2009;132(1):38-44.

[28] De Cobelli F, Esposito A, Belloni E, Pieroni M, Perseghin G, Chimenti C, Frustaci A, Del Maschio A. Delayed-enhanced cardiac MRI for differentiation of Fabry's disease from symmetric hypertrophic cardiomyopathy. *AJR Am J Roentgenol.* 2009 ;192(3):W97-102.

[29] Imbriaco M, Spinelli L, Cuocolo A, Maurea S, Sica G, Quarantelli M, Pisani A,Liuzzi R, Cianciaruso B, Sabbatini M, Salvatore M. MRI characterization of myocardial tissue in patients with Fabry's disease. *AJR Am J Roentgenol.* 2007;188(3):850-3.

[30] Germain DP. Fabry disease in 2004. *Rev Prat.* 2003;53(20):2215-20.

[31] Lidove O, Jaussaud R, Aractingi S. Dermatological and soft-tissue manifestations of Fabry disease: characteristics and response to enzyme replacement therapy. In: Mehta A, Beck M, Sunder-Plassmann G, editors. Fabry Disease: *Perspectives from 5 Years of FOS.* Oxford: Oxford PharmaGenesis; 2006. Chapter 24.

[32] Oussaud C, Dufier JL, Germain DP. Ocular manifestations in Fabry disease: a survey of 32 hemizygous male patients. *Ophtalmic genetics* 2003, Vol. 24, 3 , 129-139

[33] Hirano K, Murata K, Miyagawa A, Terasaki H, Saigusa J, Nagasaka T. et al. Histopathologic findings of cornea verticillata in a woman heterozygous for Fabry's disease. *Cornea.* 2001;20:233–6

[34] Sodi A, Sloannindis A, Metha A, Davey C, Beck Michael, Pitz Suzanne. Ocular manifestations of Fabry´s disease: data from the Fabry Outcome Survey. *Br J Ophtalmol* 2007; 91: 210-214

[35] Schiffmann R, Moore DF. Nervous system manifestations of Fabry disease: data from FOS – the Fabry Outcome Survey. In: Mehta A, Beck M, Sunder-Plassmann G, editors. Fabry Disease: Perspectives from 5 Years of FOS. Oxford: *Oxford PharmaGenesis;* 2006. Chapter 22.

[36] Dütsch M, Hilz MJ. Neurological complications in Fabry disease. *Rev Med Interne.* 2010;31 Suppl 2:S243-50.

[37] Desnick RJ. Prenatal diagnosis of Fabry disease. *Prenat Diagn;*2007; (8):693-4.

[38] Motabar O, Sidransky E, Goldin E, Zheng W. Fabry disease - current treatment and new drug development. *Curr Chem Genomics.* 2010 : 23;4:50-6.

[39] Rozenfeld PA. Fabry disease: treatment and diagnosis. *IUBMB Life.* 2009;61(11):1043-50.

[40] Weidemann F, Niemann M, Breunig F, Herrmann S, Beer M, Störk S, Voelker W, Ertl G, Wanner C, Strotmann J. Long-term effects of enzyme replacement therapy on Fabry cardiomyopathy: evidence for a better outcome with early treatment. *Circulation.* 2009;119(4):524-9.

10

The Multifaceted Complexity of Genetic Diseases: A Lesson from Pseudoxanthoma Elasticum

Daniela Quaglino, Federica Boraldi, Giulia Annovi and Ivonne Ronchetti
University of Modena and Reggio Emilia
Italy

1. Introduction

Pseudoxanthoma elasticum (PXE), also known as Grönblad-Strandberg syndrome, is an autosomal recessive disorder mainly affecting skin, eyes and the cardiovascular system due to progressive mineralization of elastic fibres (Gheduzzi et al., 2003) in the presence of normal levels of calcium and phosphorus in blood and urine.

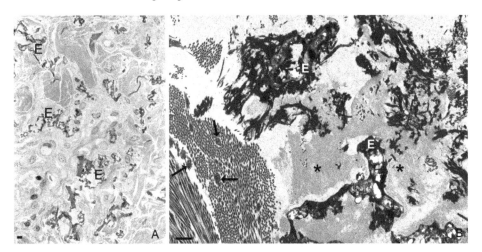

Fig. 1. Dermal biopsy from a patient affected by pseudoxanthoma elasticum (PXE).
A) Semi-thin section stained with toluidine blue and observed by light microscopy.
B) Ultrathin section stained with uranyl acetate and lead citrate visualized by transmission electron microscopy. Deformed, fragmented and mineralized elastic fibres (E) are clearly visible in the reticular dermis of the patient both at low and high magnifications. Collagen flowers (arrows) and electron-dense amorphous aggregates (*) can be recognized at the ultrastructural level. Bar= 1 μm

Although the elastic component is dramatically modified in terms of structural characteristics and functional properties, many other components of the extracellular matrix, although not calcified, appear altered. Collagen fibrils, for instance, can be laterally fused giving rise to collagen flowers, whereas glycoproteins, abnormally secreted within connective tissues, are deposited in form of large amorphous aggregates (Gheduzzi et al., 2003; Pasquali-Ronchetti et al. 1981) (Figure 1).

The disease is due to mutations in the *ABCC6* gene, encoding for a transmembrane protein (MRP6) highly expressed in liver, kidney and at a lesser extent in several other tissues, although clinically affected. The physiological substrate of MRP6 is still elusive, even though functional studies reported that the protein may be involved in the transport of complex molecules as glutathione S-conjugate leukotriene C4 and of the synthetic cyclopentapeptide BQ123 (an endothelin 1 receptor antagonist) (Belinski et al., 2002; Ilias et al., 2002). Therefore, despite the exponentially increased number of studies performed in the last decade, the pathogenesis of ectopic calcifications in PXE is a still unresolved puzzle (Uitto et al. 2010).

PXE is present in all world's populations, with an estimated prevalence of 1 in 25.000-50.000 and a 2:1 female to male ratio (Neldner & Struk, 2002). Carriers of only one mutated allele do not develop evident clinical manifestations, however they cannot be considered completely healthy carriers, since they may be, for instance, at higher risk for cardiovascular complications (Vanakker et al., 2008).

2. Clinical manifestations

The clinical expression of PXE is heterogeneous, with considerable variation in age of onset, progression and severity of the disease, even within the same family and in the presence of identical mutations (Gheduzzi et al., 2004; Hu et al., 2003a).

2.1 Skin

Patients usually develop skin lesions, mainly at puberty, starting at the posterior side of the neck and in flexural areas such as armpits, antecubital and popliteal fossae, which may later expand to the inguinal region and the periumbilical area. Alterations are usually in form of round yellowish papules, 1-3 mm in diameter, that may coalesce with time into larger protruding plaques. In a relevant number of cases, the skin becomes wrinkled and redundant hanging in folds (Neldner & Struk, 2002) (Figure 2).

In the most severely affected patients, lesions on the mucosal membranes, especially on the inner side of the lower lip, can be observed. Occasionally, calcium deposits may extrude from the skin in advanced state of the disease, a condition described as "perforating PXE" (Lund & Gilbert, 1976). Other unusual clinical presentations of PXE include acneiform lesions (Heid et al., 1980), chronic granulomatous nodules (Heyl, 1967) and brown macules in a reticulate pattern (T.H. Li et al., 1996).

2.2 Cardiovascular system

Cardiovascular manifestations, although not frequent, can be observed already before the third or fourth decade of life and are mainly related to calcium deposition and degeneration of the elastic laminae of medium sized arteries (Mendelsohn et al., 1978). The most common cardiovascular complications, in approximately 20-25% of PXE patients, are: diminished or absent peripheral vascular pulsations, early onset of reno-vascular hypertension, echographic opacities due to calcification of arteries (especially in kidneys, spleen and pancreas), arterial hypertension, angina pectoris, intermittent claudication (often regarded as the first sign of accelerated atherosclerosis), gastrointestinal haemorrhages, arteriosclerosis and increased risk of myocardial and cerebral infarction (Neldner & Struk, 2002). Marked calcification of valves and of atrial and ventricular myocardium, as well as calcified thrombi, which can result in mitral valve prolapse or stenosis and restrictive cardiomyopathy, can be clearly revealed by echocardiography (Rosenzweig et al., 1993).

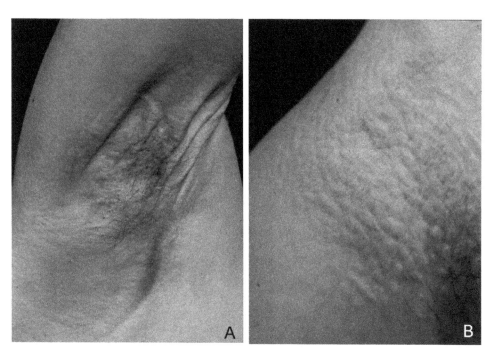

Fig. 2. Typical dermal alterations in PXE.
Papules (B) as well as wrinkled and redundant skin (A) are classical dermal lesions observed in PXE patients

About 10% of PXE patients experience bleeding complications, especially gastrointestinal haemorrhages, due to fragility of calcified submucosal vessels (Golliet-Mercier et al., 2005). Bleeding may infrequently affect other organs such as urinary tract, uterus, joints and the cerebrovascular system (Bock & Schwegler, 2008; Heaton & Wilson, 1986).

2.3 Eyes

PXE is also characterized by severe ocular alterations due to calcification of the Bruch's membrane, that is a thin layer of connective tissue bridging the pigmented retinal epithelium to the choriocapillaries and that consists of a network of interwoven elastic and collagen fibres (Booij et al., 2010). Eye abnormalities are firstly represented by peau d'orange (diffuse mottling of the fundus) that, on an average to 1 to 8 years, precedes angioid streaks (greyish irregular lines radiating outward from the optic papilla corresponding to breaks of the calcified Bruch's membrane) (Figure 3). Within 20 years from diagnosis, almost all PXE patients develop angioid streaks, that, in the course of the disease, may become pale and give way to a generalized atrophy of the adjacent tissue. In later stages, fibrovascular tissue as well as secondary choroidal neovascularization may develop. These new vessels have brittle walls, and this may cause recurrent, spontaneous, or trauma-induced retinal haemorrhages resulting in disciform scarring of the macula, which is responsible for decreased central visual acuity up to legal blindness (Georgalas et al., 2011).

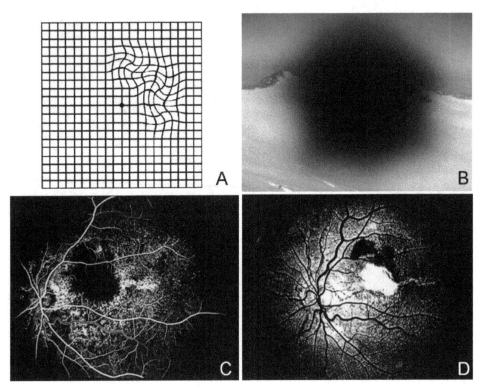

Fig. 3. Typical ocular alterations in PXE.
Elastic fibre mineralization within the Bruch's membrane, haemorrhage, neovascularization and fibrosis (C-D) are the major causes of visual abnormalities. Distortion of the Amsler grid (A) is generally the first clinical sign of ocular involvement. Progression of the disease will end up with central vision loss (B) up to legal blindness

2.4 Other organs
Interestingly, microcalcifications can be detected in several organs, as testis and breast (Bercovitch et al. 2003; Vanakker et al., 2006), as well as in liver, kidneys and spleen (59% of patients and 23.5% of healthy carriers). On renal and abdominal ultrasonography, for instance, a characteristic hyperechogenicity with dotted pattern, possibly reflecting the calcified elastic layers of arteries, has been frequently reported (Suarez et al., 1991), as well as bilateral nephrocalcinosis (Chraïbi et al., 2007). To be noted, however, that parameters of kidney and liver functions are always normal in PXE patients, suggesting that calcification does not affect the activity of these organs (Vanakker et al., 2006).

During pregnancy, the placenta is abnormal, being hypoplastic and atrophic with focal calcifications; moreover, striking anomalies of the elastic lamellae are found in the maternal vessels (Gheduzzi et al., 2001). These alterations do not negatively affect pregnancy, however early delivery can be recommended if foetus stops growing.

3. Genetics

Pseudoxanthoma elasticum is inherited in an autosomal recessive manner. As a general rule, each parent of an individual with an autosomal recessive condition carries one copy of the mutated gene, without showing or showing very mild signs and symptoms of the disorder. In a few cases, however, an affected individual may have one parent without signs and the other parent with some sign of the disease. Also these cases have to be considered autosomal recessive because the normal-appearing parent, in fact, carries an *ABCC6* gene mutation, and the affected offspring inherits two altered genes, one from each parent (Ringpfeil et al., 2006). This situation is called pseudodominance, because it resembles autosomal dominant inheritance, in which one copy of an altered gene is sufficient to cause a disorder.

Because PXE is characterized by calcification of elastic fibres, genes involved in the synthesis and assembly of the elastic fibre network were initially considered as primary candidates for mutations. These included elastin (ELN) on chromosome 7, elastin-associated microfibrillar proteins, such as fibrillin 1 and fibrillin 2 (FBN1 and FBN2) on chromosomes 15 and 5, and lysyl oxidase (LOX) also on chromosome 15. However, genetic linkage analyses excluded all these chromosomal regions (Christiano et al., 1992; Raybould et al., 1994). Subsequent studies, employing positional cloning approaches, provided strong evidence for linkage to the short arm of chromosome 16, limiting a region of approximately 500 kb (Le Saux et al., 1999).

Examination of the existing genome database revealed that this candidate region contained four genes, none of which had actually an obvious connection to elastic fibres or more generally to the extracellular matrix, but after a long systematic sequencing approach, it appeared that the *ABCC6* gene (16p.13.1) is the main site of mutations in PXE (Bergen et al., 2000; Le Saux et al., 2000; Ringpfeil et al., 2000) (Figure 4).

This gene, spanning ~73 kb genomic DNA, is composed of 31 exons, belongs to the subfamily C of the ABC genes (ATP-binding cassette) and encodes for MRP6 (a transmembrane protein of 1503 aminoacids) composed of three hydrophobic membrane segments comprising five, six, and six transmembrane spanning domains, respectively, and two evolutionary conserved intracellular nucleotide binding folds (NBFs). The NBFs contain conserved Walker A and B domains, and a C motif critical for ATP binding and transmembrane transporter functions (Chassaing et al., 2005; Hu et al., 2003b) (Figure 5).

So far, approximately 300 different mutations have been reported in *ABCC6* (Costrop et al., 2010; Gheduzzi et al., 2004; Miksch et al,. 2005; Plomp et al., 2008) and more than 80 have been detected in Italian PXE patients. The most frequent sequence changes are missense (55%) and nonsense (15%) mutations, as well as small deletions (15%), whereas less frequent alterations are represented by splicing errors, large deletions and insertions. Although the consequences of splicing mutations have not been investigated, at least 30% of all mutations cause a frameshift and the introduction of a stop-codon, which leads to premature chain termination. At protein level, the vast majority of mutations involve the cytoplasmatic domains and the carboxy-terminal end of MRP6. Mutations especially target the NBF1 and

NBF2 domains, and the 8th intracellular loop, consistent with the critical role of NBFs in ATP-driven transport. Functional studies have already shown that MRP6 transport is abolished by missense mutations located in NBF2 (Ilias et al., 2002).

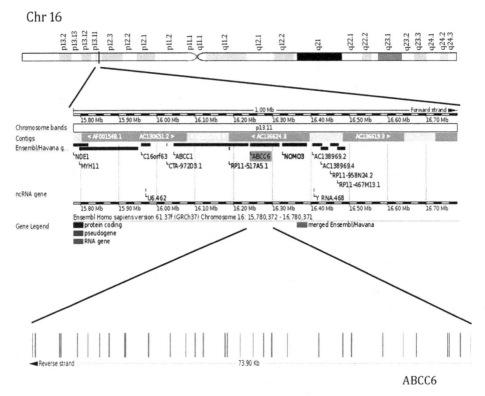

Fig. 4. Localization and structure of the *ABCC6* gene on chromosome 16

Two *ABCC6* mutations, R1141X and del (ex23_29), occur very frequently, probably due to founder effects and genetic drift. R1141X may produce an instable mRNA which is rapidly degraded by nonsense mediated RNA decay (Hu et al., 2003a; Le Saux et al., 2000). The frequency of these two recurrent mutations differs according to the population studied: of the detected mutations, ex23_29del is observed with a frequency of 28% in USA and 4% in Europe, whereas R1141X has a frequency of 4% in USA and 28% in Europe (Le Saux et al., 2001), with additional differences among European Countries, being 30% in Dutch patients (Bergen et al., 2004; Hu et al., 2003b) and about 26% and 13% in Italian and French patients, where a common founder effect was identified (Chassaing et al., 2004; Gheduzzi et al., 2004).

By contrast, in Japanese patients, neither R1141X nor ex23_29del mutations were identified, whereas mutations 2542delG and Q378X account for 53% and 25%, respectively (Noji et al., 2004). In South African families of Afrikaaners, mutation R1339C represents more than half of the detected mutations, with a common haplotype indicating, also in this case, a founder effect (Le Saux et al., 2002).

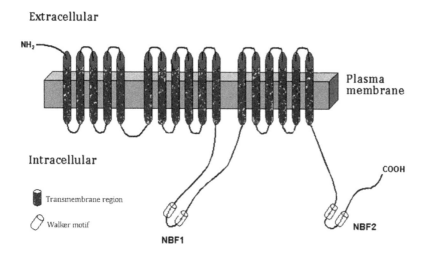

Fig. 5. Schematic drawing showing the typical transmembrane organization of the MRP6 protein

The *ABCC6* mutation detection rate is around 80-90%, since there are cases in which mutations cannot be identified in the coding region on one of the alleles, although the other allele harbours a recessive mutation (Chassaing et al., 2004; Gheduzzi et al., 2004); moreover, lack of mutation detection in some patients could reflect the occurrence of deletions (for example, deletion of exon 15 or deletion of the whole gene).

To date, no correlations have been established between the clinical phenotype and the nature or the position of the mutations (Pfender et al., 2007).

4. Pathogenesis

The physiological function and the natural substrate(s) of MRP6 are currently unknown, however, because of its homology to MRP1, it has been classified as a multidrug resistance associated protein, thus belonging to the large family of membrane proteins that transport organic anions and/or other molecules against a concentration gradient at the cost of ATP hydrolysis (Borst & Elferink, 2002; Haimeur et al., 2004). The role of MRP6 in drug resistance is actually limited to low-level resistance of a small number of chemicals, like etoposide, teniposide, doxorubicin and daunorubicin (Belinsky et al., 2002; Kool et al., 1999). Consistently with its assumed functional role, MRP6 is highly expressed in liver and kidneys being localized to the basolateral side of hepatocytes and of proximal kidney tubules, suggesting that it may transport biomolecules from cells into the blood (Bergen et al., 2000; Kool et al., 1999; Scheffer et al., 2002).

However, in spite of the high level of *ABCC6* expression, liver and kidney do not suffer from mutations in this gene. By contrast, tissues as skin, retina and vessels, which are deeply altered in PXE, express very low levels of MRP6 (Bergen et al., 2000; Kool et al., 1999). These findings raised a still unsolved dilemma concerning the pathogenesis of PXE: how do mutations in a gene expressed primarily in the liver result in the mineralization of peripheral connective tissues?

To explain the putative mechanisms leading to ectopic calcifications from *ABCC6* mutations under normal calcium and phosphorus homeostatic conditions, two theories have been reported in the literature (Uitto et al., 2010): "the liver metabolic hypothesis" and "the peripheral cell hypothesis". The metabolic hypothesis considers liver dismetabolism the only responsible for ectopic calcifications, whereas the peripheral cell hypothesis points to the role of mesenchymal cell metabolism on the homeostatic control of connective tissue calcifications in PXE.

The liver metabolic hypothesis postulates that the absence of functional MRP6 activity in hepatocytes results in deficiency of circulating factor(s) physiologically required to prevent aberrant mineralization (Jiang & Uitto, 2006; Uitto et al., 2010). In support of this hypothesis are clinical and experimental observations in PXE patients, as well as in the *Abcc6⁻/⁻* mouse (Klement et al., 2005), that serves as a model for human PXE. Firstly, clinical findings in PXE patients are rarely present at early childhood and the onset of clinical manifestations as well as the slow progression of the disease, due to continued accumulation of minerals in soft connective tissues of affected organs, can be regarded as the typical consequence of metabolic impairments that worsen with time. Secondly, serum from PXE patients, as well as from *Abcc6⁻/⁻* mice, lacks the capacity to prevent calcium/phosphate precipitation in an *in vitro* assay with smooth muscle cell cultures (Jiang et al., 2007). Furthermore, serum from PXE patients, when added to the culture medium, has been shown to modify the organization of elastic fibres without altering gene expression, thus suggesting the involvement of specific circulating factors directly acting on the assembly of elastic fibres (Le Saux et al., 2006), even if these changes occur in the absence of any *in vitro* calcification. Finally, recent skin grafting studies in wild-type and *Abcc6⁻/⁻* mice have further focused on the importance of circulating factor(s), hypothesizing that the mineralization process can be countered or even reversed by modifications of the homeostatic milieu (Jiang et al., 2009). In particular, it has been shown that the *Abcc6⁻/⁻* mouse skin graft does not develop mineralization, when placed onto the *Abcc6⁺/⁺* mouse, but calcification occurs in the skin of wild-type mouse after grafting onto the *Abcc6⁻/⁻* mouse, indicating that circulating factors in the recipient's blood could play a critical role in determining the degree of mineralization, irrespective of the graft genotype. However, in these skin graft experiments the possible modulation of fibroblast metabolism upon effect of circulating factors cannot be ruled out.

Actually, several studies have reported alterations in circulating factors in PXE patients, such as proteoglycans (Götting et al., 2005; Passi et al., 1996), plasma lipoproteins (Wang et al., 2001) and mineralization inhibitors, such as fetuin-A and Matrix Gla Protein (MGP) (Hendig et al., 2006, 2008). Moreover, a number of circulating molecules have been shown to be modified in the plasma of PXE patients by effect of a systemic altered redox balance (Garcia-Fernandez et al., 2008).

However, a number of questions remain to be elucidated. First of all, in PXE patients, despite of the absence and/or of the presence of one or more circulating factor(s), mineralization affects only a certain number of elastic fibres and only in peculiar areas of the body. Calcification seems, in fact, a rather specific phenomenon, since in PXE patients extracellular matrix components other than elastin (i.e. collagens or matrix glycoproteins) never undergo mineralization, furthermore, not all elastic fibres are calcified and not all areas of affected tissues are clinically involved (Gheduzzi et al.,2003; Pasquali-Ronchetti et al., 1981). In addition, the observation that patient's serum interferes with elastin assembly is in agreement with the above mentioned plasma modifications in PXE patients and especially with the abnormalities in glycosaminoglycan's content and species (Maccari et al., 2003, 2008;

Passi et al., 1996; Tiozzo Costa et al 1998), since it is well known that these matrix constituents are capable to greatly influence tropoelastin assembly (Gheduzzi et al., 2005; Tu & Weiss, 2008). Finally, if changes in the circulating environment can effectively modify the extent of ectopic calcifications, it is not clear why PXE mesenchymal cells, as dermal fibroblasts, maintain their abnormal phenotype even when they are cultured *in vitro* in optimal nutritional supplements and conditions far from their original environment (Boraldi et al., 2009).

Actually, in support to the "peripheral cell hypothesis", it has been demonstrated that *in vitro* skin fibroblasts isolated from PXE patients exhibit a modified biosynthetic expression profile, altered cell-cell and cell-matrix interactions associated with changes in proliferative capacity (Boraldi et al., 2009; Quaglino et al., 2000), abnormal synthesis of elastin and of glycosaminoglycan/proteoglycan complexes (Passi et al., 1996) and enhanced degradation potential due to elevated matrix metalloproteinase-2 activity (Quaglino et al., 2005). Consistently, histopathological and ultrastructural observations showed that, in PXE, mineralization occurs only on elastic fibres (Gheduzzi et al., 2003; Pasquali-Ronchetti et al., 1981), suggesting a peculiar composition and/or organization of elastic fibre components (Lebwohl et al.,1993; Sakuraoka et al., 1994). By immuno-electron microscopy, it has been demonstrated that aberrant matrix proteins known for their high affinity for calcium and normally involved in mineralization processes (such as alkaline phosphatase, vitronectin, fibronectin, bone sialoprotein, osteonectin and proteoglycans) are accumulated within PXE elastic fibres (Contri et al., 1996; Kornet et al., 2004; Passi et al., 1996).

All these data undoubtedly highlight the importance of mesenchymal cells in the pathogenesis of ectopic calcifications, never the less it is still unclear whether these changes depend or not upon the expression of the *ABCC6* gene in mesenchymal cells (Matsuzaki et al., 2005). It has to be noted, in fact, that even normal fibroblasts, possibly due to aberrant splicings, do not seem to express the full MRP6 protein (Matsuzaki et al., 2005) and that immunologically positive epitopes have been recognized only on membranes of the endoplasmic reticulum of isolated dermal fibroblasts (Boraldi et al., 2009). What could be the significance and importance of the presence of at least part of MRP6 in the endoplasmic reticulum of mesenchymal cells have not been investigated.

However, in the light of these observations, changes in membrane transport properties described in PXE cultured fibroblasts (Boraldi et al., 2003) would seem likely the result of the high level of reactive oxygen species (ROS) on the structural organization of cell membranes (Boraldi et al., 2009) and consequently on cell permeability. It has been in fact demonstrated *in vitro* (Pasquali-Ronchetti et al., 2006) and *in vivo* (Garcia-Fernandez et al., 2008) that PXE is characterized by an altered redox balance. At cellular level, the chronic oxidative stress condition is due, at least in part, to the loss of mitochondrial membrane potential ($\Delta\Psi$ (m)) with overproduction of ROS. Consistently, cultured fibroblasts produce more malondialdehyde, a product of lipid peroxidation, and accumulate higher amounts of carbonylated proteins compared to controls (Boraldi et al., 2009; Pasquali-Ronchetti et al., 2006). Likewise, in the circulation of patients, the redox unbalance leads to significantly high amount of oxidised proteins and lipids, which might have relevant effects on peripheral mesenchymal cells (Garcia-Fenandez et al., 2008).

Interestingly, among the molecular pathways which are sensitive to the redox potential is the vitamin K-cycle that, within connective tissues, is essential for the γ-glutamyl carboxylation of MGP (Matrix Gla Protein), a potent inhibitor of calcification in soft connective tissues (Schurgers et al., 2008). Consistently, in PXE fibroblasts (Gheduzzi et al., 2007) and in the *Abcc6* -/- mice (Li et al., 2007) there is a reduced carboxylation of MGP.

A recent characterization of the PXE fibroblast's protein profile revealed that numerous endoplasmic reticulum-associated proteins are differentially expressed in pathological cells. Among these proteins, calumenin and disulfide isomerase are involved in the recycling of vitamin K, leaving open the question if insufficient carboxylation of MGP in PXE cells could be due to reduced availability or to diminished recycling of vitamin K (Boraldi et al., 2009) (Figure 6).

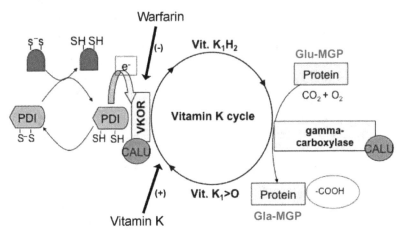

Fig. 6. Drawing illustrating the numerous factors involved in vitamin K cycle.
Vitamin K represents an important cofactor of protein carboxylation. Within the endoplasmic reticulum of mesenchymal cells, MGP (Matrix Gla protein) is activated by gamma-carboxylase from the inactive form (Glu-MGP) to the active form (Gla-MGP). Protein disulfide isomerase (PDI) and calumenin (CALU) are important modulators of these reactions. Warfarin, by inhibiting the action of vitamin K epoxide reductase, reduces the efficiency of the carboxylation process and favours the development of vascular calcifications. Modified from Wajih (Wajih et al., 2007)

To further confirm the importance of efficient MGP carboxylation in controlling the mineralization process, there are experimental evidences showing that antibodies specific for carboxylated (Gla-MGP) and non-carboxylated MGP (Glu-MGP) are differently localized within human dermal elastic fibres. In particular, both forms of MGP are rather heterogeneously distributed within elastin of control subjects, whereas in PXE patients Glu-MGP is markedly present in calcified areas and Gla-MGP is exclusively localized at the mineralization front (Gheduzzi et al., 2007). Although it has been suggested that MRP6 could function as a vitamin K transporter from the liver to the periphery, and that, in PXE, the mutated protein may prevent connective tissue from an adequate supply of the vitamin necessary for efficient carboxylation processes (Borst et al., 2008; Vanakker et al., 2010), *in vivo* and *in vitro* treatments with different forms of vitamin K do not appear to interfere and/or to inhibit the mineralization process (Jiang et al., 2011; Annovi et al., 2011).
Therefore, it could be suggested that mutated MRP6 in liver and kidney is responsible for the altered release in the circulation of factors that modify plasma components, among which proteins, lipids and, eventually, other constituents, thus contributing to produce an abnormal environment at the periphery, and to influence mesenchymal cell behaviour and

metabolism. Among peripheral alterations it would appear that there is an imbalance between production and degradation of oxidant species, abnormal protein and glycosaminoglycan synthesis, changes in post-translational protein modifications and abnormal DNA-methylation (Boraldi et al., 2009). Moreover, the alterations in the *in vitro* behaviour of PXE fibroblasts may suggest that permanent epigenetic changes have occurred, thus causing the inability of these cells to produce mature inhibitors and/or modulators of calcification (Figure 7).

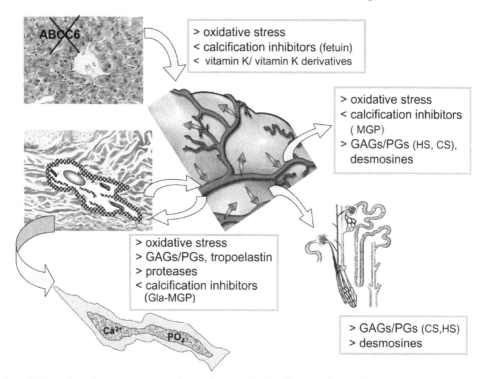

Fig. 7. Drawing that summarizes the major metabolic abnormalities observed in PXE and the relationships between organs and tissues possibly involved in the pathogenesis of elastic fibre calcification.

Absent or altered expression of the *ABCC6* gene in hepatocytes may be responsible for abnormal extrusion in the circulation of still unknown factor/s which is/are responsible for or contributing to oxidative stress, to ineffective inhibition of ectopic calcification, to reduced levels of vitamin K and/or vitamin K derivatives. Therefore, through the circulation, abnormal signals could reach mesenchymal cells epigenetically modifying their phenotype, i.e. chronic oxidative stress, altered synthesis of tropoelastin, production of glycosaminoglycans (GAGs) or proteoglycans (PGs) with peculiar physical-chemical properties, augmented proteolytic potential, lower expression of carboxylated Matrix Gla Protein (Gla-MGP), thus causing accumulation of calcium (Ca^{2+}) and phosphate (PO_4^-) mineral precipitates on elastic fibres. Abnormal products from mesenchymal cells can be found in the circulation or in the urine, i.e. parameters of redox balance, desmosines as indicators of elastin degradation, heparan sulfate (HS) and chondroitin-sulfate (CS) GAGs and inhibitors of calcification as MGP

The various levels of mineralization, even within the same tissue, could be explained by the heterogeneity of different mesenchymal cell subtypes and their peculiar functional imprinting related to structural and functional requirements of organs and tissues (Jelaska et al., 1999; Sorrell & Caplan, 2004).

On the basis of all these considerations, both "the liver metabolic" and "the peripheral cell" hypotheses, together, can actually help to understand the pathogenesis of clinical manifestations in PXE. On one side, there is the involvement of the liver that, expressing MRP6, has an important role in controlling metabolic processes and plasma composition, on the other side it cannot be underestimated the crucial role of peripheral mesenchymal cells, as fibroblasts, in regulating connective tissue homeostasis.

5. The role of modifier genes

Understanding PXE pathogenesis is further complicated by the fact that the age of disease onset and the expression of clinical symptoms are highly variable (Gonzales et al., 2009) and marked phenotypic variations have been observed in affected siblings bearing the same *ABCC6* mutation (Gheduzzi et al. 2004).

Although, there is no evidence for the involvement of other genes in the pathogenesis of PXE (Li et al., 2009), however, a number of modifying factors, both genetic and environmental, have been suggested to play a role in the phenotypic expression of the disease (Hovnanian, 2010).

One recently identified genetic factor involves polymorphisms in the promoter region of the *SPP1* gene (secreted phosphoprotein 1, also known as osteopontin) (Hendig et al., 2007). Osteopontin is a secreted, highly acidic phosphoprotein that is involved in immune cell activation, wound healing, bone morphogenenesis (Denhardt et al., 2001), thus playing a major role in regulating the mineralization process in various tissues, including skin and aorta, where osteopontin is localized to elastic fibres (Baccarani-Contri et al., 1994). Higher expression of this protein has been observed in skin biopsies from PXE patients compared to samples from unaffected regions or from healthy individuals (Contri et al., 1996) and also in mice suffering from dystrophic cardiac calcification, suggesting that its expression is influenced by the *Dyscalc1* locus on chromosome 7 (Aherrahrou et al., 2004). Although several polymorphisms in the *SPP1* gene have been described and associated with various disorders such as systemic lupus erythematosus and arteriosclerosis (Giacopelli et al., 2004), the role of osteopontin in regulating the calcification process, strongly suggested that sequence variations in the *SPP1* promoter region might account for the higher expression observed in PXE patients, thus affecting the disease outcome. Consistently, mutational screening revealed nine different sequence variations, and three *SPP1* promoter polymorphisms (c.-1748A>G, c.-155_156insG and c.244_255insTG), in particular, were significantly associated with PXE. Until now, no functional studies have been carried out with the *SPP1* promoter polymorphisms c.-1748>G, whereas the polymorphism variant c.244_245ins TG does not have a major regulatory effect. By contrast, the discovery that polymorphism c.155_156insG generates a Runx2-binding site opened a new field of investigations, since Runx2-binding sites are in fact very important for regulating *SSP1* expression in bone tissue (Giacopelli et al., 2004). A constitutive expression of Runx2, combined with a glucocorticoids' supplementation, results in a strong upregulation of *SPP1* expression and finally in a biological matrix mineralization by primary dermal fibroblasts (Phillips et al., 2006). Therefore, polymorphisms in the *SPP1* promoter may represent a genetic risk factor contributing to PXE susceptibility.

Other studies have correlated the incidence of cardiovascular complications in PXE with polymorphisms of genes encoding for xylosyltransferase 1 (*XT-1*) and xylosyltransferase 2 (*XT-2*), a set of key enzymes involved in proteoglycan biosynthesis and considered biochemical markers of fibrosis (Schön et al., 2006). The altered proteoglycan metabolism, already observed *in vitro* (Passi et al., 1996) and *in vivo* (Maccari et al., 2003), suggests that enzymes from these pathways may function as genetic co-factors in the severity of PXE. Furthermore, PXE patients have elevated serum XT-I activity. On the basis of these observations Authors suggested a connection between the severity of the disease and genetic variations in the *XYLT* genes (Schön et al., 2006).

More recent studies have shown that polymorphisms in genes associated with redox balance as catalase (*CAT*), superoxide dismutase 2 (*SOD2*) and glutathione peroxidase 1 (*GPX1*) are associated with early onset of clinical manifestations (Zarbock et al., 2007), whereas polymorphisms of the *VEGF* gene (vascular endothelial growth factor) are involved in the pathogenesis of ocular manifestations (Zarbock et al., 2009). The distribution of 10 single nucleotide polymorphisms (SNPs) in the promoter and coding region of the *VEGFA* gene has been evaluated in DNA samples from 163 German patients affected by PXE and in 163 healthy subjects. Five SNPs showed significant association with severe retinopathy. The most significant association was with polymorphism c.-460C>T. In the light of these results *VEGF* gene polymorphisms might be considered useful prognostic markers for the development of PXE-associated retinopathy, thus allowing earlier therapeutic intervention in order to prevent loss of central vision, one of the most devastating consequences of PXE (Zarbock et al., 2009).

By contrast, very few data are available on the role of *ABCC6* polymorphisms on the occurrence and/or severity of clinical manifestations in PXE patients. The *ABCC6* pR1268Q polymorphism has been associated with lower plasma triglycerides and higher plasma HDL-cholesterol, suggesting that *ABCC6* may contribute to modulate plasma lipoproteins and possibly cardiovascular complications (Wang et al., 2001). In a larger study conducted on a German cohort of PXE patients, in addition to the complete screening of the *ABCC6* gene, the *ABCC6* promoter region was also analyzed and the following polymorphisms were found: c.-127C>T, c.-132C>T and C.-219A>C. Interestingly, the difference in the c.-219A>C frequencies between PXE patients and controls was statistically significant and this polymorphism appeared located in a transcriptional activator sequence of the *ABCC6* promoter, functioning as a binding site for a transcriptional repressor predominantly found in genes involved in lipid metabolism (Schulz et al., 2006), further sustaining a possible correlation between *ABCC6* and lipid metabolism.

Surprisingly, the observation that the c.3421C>T loss-of-function mutation on one allele of *ABCC6* (R1141X) is significantly associated to coronary artery disease (CAD), in the apparently normal population (Köblös et al., 2010), was not confirmed in a cohort of Italian PXE patients (Quaglino, unpublished data), further sustaining the difficulty to perform a genotype-phenotype correlation, although not excluding the possibility that carriers of *ABCC6* loss-of-function mutations may benefit from cardiovascular prevention programs (Vanakker et al., 2008).

6. Diagnosis and treatments

In spite of the impressive progress in understanding the genetic/molecular basis of inherited diseases, also in PXE, similarly to other genetic disorders, there have been limited improvements in terms of treatment and cure. Major advances concern diagnosis, due to ability to recognize a continuously increased number of mutations (mutation detection rate varies from 80-90%). Attempts to establish genotype/phenotype correlations have yielded little clinically useful information other than the fact that, as PXE patients age, symptoms get worse, probably because of progressive accumulation of mineralized elastic fibres, associated to other age-related degenerative features (Garcia-Fernandez et al., 2008).

PXE is an important cause of blindness and of early death from cardiovascular manifestations (Neldner, 1988), therefore an early diagnosis is important in order to minimise the risk of systemic complications. One of the major problems encountered by patients affected by rare diseases, as PXE, is the difficulty to find physicians who are aware of the disorder and of the possible related complications. Therefore, strenuous efforts are necessary to spread the knowledge on these disorders not only in the scientific community, but also among practitioners, who represent the first medical reference point for patients. An additional help may derive from the definition of commonly accepted criteria for clinical diagnosis, which, in the case of PXE, include the presence of retinal angioid streaks (a fluorescein angiogram may be necessary) in combination with characteristic skin lesions (calcification of fragmented elastic fibres confirmed by von Kossa stain in a biopsy of lesional skin) (Figure 8) with or without a positive family history of PXE (two or more family members clinically diagnosed). It is however important to note that mild forms of the disorder can be easily overlooked and a negative family history does not exclude the diagnosis.

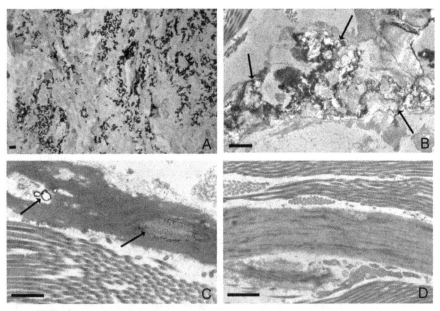

Fig. 8. Demonstration of mineralized elastic fibres is the gold standard diagnostic criteria in PXE.
A) Light microscopy of a dermal biopsy from a PXE patient stained with Von Kossa for the visualization of brownish calcified elastin. B-D) Transmission electron microscopy showing dramatically deformed and mineralized elastic fibres (arrows) in the dermis of a PXE patient (B) and small clinically irrelevant alterations (arrows) in the skin of PXE carriers (C), compared to the typical amorphous structure of normal elastic fibres (D). Bars: 1μm

Since the discovery of *ABCC6* as the PXE associated gene in 2000 (Bergen et al., 2000; Le Saux et al., 2000; Ringpfeil et al., 2000), molecular genetic testing have been rapidly developed and, although frequently limited to research laboratories or to highly specialized centres, they may represent an important diagnostic assessment. The techniques most frequently used are sequence analysis and mutation scanning, which are capable to detect missense, nonsense and frameshift mutations as well as small deletions and insertions. Testing strategies usually involve a first screening of exons in which a large number of mutations are located (i.e. exons 24 and 28), and, in case of negative results, the sequencing of the other coding regions. Moreover, since a 16.4 kb deletion involving exons 23-29 is another recurrent mutation, a specific deletion analysis can be required.

Analyses performed so far revealed that there is a considerable spectrum of genetic mutations (>300), with wide inter- and intra-familial phenotypic variations, and an extreme variability in terms of progression of the disease as well as of severity and extent of clinical manifestations. It must be reminded that PXE is a systemic disorder and therefore management of PXE requires coordinated input from a multidisciplinary team of specialists including dermatologist, primary care physician, ophthalmologist, cardiologist, vascular surgeon, plastic surgeon, genetics professional, and a nutritionist.

Moreover, once a diagnosis of PXE has been established, in order to delay and eventually manage ocular and cardiovascular complications, patients are encouraged to have clinical/instrumental examinations whose frequency may depend on the age of patient, age at diagnosis and severity of clinical manifestations. In particular, it is advisable to perform a complete dilated eye examination by a retinal specialist, particularly looking for *peau d'orange* and angioid streaks and baseline cardiovascular examination with periodic follow-up including: echocardiography, cardiac stress testing, and Doppler evaluation of peripheral vasculature.

At present, no specific treatment for PXE exists, in the sense that mineralization of elastic fibres cannot be delayed or reverted. Never the less, skin surgery has been successfully applied for cosmetic improvement (Ng et al., 1999), as well as peripheral and coronary arteries interventions in order to limit vascular complications (Donas et al., 2007; Shepherd & Rooke, 2003).

The only stage of the disease where therapy for ocular complications is possible and indicated is whenever a choroidal neovascularization (CNV) has developed (Georgalas et al., 2011). Traditional therapeutic options consist of laser photocoagulation (used to halt the progression of CNVs, although characterized by high rate of recurrence, visual loss, and central scotomas) (Pece et al., 1997) or of photodynamic therapy (PDT) (used to arrest the progression of CNVs, even though results appeared less encouraging then expected) (Heimann et al., 2005). Experimental surgical procedures, such as macular translocation or subfoveal CNV excision (Roth et al., 2005), appeared unsuccessful. More recently, taking advantage from the experience on macular degeneration, the intraocular injection of anti-angiogenic drugs, as avastin and lucentis, actually appeared to be the most effective therapeutic options for ocular complications (Verbraak, 2010).

In the absence of effective treatments specifically targeting pathways leading to ectopic calcifications, anectodical reports can be found in the literature concerning the use of drugs or of nutritional supplements. For instance, it has been suggested that pentoxifylline and cilostazol may ameliorate intermittent claudication (Muir, 2009), however, controlled studies of these drugs in PXE patients have not been performed. Interestingly, the ARED (Age Related Eye Disease) study suggested that a regimen of antioxidant vitamins could be beneficial in patients with macular degeneration. Given the similarities with PXE (i.e. ocular manifestations and altered redox balance) it is possible that the same recommendation can be valuable also for PXE (Lecerf & Desmettre, 2010), even though further investigations are required to support this hypothesis. By contrast, more promising perspectives, at least in the mouse model, seem to be represented by a diet supplemented with an excess of magnesium, although the mechanisms of reduced calcifications are still unknown (Gorgels et al., 2010; LaRusso et al, 2009) and the effects of long-term treatments with high doses of magnesium in humans have not been yet investigated.

7. PXE-like diseases

Even though no other phenotypes are known to be associated with mutations in the *ABCC6* gene, PXE-like clinical features, including aberrant mineralization of elastic fibres, have been reported in a number of apparently unrelated acquired and genetic clinical conditions (Neldner, 1988).

7.1 Acquired conditions

Among the acquired conditions, PXE-like cutaneous changes may be associated with multiple pregnancy, longstanding end-stage renal disease (Lewis et al., 2006), L-tryptophan induced eosinophilia myalgia syndrome (Mainetti et al., 1991), and amyloid elastosis (Sepp et al., 1990) as well as after D-penicillamine treatment, cutaneous exposure to calcium salts (Neldner & Martinez-Hernandez, 1979), and salpeter (Nielsen et al., 1978). In these cases, mineralization of skin may result from metabolic abnormalities affecting calcium and/or phosphate homeostasis or from direct deposition of mineral salts on collagen or elastic fibres. However, the pathomechanistic details and the role of predisposing genetic factors are unknown.

In papillary dermal elastolysis, white-yellow papules resembling PXE can be observed in aged women (60–80 years), although, in contrast to PXE, these lesions are histologically characterized by loss of elastin in the papillary dermis (Ohnishi et al., 1998).

Moreover, elastic fibres similar to those of PXE have been observed in the lesional skin of patients with a variety of inflammatory skin diseases in the absence of clinical evidence of PXE (Bowen et al., 2007), in calcific elastosis, lipedema, lipodermatosclerosis, granuloma annulare, lichen sclerosus, morphea profunda, erythema nodosum, septal panniculitis, basal cell carcinoma and fibrosing dermatitis (Bowen et al., 2007; Taylor et al., 2004).

Even though sporadically, ocular lesions similar to those typical of PXE, have also been reported in Paget's disease, Marfan's and Ehlers–Danlos syndromes (Gurwood & Mastrangelo, 1997) and calcifications of retina, retina vessels and the presence of osseous metaplasia have also been noted in patients with renal failure, Coats' disease, tuberous sclerosis and retinocytomas (Miller et al., 2004; Patel et al., 2002).

Finally it has to be mentioned that ectopic calcifications may occur in the vascular system during physiological aging, in atherosclerosis and hypercholesterolemia, hypertension, smoking, calcific aortic stenosis, Marfan syndrome, diabetes, renal failure and in smokers (Proudfoot & Shanahan, 2001). There are two types of calcifications that occur in arteries: the intimal calcification, characteristic of the atherosclerotic plaque and associated with cells and collagen, and the medial calcification (also known as Mönckeberg sclerosis) mainly associated with elastin. Patients with chronic kidney disease (CKD) frequently display both forms of calcification. Another form of vascular calcification also occurs nearly exclusively in CKD patients: calciphylaxis or calcific uremic arteriolopathy. This is a disorder of medial calcification of the small arterioles of the skin, resulting in skin necrosis (Moe & Chen, 2003).

7.2 Genetic conditions

Unexpectedly, PXE-like cutaneous changes have also been found in approximately 20% of patients with beta-thalassemia (beta-thal) and sickle cell anaemia (SCD), that are well known severe congenital forms of anemia resulting from the deficient or altered synthesis of haemoglobin beta chains (Baccarani-Contri 2001; Fabbri et al., 2009). The first report suggesting a link between beta-thal and PXE was based on the observation that angioid streaks were actually present in both diseases (Aesopos et al., 1989). Subsequent studies confirmed that PXE-like syndrome in beta-thalassemias and SCD, although less severe, is histopathologically and clinically identical to inherited PXE consisting of indistinguishable cutaneous, ocular and vascular abnormalities due to elastic fibre calcification (Baccarani-Contri et al., 2001; Bercovitch & Terry, 2004; Hamlin et al., 2003) (Figure 9). In particular, it has been observed that beta-thal patients have calcifications of the posterior tibial artery (55%), typical skin lesions (20%), angioid streaks (52%) and that one or more of the three manifestations are actually present in 85% of the patients (Aesopos et al., 1998). Cardiovascular complications have been only sporadically observed, although they include intracranial haemorrhages, ischemic strokes, coronary arterial calcification complicated by unstable angina, myocardial infarction, mitral valve prolapse, valve calcification and leaflet thickening, pericardial thickening, renal artery calcification with arterial hypertension and peripheral arterial abnormalities complicated by gastric haemorrhage and intestinal infarcts (Aessopos et al., 1997,1998, 2001; Cianciulli et al., 2002; Farmakis et al., 2003).

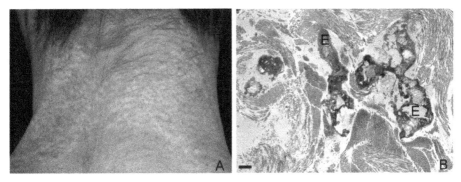

Fig. 9. PXE-like alterations in a patient affected by beta-thalassemia.
In these patients, papules and skin folds in typical areas of the neck (A) are associated to mineralized elastic fibres (E) in the dermis, as visualized by transmission electron microscopy (B). Bar: 1 μm

A genetic link between beta-thalassemia or SCDs and PXE is unlikely. In first instance, no mutations in the *ABCC6* gene were found in a cohort of beta-thal patients (Hamlin et al., 2003), moreover, *ABCC6* as well as other genes encoding for elastin or elastin associated molecules (i.e. fibrillins 1 and 2, elastin-related glycoproteins and lysyl-oxidase) are located on chromosomes different from that of the β-globin gene (Ringpfeil et al., 2000) and family members who do not have a haemoglobinopathies fail to show any PXE stigmata (Aessopos et al., 1994).

Never the less, in a study by Martin and coworkers (2006), fifty PXE patients have been investigated with the aim to determine the incidence of haemoglobin abnormalities typical of thalassemia. No cases of beta thalassemia were diagnosed in this cohort of patients, however in 20% of cases a significant but isolated (i.e. without microcytic anemia) increase of haemoglobin A2 (HbA2) was observed. The severity of clinical manifestations, other than the extent of cutaneous involvement, appeared independent from levels of haemoglobin. Therefore, ABCC6 plus beta-globin digenism was ruled out of the pathogenesis of PXE, but it could be hypothesized a functional epigenetic reaction between ABCC6 and the beta-globin locus, even though reciprocal interactions are clearly unequal since the change in ABCC6 transcription occurring during the course of beta thalassaemia is responsible for a PXE phenotype, while increased HbA2 during the course of PXE has no haematological clinical consequences.

Interestingly, it has been recently demonstrated that a mouse model of beta-thal (Hbb(th3/+)) exhibits a NF-E2-induced transcriptional down-regulation of liver ABCC6 (Martin et al., 2011), even though there are no evidence for spontaneous calcifications. It has been therefore suggested that decreased expression of mrp6 occurring later in life is probably insufficient to promote mineralization in the Hbb(th3/+) mouse C57BL/6J genetic background. However, these data may indicate that i) other factors, beside ABCC6 expression are involved in the pathogenesis of calcifications, ii) responsive fibroblasts or other mesenchymal cells are required in order to modify connective tissue homeostasis, and iii) independently from the primary gene defect, common pathways may be involved in these disorders.

Within this context, it has been suggested that the elastic tissue injury in these patients may be the result of an oxidative process, induced by the combined and interactive effects of different factors (Aessopos et al., 1998; Garcia-Fernandez et al., 2008; Pasquali-Ronchetti et al., 2006). Plasma membrane microparticles, derived from the oxidative damage of red cell membranes by the effect of denatured hemoglobin products and free iron (Olivieri, 1999), as well as unbound fractions of hemoglobin and haem, which exceed the binding capacity of haptoglobin and hemopexin in the context of chronic hemolysis, have been considered to elicit inflammatory and oxidative reactions (Belcher et al., 2000; Gutteridge & Smith, 1988). The accumulated and prolonged effects of ROS/free radicals may result in disturbance of mesenchymal cell metabolism with structural deterioration of elastic fibres (Bunda et al., 2005). Accordingly, oxidative stress constitutes a potential acquired mechanism affecting the same molecular pathways, which are implicated in the pathogenesis of hereditary PXE.

The recent observation that a PXE-like phenotype can be observed in patients with pronounced deficiency of the vitamin K-dependent clotting factors raises the intriguing and exiting possibility that there might an additional pathway, independent of ABCC6, leading to the PXE phenotype (Vanakker et al. 2007).

Congenital deficiency of the vitamin K-dependent factors (VKCFD) is a rare bleeding disorder that can be caused either by mutation in the gamma-glutamyl carboxylase gene (GGCX) or in the vitamin K epoxide reductase complex(VKORC) (Oldenburg et al, 2000; Pauli et al, 1987). Moreover, acquired forms of the disorder can occur more frequently due to intestinal malabsorption of vitamin K (Djuric et al., 2007) or after prolonged treatments with vitamin K antagonists as warfarin (Palaniswamy et al., 2011). Vitamin K undergoes oxidation-reduction cycling within the endoplasmic reticulum, donating electrons to activate specific proteins via enzymatic gamma-carboxylation of glutamate groups before being enzymatically re-reduced (Figure 6).

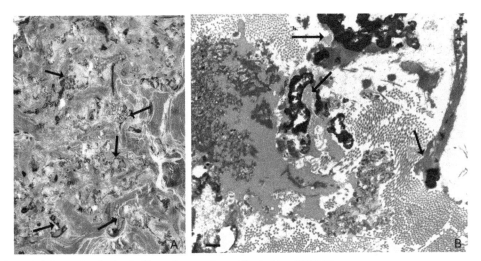

Fig. 10. Mineralized elastic fibres in a patient affected by VKFCD.
A) Light and B) transmission electron microscopy of a skin biopsy. Heavy mineralized
elastic fibres (arrows) can be seen. Bar: 1μm

In addition to coagulation factors (II, VII, IX, X, and prothrombin) vitamin K activates
protein C and protein S, osteocalcin (OC), matrix Gla protein (MGP), periostin, Gas6, and
other vitamin K-dependent (VKD) proteins that, within bones, support calcium homeostasis
and the mineralization process, whereas in vessel walls, and possibly in other peripheral
soft connective tissues, they inhibit calcification, favouring endothelial integrity, cell growth
and tissue renewal (Kidd, 2010).

Clinical overlap of PXE and VKCFD was obvious from the skin manifestations of yellowish
papules or leathery plaques, with dot-like depressions, angioid streaks and/or ocular *peau
d'orange*, as well as fragmentation and calcification of elastic fibres in the dermis. Important
phenotypic differences from PXE included much more severe skin laxity with involvement
of the trunk and limbs with thick, leathery skin folds rather than confinement to flexural
areas, and no decrease in visual acuity. By light microscopy, changes in the reticular dermis
were identical to those typical of PXE, consisting in polymorphous, fragmented, and
mineralized elastic fibres, as shown by von Kossa stain. At the ultrastructural level,
however, elastin had a more fragmented and mottled appearance than that typically
observed in PXE (Vanakker et al., 2007) (Figure 10). In the light of these observations, it has
been demonstrated *in vitro* (Gheduzzi et al., 2007) and *in vivo* (Li et al., 2007) that PXE is
characterized by low levels of carboxylated-Matrix Gla Protein (Gla-MGP), thus suggesting
that these changes may play a role in the pathogenesis of PXE, as described in more details
in paragraph 4.

8. Conclusions

Pseudoxanthoma elasticum (PXE) is a rare genetic disorder characterized by mineralization
of elastic fibres within all connective tissues, although the most important clinical
manifestations affect skin, eyes and the cardiovascular system. Despite the dramatic
involvement of the extracellular matrix, the first attempts made by researchers to find out

the gene defect among those coding for matrix molecules failed and in 2000 three groups, independently, demonstrated that PXE is due to mutations in the *ABCC6* gene, that belongs to the ABC membrane transporters. To date the physiological substrate of this transporter is not known and still elusive are the pathogenetic mechanisms linking a defective cellular transporter, mainly expressed in liver and kidney, to ectopic calcification of connective tissues. This disease may therefore represent a very interesting example for investigating the complexity that regulates molecular pathways and the influence of metabolism on several organs/systems. Moreover, there is also evidence that similar endpoints (i.e. clinical and histological alterations) can be observed in some patients starting from gene defects different from *ABCC6* (i.e. beta-thalassemia, vitamin-K dependent coagulation deficiency). These data support the importance of using wide-spread technologies as transcriptomic or proteomic analyses to have a broader view of the molecular pathways that may be involved in the pathogenesis of elastic fibre calcification. Moreover recent findings in the literature highlights the role of polymorphisms in other genes that could be responsible for phenotypic changes and for a different severity of clinical manifestations in this monogenic disorder.

9. Acknowledgments

Authors gratefully acknowledge FCRM (EctoCal), PXE International and PXE Italia Onlus for their support.

10. References

Aesopos, A., Stamatelos, G., Savvides, P., Rombos, I., Tassiopoulos, T., & Kaklamanis, P. (1989). Pseudoxanthoma elasticum and angioid streaks in two cases of beta-thalassaemia. *Clin Rheumatol*, Vol. 8, No 4, pp. 522-527, ISSN 0770-3198

Aessopos, A., Voskaridou, E., Kavouklis, E., Vassilopoulos, G., Rombos, Y., Gavriel, L., & Loukopoulos, D. (1994). Angioid streaks in sickle-thalassemia. *Am J Ophthalmol*, Vol. 117, No 5, pp. 589-592, ISSN 0002-9394

Aessopos, A., Farmakis, D., Karagiorga, M., Rombos, I., & Loucopoulos, D. (1997). Pseudoxanthoma elasticum lesions and cardiac complications as contributing factors for strokes in beta-thalassemia patients. *Stroke*, Vol. 28, No 12, pp. 2421-2424, ISSN 0039-2499

Aessopos, A., Samarkos, M., Voskaridou, E., Papaioannou, D., Tsironi, M., Kavouklis, E., Vaiopoulos, G., Stamatelos, G., & Loukopoulos, D. (1998). Arterial calcifications in beta-thalassemia. *Angiology*, Vol. 49, No 2, pp. 137-143, ISSN 0003-3197

Aessopos, A., Farmakis, D., Karagiorga, M., Voskaridou, E., Loutradi, A., Hatziliami, A., Joussef, J., Rombos, J., & Loukopoulos, D. (2001). Cardiac involvement in thalassemia intermedia: a multicenter study. *Blood*, Vol. 97, No 11, pp. 3411-3416, ISSN 0006-4971

Aherrahrou, Z., Axtner, S.B., Kaczmarek, P.M., Jurat, A., Korff, S., Doehring, L.C., Weichenhan, D., Katus, H.A., & Ivandic, B.T. (2004). A locus on chromosome 7 determines dramatic up-regulation of osteopontin in dystrophic cardiac calcification in mice. *Am J Pathol*, Vol. 164, No 4, pp. 1379-1387, ISSN 0002-9440

Annovi, G., Boraldi, F., Guerra, D., Schurgers, L.J., Tiozzo, R., Pasquali-Ronchetti, I., & Quaglino, D. (2011). Does Vitamin K Supplementation Affects Vitamin K Cycle in

Control and PXE Fibroblasts? In: XXX Italian Society for the Study of Connective Tissues (SISC) Meeting, October 27-29, 2010, Palermo, Italy. *Connect. Tissue Res*, vol.52, No 4, pp.255-289, ISSN 0300-8207

Baccarani-Contri, M., Vincenti, D., Cicchetti, F., Mori, G., & Pasquali-Ronchetti, I. (1994). Immunochemical identification of abnormal constituents in the dermis of pseudoxanthoma elasticum patients. *Eur J Histochem*, Vol. 38, No 2, pp. 111-123, ISSN 1121-760X

Baccarani-Contri, M., Bacchelli, B., Boraldi, F., Quaglino, D., Taparelli, F., Carnevali, E., Francomano, M.A., Seidenari, S., Bettoli, V., De Sanctis, V., & Pasquali-Ronchetti, I. (2001). Characterization of pseudoxanthoma elasticum-like lesions in the skin of patients with beta-thalassemia. *J Am Acad Dermatol*, Vol. 44, No 1, pp. 33-39, ISSN 0190-9622

Belcher, J.D., Marker, P.H., Weber, J.P., Hebbel, R.P., & Vercellotti, G.M. (2000). Activated monocytes in sickle cell disease: potential role in the activation of vascular endothelium and vaso-occlusion. *Blood*, Vol. 96, No 7, pp. 2451-2459, ISSN 0006-4971

Belinsky, M.G., Chen, Z.S., Shchaveleva, I., Zeng, H., & Kruh, G.D. (2002). Characterization of the drug resistance and transport properties of multidrug resistance protein 6 (MRP6, ABCC6). *Cancer Res*, Vol. 62, No 21, pp. 6172-6177, ISSN 0008-5472

Bercovitch, L., Schepps, B., Koelliker, S., Magro, C., Terry, S., & Lebwohl, M. (2003). Mammographic findings in pseudoxanthoma elasticum. *J Am Acad Dermatol*, Vol. 48, No 3, pp. 359-366, ISSN 0190-9622

Bercovitch, L., & Terry, P. (2004). Pseudoxanthoma elasticum 2004. *J Am Acad Dermatol*, Vol. 51, No 1 Suppl, pp. S13-14, ISSN 0190-9622

Bergen, A.A., Plomp, A.S., Schuurman, E.J., Terry, S., Breuning, M., Dauwerse, H., Swart, J., Kool, M., van Soest, S., Baas, F., ten Brink, J.B., & de Jong, P.T. (2000). Mutations in ABCC6 cause pseudoxanthoma elasticum. *Nat Genet*, Vol. 25, No 2, pp. 228-231, ISSN 1061-4036

Bergen, A.A., Plomp, A.S., Gorgels, T.G., & de Jong, P.T. (2004). From gene to disease; pseudoxanthoma elasticum and the ABCC6 gene. *Ned Tijdschr Geneeskd*, Vol. 148, No 32. pp. 1586-1589, ISSN 0028-2162

Bock, A., & Schwegler, G. (2008). Intracerebral haemorrhage as first manifestation of pseudoxanthoma elasticum. *Clin Neurol Neurosurg*. Vol. 110, No 3, pp. 262-264, ISSN 0303-8467

Booij, J.C., Baas, D.C., Beisekeeva, J., Gorgels, T.G., & Bergen, A.A. (2010). The dynamic nature of Bruch's membrane. *Prog Retin Eye Res*, Vol. 29, No 1, pp. 1-18, ISSN 1350-9462

Boraldi, F., Quaglino, D., Croce, M.A., Garcia Fernandez, M.I., Tiozzo, R., Gheduzzi, D., Bacchelli, B., & Pasquali Ronchetti, I. (2003). Multidrug resistance protein-6 (MRP6) in human dermal fibroblasts. Comparison between cells from normal subjects and from Pseudoxanthoma elasticum patients. *Matrix Biol*, Vol. 22, No 6, pp. 491-500, ISSN 0945-053X

Boraldi, F., Annovi, G., Guerra, D., Paolinelli Devincenzi, C., Garcia-Fernandez, M.I., Panico, F., De Santis, G., Tiozzo, R., Ronchetti, I., & Quaglino, D. (2009). Fibroblast protein profile analysis highlights the role of oxidative stress and vitamin K recycling in the pathogenesis of pseudoxanthoma elasticum. *Proteomics Clin Appl*, Vol. 3, No 9, pp. 1084-1098, ISSN 1862-8346

Borst, P., & Elferink, R.O. (2002). Mammalian ABC transporters in health and disease. *Annu Rev Biochem*, Vol. 71, pp. 537-592, ISSN 0066-4154

Borst, P., van de Wetering, K., & Schlingemann, R. (2008). Does the absence of ABCC6 (multidrug resistance protein 6) in patients with Pseudoxanthoma elasticum prevent the liver from providing sufficient vitamin K to the periphery? *Cell Cycle*, Vol. 7, No 11, pp. 1575-1579, ISSN 1538-4101

Bowen, A.R., Götting, C., LeBoit, P.E., & McCalmont, T.H. (2007). Pseudoxanthoma elasticum-like fibers in the inflamed skin of patients without pseudoxanthoma elasticum. *J Cutan Pathol*, Vol. 34, No 10, pp. 777-781, ISSN 0303-6987

Bunda, S., Kaviani, N., & Hinek, A. (2005). Fluctuations of intracellular iron modulate elastin production. *J Biol Chem*, Vol. 280, No 3, pp. 2341-2351, ISSN 0021-9258

Chassaing, N., Martin, L., Mazereeuw, J., Barrié, L., Nizard, S., Bonafé, J.L., Calvas, P., & Hovnanian, A. (2004). Novel ABCC6 mutations in pseudoxanthoma elasticum. *J Invest Dermatol*, Vol. 122, No 3, pp. 608-613, ISSN 0022-202X

Chassaing, N., Martin, L., Calvas, P., Le Bert, M., & Hovnanian, A. (2005). Pseudoxanthoma elasticum: a clinical, pathophysiological and genetic update including 11 novel ABCC6 mutations. *J Med Genet*, Vol. 42, No 12, pp. 881-892, ISSN 0022-2593

Chraïbi, R., Ismaili, N., Belgnaoui, F., Akallal, N., Bouhllab, J., Senouci, K., & Hassam, B. (2007). Pseudoxanthoma elasticum and nephrocalcinosis. *Ann Dermatol Venereol*, Vol. 134, No 10 Pt 1, pp. 764-766, ISSN 0151-9638

Christiano, A.M., Lebwohl, M.G., Boyd, C.D., & Uitto, J. (1992). Workshop on pseudoxanthoma elasticum: molecular biology and pathology of the elastic fibers. Jefferson Medical College, Philadelphia, Pennsylvania, June 10, 1992. *J Invest Dermatol*, Vol. 99, No 5, pp. 660-663, ISSN 0022-202X

Cianciulli, P., Sorrentino, F., Maffei, L., Amadori, S., Cappabianca, M.P., Foglietta, E., Carnevali, E., & Pasquali-Ronchetti, I. (2002). Cardiovascular involvement in thalassaemic patients with pseudoxanthoma elasticum-like skin lesions: a long-term follow-up study. *Eur J Clin Invest*, Vol. 32, No. 9, pp. 700-706, ISSN 0014-2972

Contri, M.B., Boraldi, F., Taparelli, F., De Paepe, A., & Pasquali Ronchetti, I. (1996). Matrix proteins with high affinity for calcium ions are associated with mineralization within the elastic fibers of pseudoxanthoma elasticum dermis. *Am J Pathol*, Vol. 148, No 2, pp. 569-567, ISSN 0002-9440

Costrop, L.M., Vanakker, O.O., Van Laer, L., Le Saux, O., Martin, L., Chassaing, N., Guerra, D., Pasquali-Ronchetti, I., Coucke. P.J., & De Paepe, A. (2010). Novel deletions causing pseudoxanthoma elasticum underscore the genomic instability of the ABCC6 region. *J Hum Genet*, Vol. 55, No 2, pp. 112-117, ISSN 1434-5161

Denhardt, D.T., Giachelli, C.M., & Rittling, S.R. (2001). Role of osteopontin in cellular signaling and toxicant injury. *Annu Rev Pharmacol Toxicol*, Vol. 41, pp. 723-749, ISSN 0362-1642

Djuric, Z., Zivic, S., & Katic, V. (2007). Celiac disease with diffuse cutaneous vitamin K-deficiency bleeding. *Adv Ther*, Vol. 24, No 6, pp. 1286-1289, ISSN 0741-238X

Donas, K.P., Schulte, S., & Horsch, S. (2007). Balloon angioplasty in the treatment of vascular lesions in pseudoxanthoma elasticum. *J Vasc Interv Radiol*, Vol. 18, No 3, pp. 457-459, ISSN 1051-0443

Fabbri, E., Forni, G.L., Guerrini, G., & Borgna-Pignatti, C. (2009). Pseudoxanthoma-elasticum-like syndrome and thalassemia: an update. *Dermatol Online J*, Vol. 15, No 7, pp. 7, ISSN 1087-2108

Farmakis, D., Moyssakis, I., Perakis, A., Rombos, Y., Deftereos, S., Giakoumis, A., Polymeropoulos, E., & Aessopos, A. (2003). Unstable angina associated with coronary arterial calcification in a thalassemia intermedia patient with a pseudoxanthoma elasticum-like syndrome. *Eur J Haematol*, Vol. 70, No 1, pp. 64-66, ISSN 0902-4441

Garcia-Fernandez, M.I., Gheduzzi, D., Boraldi, F., Paolinelli DeVincenzi, C., Sanchez, P., Valdivielso, P., Morilla, M.J., Quaglino, D., Guerra, D., Casolari, S., Bercovitch, L., & Pasquali-Ronchetti, I. (2008). Parameters of oxidative stress are present in the circulation of PXE patients. *Biochim Biophys Acta*, Vol. 1782, No 7-8, pp. 474-481, ISSN 0925-4439

Georgalas, I., Tservakis, I., Papaconstaninou, D., Kardara, M., Koutsandrea, C., & Ladas, I. (2011). Pseudoxanthoma elasticum, ocular manifestations, complications and treatment. *Clin Exp Optom*, Vol. 94, No 2, pp. 169-180, ISSN 0816-4622

Gheduzzi, D., Taparelli, F., Quaglino, D. Jr, Di Rico, C., Bercovitch, L., Terry, S., Singer, D.B., & Pasquali-Ronchetti, I. (2001). The placenta in pseudoxanthoma elasticum: clinical, structural and immunochemical study. *Placenta*, Vol. 22, No 6, pp. 580-590, ISSN 0143-4004

Gheduzzi, D., Sammarco, R., Quaglino, D., Bercovitch, L., Terry, S., Taylor, W., & Pasquali Ronchetti, I. (2003). Extracutaneous ultrastructural alterations in pseudoxanthoma elasticum. *Ultrastruct Pathol*, Vol. 27, No 6, pp. 375-384, ISSN 0191-3123

Gheduzzi, D., Guidetti, R., Anzivino, C., Tarugi, P., Di Leo, E., Quaglino, D., & Ronchetti, I.P. (2004). ABCC6 mutations in Italian families affected by pseudoxanthoma elasticum (PXE). *Hum Mutat*, Vol. 24, No 5, pp. 438-439, ISSN 1059-7794

Gheduzzi, D., Guerra, D., Bochicchio, B., Pepe, A., Tamburo, A.M., Quaglino, D., Mithieux, S., Weiss, A.S., & Pasquali Ronchetti, I. (2005). Heparan sulphate interacts with tropoelastin, with some tropoelastin peptides and is present in human dermis elastic fibers. *Matrix Biol*, Vol. 24, No 1, pp.15-25, ISSN 0945-053X

Gheduzzi, D., Boraldi, F., Annovi, G., Paolinelli DeVincenzi, C., Schurgers, L.J., Vermeer, C., Quaglino, D., & Pasquali Ronchetti, I. (2007). Matrix Gla protein is involved in elastic fiber calcification in the dermis of pseudoxanthoma elasticum patients. *Lab Invest*, Vol. 87, No 10, pp. 998-1008, ISSN 0023-6837

Giacopelli, F., Marciano, R., Pistorio, A., Catarsi, P., Canini, S., Karsenty, G., & Ravazzolo, R. (2004). Polymorphisms in the osteopontin promoter affect its transcriptional activity. *Physiol Genomics*, Vol. 20, No 1, pp. 87-96, ISSN 0888-7543

Golliet-Mercier, N., Allaouchiche, B., & Monneuse, O. (2005). Pseudoxanthoma elasticum with severe gastrointestinal bleeding. *Ann Fr Anesth Reanim*, Vol. 24, No 7, pp. 833-834, ISSN 0750-7658

Gonzalez, M.E., Votava, H.J., Lipkin, G., & Sanchez, M. (2009). Pseudoxanthoma elasticum. *Dermatol Online J*, Vol. 15, No 8, pp. 17, ISSN 1087-2108

Gorgels, T.G., Waarsing, J.H., de Wolf, A., ten Brink, J.B., Loves, W.J., & Bergen, A.A. (2010). Dietary magnesium, not calcium, prevents vascular calcification in a mouse model for pseudoxanthoma elasticum. *J Mol Med*, Vol. 88, No 5. pp. 467-475, ISSN 0946-2716

Götting. C,, Hendig, D., Adam, A., Schön, S., Schulz, V., Szliska, C., Kuhn, J., & Kleesiek, K. (2005). Elevated xylosyltransferase I activities in pseudoxanthoma elasticum (PXE)

patients as a marker of stimulated proteoglycan biosynthesis. *J Mol Med*, Vol. 83, No 12, pp. 984-992, ISSN 0946-2716

Gurwood, A.S., & Mastrangelo, D.L. (1997). Understanding angioid streaks. *J Am Optom Assoc*, Vol. 68, No 5, pp. 309-324, ISSN 0003-0244

Gutteridge, J.M., & Smith, A. (1988). Antioxidant protection by haemopexin of haem-stimulated lipid peroxidation. *Biochem J*, Vol. 256, No 3, pp. 861-865, ISSN 0264-6021

Haimeur, A., Conseil, G., Deeley, R.G., & Cole, S.P. (2004). Mutations of charged amino acids in or near the transmembrane helices of the second membrane spanning domain differentially affect the substrate specificity and transport activity of the multidrug resistance protein MRP1 (ABCC1). *Mol Pharmacol*, Vol. 65, No 6, pp. 1375-1385, ISSN 0026-895X

Hamlin, N., Beck, K., Baccelli, B., Cianciulli, P., Pasquali-Ronchetti, I., & Le Saux, O. (2003). Acquired Pseudoxanthoma elasticum-like syndrome in beta-thalassaemia patients. *Br J Haematol*, Vol. 122, No 5, pp. 852-854, ISSN 0007-1048

Heaton, J.P., & Wilson, J.W. (1986). Pseudoxanthoma elasticum and its urological implications. *J Urol, Vol* 135, No 4, pp. 776-777, ISSN 0022-5347

Heid, E., Eberst, E., Lazrak, B., & Basset, A. (1980). Pseudoxanthoma elasticum and acneiform lesions. *Ann Dermatol Venereol*, Vol. 107, No. 6, pp. 569-567, ISSN 0151-9638

Heimann, H., Gelisken, F., Wachtlin, J., Wehner, A., Völker, M., Foerster, M.H., & Bartz-Schmidt, K.U. (2005) Photodynamic therapy with verteporfin for choroidal neovascularization associated with angioid streaks. *Graefes Arch Clin Exp Ophthalmol*, Vol. 243, No 11, pp. 1115-1123, ISSN 0721-832X

Hendig, D., Schulz, V., Arndt, M., Szliska, C., Kleesiek, K., & Götting, C. (2006). Role of serum fetuin-A, a major inhibitor of systemic calcification, in pseudoxanthoma elasticum. *Clin Chem*, Vol. 52, No 2, pp. 227-234, ISSN 0009-9147

Hendig, D., Arndt, M., Szliska, C., Kleesiek, K., & Götting, C. (2007). SPP1 promoter polymorphisms: identification of the first modifier gene for pseudoxanthoma elasticum. *Clin Chem*, Vol. 53, No 5, pp. 829-836, ISSN 0009-9147

Hendig, D., Zarbock, R., Szliska, C., Kleesiek, K., & Götting, C. (2008). The local calcification inhibitor matrix Gla protein in pseudoxanthoma elasticum. *Clin Biochem*, Vol. 41, No 6, pp. 407-412, ISSN 0009-9120

Heyl T. (1967). Psedoxanthoma elasticum with granulomatous skin lesions. *Arch Dermatol*, Vol 96, No 5, pp.528-531, ISSN 0003-987X

Hovnanian, A. (2010). Modifier genes in pseudoxanthoma elasticum: novel insights from the Ggcx mouse model. *J Mol Med*, Vol. 88, No 2, pp. 149-153, ISSN 0946-2716

Hu, X., Peek, R., Plomp, A., ten Brink, J., Scheffer, G., van Soest, S., Leys, A., de Jong, P.T., & Bergen, A.A. (2003a). Analysis of the frequent R1141X mutation in the ABCC6 gene in pseudoxanthoma elasticum. *Invest Ophthalmol Vis Sci*, Vol. 44, No 5, pp. 1824-1829, ISSN 0146-0404

Hu, X., Plomp, A., Wijnholds, J., Ten Brink, J., van Soest, S., van den Born, L.I., Leys, A., Peek, R., de Jong, P.T., & Bergen, A.A. (2003b). ABCC6/MRP6 mutations: further insight into the molecular pathology of pseudoxanthoma elasticum. *Eur J Hum Genet*, Vol. 11, No 3, pp. 215-224, ISSN 1018-4813

Iliás, A., Urbán, Z., Seidl, T.L., Le Saux, O., Sinkó, E., Boyd, C.D., Sarkadi, B., & Váradi, A. (2002). Loss of ATP-dependent transport activity in pseudoxanthoma elasticum-associated mutants of human ABCC6 (MRP6). *J Biol Chem*, Vol. 277, No 19, pp. 16860-16867, ISSN 0021-9258

Jelaska, A., Strehlow, D., & Korn, J.H. (1999). Fibroblast heterogeneity in physiological conditions and fibrotic disease. *Springer Semin Immunopathol*, Vol. 21, No 4, pp. 385-395, ISSN 0344-4325

Jiang, Q., & Uitto, J. (2006). Pseudoxanthoma elasticum: a metabolic disease? *J Invest Dermatol*, Vol. 126, No 7, pp. 1440-1441, ISSN 0022-202X

Jiang, Q., Li, Q., & Uitto, J. (2007). Aberrant mineralization of connective tissues in a mouse model of pseudoxanthoma elasticum: systemic and local regulatory factors. *J Invest Dermatol*, Vol. 127, No 6, pp. 1392-1402, ISSN 0022-202X

Jiang, Q., Endo, M., Dibra, F., Wang, K., & Uitto, J. (2009). Pseudoxanthoma elasticum is a metabolic disease. *J Invest Dermatol*, Vol. 129, No 2, pp. 348-354, ISSN 0022-202X

Jiang, Q., Li, Q., Grand-Pierre, A.E., Schurgers, L.J., & Uitto, J. (2011). Administration of vitamin K does not counteract the ectopic mineralization of connective tissues in Abcc6 (-/-) mice, a model for pseudoxanthoma elasticum. *Cell Cycle*, Vol. 10, No 4, pp. 701-707, ISSN 1538-4101

Kidd, P.M. (2010). Vitamins D and K as pleiotropic nutrients: clinical importance to the skeletal and cardiovascular systems and preliminary evidence for synergy. *Altern Med Rev*, Vol. 15, No 3, pp.199-222, ISSN 1089-5159

Klement, J.F., Matsuzaki, Y., Jiang, Q.J., Terlizzi, J., Choi, H.Y., Fujimoto, N., Li, K., Pulkkinen, L., Birk, D.E., Sundberg, J.P., & Uitto, J. (2005). Targeted ablation of the abcc6 gene results in ectopic mineralization of connective tissues. *Mol Cell Biol*, Vol. 25, No 18, pp. 8299-8310, ISSN 0270-7306

Köblös, G., Andrikovics, H., Prohászka, Z., Tordai, A., Váradi, A., & Arányi, T. (2010). The R1141X loss-of-function mutation of the ABCC6 gene is a strong genetic risk factor for coronary artery disease. *Genet Test Mol Biomarkers*, Vol. 14, No 1, pp. 75-78, ISSN 1945-0265

Kool, M., van der Linden, M., de Haas, M., Baas, F., & Borst, P. (1999). Expression of human MRP6, a homologue of the multidrug resistance protein gene MRP1, in tissues and cancer cells. *Cancer Res*, Vol. 59, No 1, pp. 175-182, ISSN 0008-5472

Kornet, L., Bergen, A.A., Hoeks, A.P., Cleutjens, J.P., Oostra, R.J., Daemen, M.J., van Soest, S., & Reneman, R.S. (2004). In patients with pseudoxanthoma elasticum a thicker and more elastic carotid artery is associated with elastin fragmentation and proteoglycans accumulation.*Ultrasound Med Biol*, Vol. 30, No 8, pp. 1041-1048, ISSN 0301-5629

LaRusso, J., Li, Q., Jiang, Q., & Uitto, J. (2009). Elevated dietary magnesium prevents connective tissue mineralization in a mouse model of pseudoxanthoma elasticum (Abcc6(-/-)). *J Invest Dermatol*, Vol. 129, No 6, pp. 1388-1394, ISSN 0022-202X

Le Saux, O., Urban, Z., Göring, H.H., Csiszar, K., Pope, F.M., Richards, A., Pasquali-Ronchetti, I., Terry, S., Bercovitch, L., Lebwohl, M.G., Breuning, M., van den Berg, P., Kornet, L., Doggett, N., Ott, J., de Jong, P.T., Bergen, A.A., & Boyd, C.D. (1999). Pseudoxanthoma elasticum maps to an 820-kb region of the p13.1 region of chromosome 16. *Genomics*, Vol. 62, No 1, pp. 1-10, ISSN 0888-7543

Le Saux, O., Urban, Z., Tschuch, C., Csiszar, K., Baccelli, B., Quaglino, D., Pasquali-Ronchetti, I., Pope, F.M., Richards, A., Terry, S., Bercovitch, L., de Paepe, A., & Boyd, C.D. (2000). Mutations in a gene encoding an ABC transporter cause pseudoxanthoma elasticum. *Nat Genet*, Vol. 25, No 2, pp. 223-227, ISSN 1061-4036

Le Saux, O., Beck, K., Sachsinger, C., Silvestri, C., Treiber, C., Göring, H.H., Johnson, E.W., De Paepe, A., Pope, F.M., Pasquali-Ronchetti, I., Bercovitch, L., Marais, A.S.,

Viljoen, D.L., Terry, S.F., & Boyd, C.D. (2001). A spectrum of ABCC6 mutations is responsible for pseudoxanthoma elasticum. *Am J Hum Genet*, Vol. 69, No 4, pp. 749-764, ISSN 0002-9297

Le Saux, O., Beck, K., Sachsinger, C., Treiber, C., Göring, H.H., Curry, K., Johnson, E.W., Bercovitch, L., Marais, A.S., Terry, S.F., Viljoen, D.L., & Boyd, C.D. (2002). Evidence for a founder effect for pseudoxanthoma elasticum in the Afrikaner population of South Africa. *Hum Genet*, Vol. 111, No 4-5, pp. 331-338, ISSN 0340-6717

Le Saux, O., Bunda, S., VanWart, C.M., Douet, V., Got, L., Martin, L., & Hinek, A. (2006). Serum factors from pseudoxanthoma elasticum patients alter elastic fiber formation in vitro. *J Invest Dermatol*, Vol. 126, No 7, pp. 1497-1505, ISSN 0022-202X

Lebwohl, M., Schwartz, E., Lemlich, G., Lovelace, O., Shaikh-Bahai, F., & Fleischmajer, R. (1993). Abnormalities of connective tissue components in lesional and non-lesional tissue of patients with pseudoxanthoma elasticum. *Arch Dermatol Res*, Vol. 285, No 3, pp. 121-126, ISSN 0003-987X

Lecerf, J.M., & Desmettre, T. (2010). Nutrition and age-related macular degeneration. *J Fr Ophtalmol*, Vol. 33, No 10, pp. 749-757, ISSN 0181-5512

Lewis, K.G., Lester, B.W., Pan, T.D., & Robinson-Bostom, L. (2006). Nephrogenic fibrosing dermopathy and calciphylaxis with pseudoxanthoma elasticum-like changes. *J Cutan Pathol*, Vol. 33, No 10, pp. 695-700, ISSN 0303-6987

Li, Q., Jiang, Q., Schurgers, L.J., & Uitto, J. (2007). Pseudoxanthoma elasticum: reduced gamma-glutamyl carboxylation of matrix gla protein in a mouse model (Abcc6-/-). *Biochem Biophys Res Commun*, Vol. 364, No 2, pp. 208-213, ISSN 0006-291X

Li, Q., Jiang, Q., Pfendner, E., Váradi, A., & Uitto, J. (2009). Pseudoxanthoma elasticum: clinical phenotypes, molecular genetics and putative pathomechanisms. *Exp Dermatol*, Vol. 18, No 1, pp. 1-11, ISSN 0906-6705

Li, T.H., Tseng, C.R., Hsiao, G.H., & Chiu, H.C. (1996). An unusual cutaneous manifestation of pseudoxanthoma elasticum mimicking reticulate pigmentary disorders. *Br J Dermatol*, Vol. 134, No 6, pp. 1157-1159, ISSN 0007-0963

Lund, H.Z., & Gilbert, C.F. (1976). Perforating pseudoxanthoma elasticum. Its distinction from elastosis perforans serpiginosa. *Arch Pathol Lab Med*, Vol. 100, No 10, pp. 544-546, ISSN 0003-9985

Maccari, F., Gheduzzi, D., & Volpi, N. (2003). Anomalous structure of urinary glycosaminoglycans in patients with pseudoxanthoma elasticum. *Clin Chem*, Vol. 49, No 3, pp. 380-388, ISSN 0009-9147

Maccari, F., & Volpi, N. (2008). Structural characterization of the skin glycosaminoglycans in patients with pseudoxanthoma elasticum. *Int J Dermatol*, Vol. 47, No 10, pp. 1024-1027, ISSN 0011-9059

Mainetti, C., Masouyé, I., & Saurat, J.H. (1991). Pseudoxanthoma elasticum-like lesions in the L-tryptophan-induced eosinophilia-myalgia syndrome. *J Am Acad Dermatol*, Vol. 24, No. 4, pp. 657-658, ISSN 0190-9622

Martin, L., Pissard, S., Blanc, P., Chassaing, N., Legac, E., Briault, S., Le Bert, M., & Le Saux, O. (2006). Increased haemoglobin A2 levels in pseudoxanthoma elasticum. *Ann Dermatol Venereol*, Vol. 133, No 8-9 Pt 1, pp. 645-651, ISSN 0151-9638

Martin, L., Douet, V., VanWart, C.M., Heller, M.B., & Le Saux, O. (2011). A mouse model of β-thalassemia shows a liver-specific down-regulation of Abcc6 expression. *Am J Pathol*, Vol. 178, No 2, pp. 774-783, ISSN 0002-9440

Matsuzaki, Y., Nakano, A., Jiang, Q.J., Pulkkinen, L., & Uitto, J. (2005). Tissue-specific expression of the ABCC6 gene. *J Invest Dermatol*, Vol. 125, No 5, pp. 900-905, ISSN 0022-202X

Mendelsohn, G., Bulkley, B.H., & Hutchins, G.M. (1978). Cardiovascular manifestations of Pseudoxanthoma elasticum. *Arch Pathol Lab Med*, Vol. 102, No 6, pp. 298-302, ISSN 0003-9985

Miksch, S., Lumsden, A., Guenther, U.P., Foernzler, D., Christen-Zäch, S., Daugherty, C., Ramesar R.K., Lebwohl, M., Hohl, D., Neldner, K.H., Lindpaintner, K., Richards, R.I., & Struk, B. (2005). Molecular genetics of pseudoxanthoma elasticum: type and frequency of mutations in ABCC6. *Hum Mutat*, Vol. 26, No 3, pp. 235-248, ISSN 1059-7794

Miller, D.M., Benz, M.S., Murray, T.G., & Dubovy, S.R. (2004). Intraretinal calcification and osseous metaplasia in coats disease. *Arch Ophthalmol*, Vol. 122, No 11, pp. 1710-1712, ISSN 0003-9950

Moe, S.M., & Chen, N.X. (2003). Calciphylaxis and vascular calcification: a continuum of extra-skeletal osteogenesis. *Pediatr Nephrol*, Vol. 18, No 10, pp. 969-975, ISSN 0931-041X

Muir, R.L. (2009). Peripheral arterial disease: Pathophysiology, risk factors, diagnosis, treatment, and prevention. *J Vasc Nurs*, Vol. 27, No 2, pp. 26-30, ISSN 1062-0303

Neldner, K.H., & Martinez-Hernandez, A. (1979). Localized acquired cutaneous pseudoxanthoma elasticum. *J Am Acad Dermatol*, Vol. 1, No 6, pp. 523-530, ISSN 0190-9622

Neldner, K.H. (1988). Pseudoxanthoma elasticum. *Int J Dermatol*, Vol. 27, No 2, pp. 98-100, ISSN 0011-9059

Neldner, K.H. & Struk, B. (2002). Pseudoxanthoma elasticum. In : *Connective Tissue and ist heritable disorders. Molecular, Genetic and medical aspects*, Royce, P.M., Steinmann, B., pp. 561-583, Wiley-Liss & Sons, ISBN 9780471251859, New York

Ng, A.B., O'Sullivan, S.T., & Sharpe, D.T. (1999). Plastic surgery and pseudoxanthoma elasticum. *Br J Plast Surg*, Vol. 52, No 7, pp. 594-596, ISSN 0007-1226

Nielsen, A.O., Christensen, O.B., Hentzer, B., Johnson, E., & Kobayasi, T. (1978). Salpeter-induced dermal changes electron-microscopically indistinguishable from pseudoxanthoma elasticum. *Acta Derm Venereol*, Vol. 58, No 4, pp. 323-327, ISSN 0001-5555

Noji, Y., Inazu, A., Higashikata, T., Nohara, A., Kawashiri, M.A., Yu, W., Todo, Y., Nozue, T., Uno, Y., Hifumi, S., & Mabuchi, H. (2004). Identification of two novel missense mutations (p.R1221C and p.R1357W) in the ABCC6 (MRP6) gene in a Japanese patient with pseudoxanthoma elasticum (PXE). *Intern Med*, Vol. 43, No 12, pp. 1171-1176, ISSN 1349-7235

Ohnishi, Y., Tajima, S., Ishibashi, A., Inazumi, T., Sasaki, T., & Sakamoto, H. (1998). Pseudoxanthoma elasticum-like papillary dermal elastolysis: report of four Japanese cases and an immunohistochemical study of elastin and fibrillin-1. *Br J Dermatol*, Vol. 139, No 1, pp. 141-144, ISSN 0007-0963

Oldenburg, J., von Brederlow, B., Fregin, A., Rost, S., Wolz, W., Eberl, W., Eber, S., Lenz, E., Schwaab, R., Brackmann, H.H., Effenberger, W., Harbrecht, U., Schurgers, L.J., Vermeer, C., & Müller, C.R. (2000). Congenital deficiency of vitamin K dependent coagulation factors in two families presents as a genetic defect of the vitamin K-epoxide-reductase-complex. *Thromb Haemost*, Vol. 84, No 6, pp. 937-941, ISSN 0340-6245

Olivieri, N.F. (1999). The beta-thalassemias. *N Engl J Med*, Vol. 341, No 2, pp. 99-109, ISSN 0028-4793

Palaniswamy, C., Sekhri, A., Aronow, W.S., Kalra, A., & Peterson, S.J. (2011). Association of warfarin use with valvular and vascular calcification: a review. *Clin Cardiol*, Vol. 34, No 2, pp. 74-81, ISSN 0160-9289

Pasquali-Ronchetti, I., Volpin, D., Baccarani-Contri, M., Castellani, I., & Peserico, A. (1981). Pseudoxanthoma elasticum. Biochemical and ultrastructural studies. *Dermatology*, Vol. 163, No 4, pp. 307-325, ISSN 1018-8665

Pasquali-Ronchetti, I., Garcia-Fernandez, M.I., Boraldi, F., Quaglino, D., Gheduzzi, D., De Vincenzi Paolinelli, C. Tiozzo, R., Bergamini, S., Ceccarelli, D., & Moscatello, U. (2006). Oxidative stress in fibroblasts from patients with pseudoxanthoma elasticum: possible role in the pathogenesis of clinical manifestations. *J Pathol*, Vol. 208, No 1, pp. 54-61, ISSN 0022-3417

Passi, A., Albertini, R., Baccarani Contri, M., de Luca, G., de Paepe, A., Pallavicini, G., Pasquali Ronchetti, I., & Tiozzo, R. (1996). Proteoglycan alterations in skin fibroblast cultures from patients affected with pseudoxanthoma elasticum. *Cell Biochem Funct*, Vol. 14, No 2, pp. 111-120, ISSN 0263-6484

Patel, D.V., Snead, M.P., & Satchi, K. (2002). Retinal arteriolar calcification in a patient with chronic renal failure. *Br J Ophthalmol*, Vol. 86, No 9, pp. 1063, ISSN 0007-1161

Pauli, R.M., Lian, J.B., Mosher, D.F., & Suttie, J.W. (1987). Association of congenital deficiency of multiple vitamin K-dependent coagulation factors and the phenotype of the warfarin embryopathy: clues to the mechanism of teratogenicity of coumarin derivatives. *Am J Hum Genet*, Vol. 41, No 4, pp. 566-583, ISSN 0002-9297

Pece, A., Avanza, P., Galli, L., & Brancato, R. (1997). Laser photocoagulation of choroidal neovascularization in angioid streaks. *Retina*, Vol. 17, No 1, pp. 12-16, ISSN 0275-004X

Pfendner, E.G., Vanakker, O.M., Terry, S.F., Vourthis, S., McAndrew, P.E., McClain, M.R., Fratta, S., Marais, A.S., Hariri, S., Coucke, P.J., Ramsay, M., Viljoen, D., Terry, P.F., De Paepe, A., Uitto, J., & Bercovitch, L.G. (2007). Mutation detection in the ABCC6 gene and genotype-phenotype analysis in a large international case series affected by pseudoxanthoma elasticum. *J Med Genet*, Vol. 44, No 10, pp. 621-628, ISSN 0022-2593

Phillips, J.E., Hutmacher, D.W., Guldberg, R.E., & García, A.J. (2006). Mineralization capacity of Runx2/Cbfa1-genetically engineered fibroblasts is scaffold dependent. *Biomaterials*, Vol. 27, No 32, pp. 5535-5545, ISSN 0142-9612

Plomp, A.S., Florijn, R.J., Ten Brink, J., Castle, B., Kingston, H., Martín-Santiago, A., Gorgels, T.G., de Jong, P.T., & Bergen, A.A. (2008). ABCC6 mutations in pseudoxanthoma elasticum: an update including eight novel ones. *Mol Vis*, Vol. 24, No 14, pp. 18-24, ISSN 1090-0535

Proudfoot, D., & Shanahan, C.M. (2001).Biology of calcification in vascular cells: intima versus media. *Herz*, Vol. 26, No 4, pp. 245-251, ISSN 0340-9937

Quaglino, D., Boraldi, F., Barbieri, D., Croce, A., Tiozzo, R., & Pasquali Ronchetti, I. (2000). Abnormal phenotype of in vitro dermal fibroblasts from patients with Pseudoxanthoma elasticum (PXE). *Biochim Biophys Acta*, Vol. 1501, No 1, pp. 51-62, ISSN 0925-4439

Quaglino, D., Sartor, L., Garbisa, S., Boraldi, F., Croce, A., Passi, A., De Luca, G., Tiozzo, R., & Pasquali-Ronchetti, I. (2005). Dermal fibroblasts from pseudoxanthoma elasticum patients have raised MMP-2 degradative potential. *Biochim Biophys Acta*, Vol. 1741, No 1-2, pp. 42-47, ISSN 0925-4439

Raybould, M.C., Birley, A.J., Moss, C., Hultén, M., & McKeown, C.M. (1994). Exclusion of an elastin gene (ELN) mutation as the cause of pseudoxanthoma elasticum (PXE) in one family. *Clin Genet*, Vol. 45, No 1, pp. 48-51, ISSN 0009-9163

Ringpfeil, F., Lebwohl, M.G., Christiano, A.M., & Uitto, J. (2000). Pseudoxanthoma elasticum: mutations in the MRP6 gene encoding a transmembrane ATP-binding cassette (ABC) transporter. *Proc Natl Acad Sci U S A*, Vol. 97, No 11, pp. 6001-6006, ISSN 0027-8424

Ringpfeil, F., McGuigan, K., Fuchsel, L., Kozic, H., Larralde, M., Lebwohl, M., & Uitto, J. (2006). Pseudoxanthoma elasticum is a recessive disease characterized by compound heterozygosity. *J Invest Dermatol*, Vol. 126, No 4, pp. 782-786, ISSN 0022-202X

Rosenzweig, B.P., Guarneri, E., & Kronzon, I. (1993). Echocardiographic manifestations in a patient with pseudoxanthoma elasticum. *Ann Intern Med*, Vol. 119, No 6, pp. 487-490, ISSN 0003-4819

Roth, D.B., Estafanous, M., & Lewis, H. (2005). Macular translocation for subfoveal choroidal neovascularization in angioid streaks. *Am J Ophthalmol*, Vol. 131, No 3, pp. 390-392, ISSN 0002-9394

Sakuraoka, K., Tajima, S., Nishikawa, T., & Seyama, Y. (1994). Biochemical analyses of macromolecular matrix components in patients with pseudoxanthoma elasticum. *J Dermatol*, Vol. 21, No 2, pp. 98-101, ISSN 0385-2407

Scheffer, G.L., Hu, X., Pijnenborg, A.C., Wijnholds, J., Bergen, A.A., & Scheper, R.J. (2002). MRP6 (ABCC6) detection in normal human tissues and tumors. *Lab Invest*, Vol. 82, No 4, pp. 515-518, ISSN 0023-6837

Schön, S., Schulz, V., Prante, C., Hendig, D., Szliska, C., Kuhn, J., Kleesiek, K., & Götting, C.(2006). Polymorphisms in the xylosyltransferase genes cause higher serum XT-I activity in patients with pseudoxanthoma elasticum (PXE) and are involved in a severe disease course. *J Med Genet*, Vol. 43, No 9, pp. 745-749, ISSN 0022-2593

Schulz, V., Hendig, D., Henjakovic, M., Szliska, C., Kleesiek, K., & Götting, C. (2006). Mutational analysis of the ABCC6 gene and the proximal ABCC6 gene promoter in German patients with pseudoxanthoma elasticum (PXE). *Hum Mutat*, Vol. 27, No 8, pp. 831, ISSN 1059-7794

Schurgers, L.J., Cranenburg, E.C., & Vermeer, C. (2008). Matrix Gla-protein: the calcification inhibitor in need of vitamin K. *Thromb Haemost*, Vol. 100, No 4, pp. 593-603, ISSN 0340-6245

Sepp, N., Pichler, E., Breathnach, S.M., Fritsch, P., & Hintner, H. (1990). Amyloid elastosis: analysis of the role of amyloid P component. *J Am Acad Dermatol*, Vol. 22, No 1, pp. 27-34, ISSN 0190-9622

Shepherd, R.F., & Rooke, T. (2003). Uncommon arteriopathies: what the vascular surgeon needs to know. *Semin Vasc Surg*, Vol. 16, No 3, pp. 240-251, ISSN 0895-7967

Sorrell, J.M., & Caplan, A.I. (2004). Fibroblast heterogeneity: more than skin deep. *J Cell Sci*, Vol. 117, No Pt 5, pp. 667-675, ISSN 0021-9533

Suarez, M.J., Garcia, J.B., Orense, M., Raimunde, E., Lopez, M.V., & Fernandez, O. (1991). Sonographic aspects of pseudoxanthoma elasticum. *Pediatr Radiol*, Vol. 21, No 7, pp. 538-539, ISSN 0301-0449

Taylor, N.E., Foster, W.C., Wick, M.R., & Patterson, J.W. (2004). Tumefactive lipedema with pseudoxanthoma elasticum-like microscopic changes. *J Cutan Pathol*, Vol. 31, No 2, pp. 205-209, ISSN 0303-6987

Tiozzo Costa, R., Baccarani Contri, M., Cingi, M.R., Pasquali Ronchetti, I., Salvini, R., Rindi, S., & De Luca, G. (1988). Pseudoxanthoma elasticum (PXE): ultrastructural and biochemical study on proteoglycan and proteoglycan-associated material produced by skin fibroblasts in vitro. *Coll Relat Res*, Vol. 8, No 1, pp. 49-64, ISSN 0174-173X

Tu, Y., Weiss, A.S. (2008). Glycosaminoglycan-mediated coacervation of tropoelastin abolishes the critical concentration, accelerates coacervate formation, and facilitates spherule fusion: implications for tropoelastin microassembly. *Biomacromolecules*, Vol. 9, No 7, pp. 1739-1744, ISSN 1525-7797

Uitto, J., Li, Q., & Jiang, Q. (2010). Pseudoxanthoma elasticum: molecular genetics and putative pathomechanisms. *J Invest Dermatol*, Vol. 130, No 3, pp. 661-670, ISSN 0022-202X

Vanakker, O.M., Voet, D., Petrovic, M., van Robaeys, F., Leroy, B.P., Coucke, P., & de Paepe, A. (2006). Visceral and testicular calcifications as part of the phenotype in pseudoxanthoma elasticum: ultrasound findings in Belgian patients and healthy carriers. *Br J Radiol*, Vol. 79, No 939, pp. 221-225, ISSN 0007-1285

Vanakker, O.M., Martin, L., Gheduzzi, D., Leroy, B.P., Loeys, B.L., Guerci, V.I., Matthys, D., Terry, S.F., Coucke, P.J., Pasquali-Ronchetti, I., & De Paepe, A. (2007). Pseudoxanthoma elasticum-like phenotype with cutis laxa and multiple coagulation factor deficiency represents a separate genetic entity. *J Invest Dermatol*, Vol. 127, No 3, pp. 581-587, ISSN 0022-202X

Vanakker, O.M., Leroy, B.P., Coucke, P., Bercovitch, L.G., Uitto, J., Viljoen, D., Terry, S.F., Van Acker, P., Matthys, D., Loeys, B., & De Paepe, A. (2008). Novel clinico-molecular insights in pseudoxanthoma elasticum provide an efficient molecular screening method and a comprehensive diagnostic flowchart. *Hum Mutat*. Vol. 29, No 1, pp. 205, ISSN 1059-7794

Vanakker, O.M., Martin, L., Schurgers, L.J., Quaglino, D., Costrop, L., Vermeer, C., Pasquali-Ronchetti, I., Coucke, P.J., & De Paepe, A. (2010). Low serum vitamin K in PXE results in defective carboxylation of mineralization inhibitors similar to the GGCX mutations in the PXE-like syndrome. *Lab Invest*, Vol. 90, No 6, pp. 895-905, ISSN 0023-6837

Verbraak, F.D. (2010). Antivascular endothelial growth factor treatment in pseudoxanthoma elasticum patients. *Dev Ophthalmol*, Vol. 46, pp. 96-106, ISSN 0250-3751

Wang, J., Near, S., Young, K., Connelly, P.W., & Hegele, R.A. (2001). ABCC6 gene polymorphism associated with variation in plasma lipoproteins. *J Hum Genet*, Vol. 46, No 12, pp. 699-705, ISSN 1434-5161

Wajih, N., Hutson, S.M., & Wallin, R. (2007). Disulfide-dependent protein folding is linked to operation of the vitamin K cycle in the endoplasmic reticulum. A protein disulfide isomerase-VKORC1 redox enzyme complex appears to be responsible for vitamin K1 2,3-epoxide reduction. *J Biol Chem*, Vol. 282, No 4, pp. 2626-2635, ISSN 0021-9258

Zarbock, R., Hendig, D., Szliska, C., Kleesiek, K., & Götting, C. (2007). Pseudoxanthoma elasticum: genetic variations in antioxidant genes are risk factors for early disease onset. *Clin Chem*, Vol. 53, No 10, pp.1734-1740, ISSN 0009-9147

Zarbock, R., Hendig, D., Szliska, C., Kleesiek, K., & Götting, C. (2009). Vascular endothelial growth factor gene polymorphisms as prognostic markers for ocular manifestations in pseudoxanthoma elasticum. *Hum Mol Genet*, Vol. 18, No 17, pp. 3344-3351, ISSN 0964-6906

Permissions

The contributors of this book come from diverse backgrounds, making this book a truly international effort. This book will bring forth new frontiers with its revolutionizing research information and detailed analysis of the nascent developments around the world.

We would like to thank Kenji Ikehara, for lending his expertise to make the book truly unique. He has played a crucial role in the development of this book. Without his invaluable contribution this book wouldn't have been possible. He has made vital efforts to compile up to date information on the varied aspects of this subject to make this book a valuable addition to the collection of many professionals and students.

This book was conceptualized with the vision of imparting up-to-date information and advanced data in this field. To ensure the same, a matchless editorial board was set up. Every individual on the board went through rigorous rounds of assessment to prove their worth. After which they invested a large part of their time researching and compiling the most relevant data for our readers. Conferences and sessions were held from time to time between the editorial board and the contributing authors to present the data in the most comprehensible form. The editorial team has worked tirelessly to provide valuable and valid information to help people across the globe.

Every chapter published in this book has been scrutinized by our experts. Their significance has been extensively debated. The topics covered herein carry significant findings which will fuel the growth of the discipline. They may even be implemented as practical applications or may be referred to as a beginning point for another development. Chapters in this book were first published by InTech; hereby published with permission under the Creative Commons Attribution License or equivalent.

The editorial board has been involved in producing this book since its inception. They have spent rigorous hours researching and exploring the diverse topics which have resulted in the successful publishing of this book. They have passed on their knowledge of decades through this book. To expedite this challenging task, the publisher supported the team at every step. A small team of assistant editors was also appointed to further simplify the editing procedure and attain best results for the readers.

Our editorial team has been hand-picked from every corner of the world. Their multi-ethnicity adds dynamic inputs to the discussions which result in innovative outcomes. These outcomes are then further discussed with the researchers and contributors who give their valuable feedback and opinion regarding the same. The feedback is then collaborated with the researches and they are edited in a comprehensive manner to aid the understanding of the subject.

Apart from the editorial board, the designing team has also invested a significant amount of their time in understanding the subject and creating the most relevant covers. They scrutinized every image to scout for the most suitable representation of the subject and create an appropriate cover for the book.

The publishing team has been involved in this book since its early stages. They were actively engaged in every process, be it collecting the data, connecting with the contributors or procuring relevant information. The team has been an ardent support to the editorial, designing and production team. Their endless efforts to recruit the best for this project, has resulted in the accomplishment of this book. They are a veteran in the field of academics and their pool of knowledge is as vast as their experience in printing. Their expertise and guidance has proved useful at every step. Their uncompromising quality standards have made this book an exceptional effort. Their encouragement from time to time has been an inspiration for everyone.

The publisher and the editorial board hope that this book will prove to be a valuable piece of knowledge for researchers, students, practitioners and scholars across the globe.

List of Contributors

Saovaros Svasti, Orapan Sripichai, Manit Nuinoon, Pranee Winichagoon and Suthat Fucharoen
Thalassemia Research Center, Institute of Molecular Biosciences, Mahidol University, Phutthamonthon, Nakhonpathom, Thailand

Beatriz Puisac, María Arnedo, M Concepción Gil-Rodríguez, Esperanza Teresa, Angeles Pié, Gloria Bueno, Feliciano J. Ramos, Paulino Goméz-Puertas and Juan Pié
Unit of Clinical Genetics and Functional Genomics School of Medicine, University of Zaragozam, Spain

María Arnedo, Mónica Ramos, Beatriz Puisac, Mª Concepción Gil-Rodríguez, Esperanza Teresa, Ángeles Pié, Gloria Bueno, Feliciano J. Ramos, Paulino Gómez-Puertas and Juan Pié
Unit of Clinical Genetics and Functional Genomics, School of Medicine, University of Zaragoza, Spain

Yoshinari Uehara
Department of Cardiology, Fukuoka University Faculty of Medicine, Nanakuma, Jonan-ku, Fukuoka, Japan

Bo Zhang
Department of Biochemistry, Fukuoka University Faculty of Medicine, Nanakuma, Jonan-ku, Fukuoka, Japan

Keijiro Saku
Department of Cardiology, Fukuoka University Faculty of Medicine, Nanakuma, Jonan-ku, Fukuoka, Japan

Tangvarasittichai Surapon
Chronic Diseases Research Unit, Department of Medical Technology, Naresuan University, Phitsanulok, Thailand

Cristina Maria Mihai
"Ovidius" University, Faculty of Medicine, Constanta, Romania

Jan D. Marshall
The Jackson Laboratory, Bar Harbor, ME, USA

Ramona Mihaela Stoicescu
"Ovidius" University, Faculty of Pharmacy, Constanta, Romania

Michael Sjoding and D. Kyle Hogarth
University of Chicago, U.S.A.

Jonay Poveda Nuñez and Alberto Ortiz
IIS-Fundacion Jimenez Diaz and Universidad Autonoma de Madrid, Madrid, Spain

Ana Belen Sanz and Maria Dolores Sanchez Niño
IdiPaz, Madrid, Spain

Rocio Toro Cebada, Alipio Magnas and Jose Luis Zamorano
Departamento de Medicina de la Universidad de Cadiz, c/DR Marañon S/N, Cadiz, Spain

Daniela Quaglino, Federica Boraldi, Giulia Annovi and Ivonne Ronchetti
University of Modena and Reggio Emilia, Italy

Printed in the USA
CPSIA information can be obtained
at www.ICGtesting.com
JSHW011419221024
72173JS00004B/596

9 781632 412379